MADMEN

A SOCIAL HISTORY OF
MADHOUSES, MAD-DOCTORS & LUNATICS

4 3 3 9 5 0 1 0 0 3 0 9 8 4 4 2 7 7 2 6 0 1 2

ROY PORTER

D1351109

TEMPUS

Cover pictures:

Front: Coloured etching by George Cruickshank, 1819, after W. Hogarth. Wellcome Library, London.

Back: An affluent man receiving electric therapy, coloured etching. Wellcome Library, London.

This edition first published 2006
First published as *Mind Forg'd Manacles* in 1987 by The Athlone Press Ltd

Tempus Publishing Limited
The Mill, Brimscombe Port,
Stroud, Gloucestershire, GL5 2QG
www.tempus-publishing.com

British Library Cataloguing in Publication Data.
A catalogue record for this book is available from the British Library.

ISBN 0 7524 3730 5

Typesetting and origination by Tempus Publishing Limited
Printed and bound in Great Britain

Contents

Introduction

My basic aims in this book are those of exposition and synthesis. There is much to be said about mad people, and how they were regarded and treated in England before the nineteenth century. Who were they? Were they hailed, hated or harassed? How and why did the handling of mentally abnormal people change? There have been, however, surprisingly few attempts to address these questions in a broad way, integrating the mass of available information within a framework of analysis and interpretation. Combining exact scholarship with chronological sweep, Basil Clarke's *Mental Disorder in Earlier Britain* does just that for the medieval period. The Tudor and Stuart epochs remain curiously ill-researched as a whole, despite the brilliant close-up illumination offered by Michael MacDonald's study of Richard Napier. Here I attempt to survey developments spanning the period roughly from the Civil War to the dawn of the nineteenth century.

For this era, there has been much first-rate research in particular specialised sectors. For instance, William Ll. Parry-Jones' *The Trade in Lunacy* deals definitively with the first century of private lunatic asylums; similarly, accounts such as Max Byrd's *Visits to Bedlam* and Michael V. DePorte's *Nightmares and Hobbyhorses* offer stimulating analysis of attitudes towards insanity among the literary elite, and how they changed. As will be obvious, I have relied heavily, and with great gratitude, upon these works and others like them. Above all – though nowadays it seems heretical for a historian to confess this – I am deeply indebted to the psychiatrists Ida Macalpine and Richard Hunter, whose anthology, *Three Hundred Years of Psychiatry*, and monograph, *George III and the Mad Business*, remain models of accurate and tireless scholarship.

In the text which follows, I have principally attempted to weave the information and insights already available in printed sources into a more comprehensive interpretation, highlighting the intimate yet complex relationships between lunacy, literature and the law, between mad people, madhouses and mad-doctors, between attitudes and action, society and psychiatry. Such originality as this book may possess lies less in presenting a body of fundamentally novel research (by contrast, say, to Michael MacDonald's *Mystical Bedlam*) than in seeking to establish a coherent narrative and integrated analysis, conceived in the light of critical currents within the history, philosophy and politics of psychiatry. Though these issues are complex and controversial, I have tried to produce a text simple enough to be used in student courses.

I am acutely aware that this book does little more than skim the surface of many critical topics. No substantial body of research has yet been produced on numerous fundamental issues, such as how mad people were treated by the parochial Poor Law system during this period, or upon basic source materials, such as patients' casebooks as kept by mad-doctors. Then again, compared to the abundance of recent scholarship on women and madness in the nineteenth century, we remain sadly ignorant about what was happening to mad women in earlier centuries. I myself aspire to fill in some of these gaps in later, more specialised studies, currently in progress. From close examination of sick people's own written remains, I aim to add to my discussion in Chapter 5 of the state of 'minds diseased', just as I hope to be able to make a contribution to a desperately needed new history of Bethlem Hospital.

Until the seventeenth and eighteenth centuries receive the concentrated attention hitherto commonly lavished only on the nineteenth, many of the generalisations I shall be advancing must, however, rest on somewhat shaky foundations, which future research will surely undermine. At least, I trust, this book will bring some of these areas of ignorance more sharply into focus. With luck, it might even encourage some sorely needed cross-cultural research. This book treats the shaping of psychiatry in England, with only the barest of glimpses at parallel, but often significantly different, developments in other nations. Even if it avoids the dangers of chauvinism, this approach must be blinkered, lacking an assured grasp of what is common and what unique. A proper comparative history is a high priority.

I have tried to avoid looking at my sources through the psychiatric eyes of today, neither have I attempted a psycho-historical reconstruction of the eighteenth-century psychic underground, individual or collective, in the manner perhaps of Norman O. Brown's *Life Against Death* or even as advocated in Peter Gay's *Freud for Historians*. I am not much concerned with passing clinical judgements on who was truly 'sane' or 'mad'. Neither do I translate the diagnostic categories of old mad-doctors into modern psychiatric jargon. Indeed, I have largely avoided even using such terms as 'psychiatry' for the period before they came into use right at the end of my study. There is a place for such approaches – Macalpine and Hunter actually entitled one of their books *Schizophrenia 1677* – but my concern here is rather different, attempting principally to recover the internal coherence of now unfamiliar beliefs about the mind and madness, and to set them in their wider frames of meaning. I have largely abstained from the anachronistic use of terminology, but have not followed that plan rigidly where it would make the result cumbersome.

I have, however, made very copious use in my text of quotations from original sources, in the hope that the immersion and absorption in alien thought-worlds which they facilitate will challenge some of the glib generalisations which have been flung around in some recent histories of psychiatry. Given that this book is centrally about confrontations between alien thought-worlds, it is valuable for us today to be forced to undergo a comparable experience. Many of the people featured in this book – those conventionally labelled mad, their doctors, and not least the public at large – found their every encounter with 'madness' profoundly disorientating, an endless reconnaissance of the unfamiliar. I hope that this book might produce a similar defamiliarising effect.

It might be helpful to indicate here how this book has been conceived and organised. During the seventeenth and eighteenth centuries madness was an extremely broad sociocultural category, with many manifestations and meanings. Madness could be seen as medical, or moral, or religious, or, indeed, Satanic. It could be sited in the mind or the soul, in the brain or the body. It could be good or bad. No clear-cut and rigid boundaries were generally recognised between what we might call clinical insanity proper and a variety of other, possibly less severe, peculiarities of thought and behaviour, such as melancholy or hypochondria, or just being 'cracked'. And the language of madness and all its related synonyms, formal and colloquial, served not merely to diagnose desperately disturbed individuals but also, more metaphorically, to express wider moral and political values. One of the key tasks of this book is to map these meanings of madness, to show how such meanings were disputed and negotiated, and to analyse the ideological implications they carried.

These configurations changed markedly during the century and a half under consideration; and the book sets out to explore what brought about such changes: political pressures, reorientations of religious temper, new philosophies of mind and medical researches, and so forth. I do not believe that in this period (unlike perhaps later) these changing attitudes and practices towards the disturbed (and the disturbing) overwhelmingly stemmed from the medical profession. Hence doctors are

neither the heroes nor the villains of my story. Rather, I have
tried to show how the subtle shifts in evaluations of madness
– some sorts being seen as good, others as bad; some as curable,
others as hopeless; some as culpable, others as blameless, and
so forth – arose from influential elements in the community
at large, among whom doctors formed just a part. In any case
these were often contested; there was a plurality of frequently
competing views about madness.

Thomas Szasz has written of the 'manufacture of madness',
seeing that process as a rather conspiratorial form of scapegoating.
It seems to me that in the period under discussion madness was
manufactured in precisely the sense that all other dimensions of
life – morals, religion, the law etc. – are of human making: society
moulds basic human needs, wants, expressions into culture. And
that culture had its victims. I chose the quotation from Blake for
my original title – 'Mind Forg'd Manacles' – to convey the sense
in which that society first created instruments of cultural torture,
such as a theology of eternal damnation, which drove some out
of their minds, and then additionally frequently stigmatised the
mad as evil and dangerous. I do not, however, see the shaping of
madness in this period as a kind of plot, engineered by sinister
professional interests and consistently serving well-defined functions of social control.

What is at stake here is not a matter of whether those who
dealt with the mad were men of good will or not; nor even
whether the treatment of the mad got better or worse (in some
ways it became more repressive; in others, less so). It is simply that
before the nineteenth century, the resources and institutions had
not yet been developed which would have permitted a single
professional group to assume full legal control of the mad.

To say this shifts the focus from the 'manufacture of madness' to the 'manufacture of psychiatry'. Throughout the period
covered by this book various people – some doctors, some not
– treated the mad and theorised about insanity and a whole
range of cognate and mysterious disorders of consciousness and
conduct. But I have also been concerned to show that particularly

in the latter half of the eighteenth century specialists in treating mental disorders began to grow in prominence, linked above all to the increase in institutional provision for the disturbed. I have tried to relate the rise of this occupation (the 'proto-psychiatrist') to its institution (the asylum) and to its material practice (management). A full study of the emergence of the practice and profession of psychiatry in Britain is needed; here I offer some account of its gestation. The cut-off point chosen for this study may approximately mark an important moment of transition, from a time when the politics of madness lay in the public domain in the widest sense, to an age in which madness came under the dominion of psychological medicine and its institutions.

I

Orientations

HISTORIOGRAPHICAL

When Polonius judged that to 'define true madness, What is't but to be nothing else but mad', he struck a mighty chord. For the one thing commentators from Shakespeare onwards were able to agree upon was that insanity was a veritable Proteus. How infinite its varieties! How mercurial its qualities! How artfully could lunacy ape sanity! (Perfect mimicry of normalcy was later to become one of the giveaways of madness.) Was there not reason in madness; was not folly jumbled with wisdom? Just how thin were the partitions! After all, as the young Charles Darwin was to remark, 'My Father says there is perfect gradation between sound people and insane – that everybody is insane at some time.'

Early in the nineteenth century, the psychiatric doctor James Parkinson recorded an incident typifying this maddening anarchy:

A lunatic having committed in his own house several acts of violence, the family obtained a police officer from a neighbouring office to restrain him until the keeper from the madhouse arrived. When the keeper came, he inquired particularly how he should know the patient, on his first entering the room, that he might immediately secure him with the waist coat, to prevent any dangerous struggle. He was told that he had on a brown coat, and that he would know him by his raving. He therefore glided into the room, where the police officer, who also had a brown coat on, sat with his back towards the door, remonstrating with the patient, who in seeing the keeper enter, with the waistcoat in his hand, became immediately calm, and with a wink and a nod, so completely misled the keeper, that in half a minute the police officer in spite of his resistance, was completely invested with the strait jacket.[1]

For Parkinson, the moral of the tale was the indispensability of psychiatric expertise: otherwise madness in masquerade would never be exposed. For others, it would have been that madness was a lord of misrule. For today's anti-psychiatrists, the madman's victory over the police might seem like the tables turned, madness' revenge in captivating its captor. Indeed, the ancient perception of insanity as a mocker or anarch, turning normality topsy-turvy, has been widely co-opted by today's radical critics of psychiatry for their own purposes. For them, insanity is Reason's jester, mental abnormality civilisation's monster yet mirror. Some critics would go so far as to altogether deny its independent reality as a disease condition, arguing that 'madness' is just a scapegoating stigma which power uses to patrol its own boundaries and validate itself. Nathaniel Lee, the Restoration poet confined to Bethlem, long ago put the politics of that view in a nutshell: 'They said I was mad; and I said they were mad; damn them, they outvoted me.'

Despite this vision of madness as a will-o'-the-wisp, a cunning devil shimmering down from Burton's *Anatomy of Melancholy* (1621) to current anti-psychiatry, there is a remarkable consensus among scholars as to the path which the history of insanity ought to be treading. Of course, leading surveyors of English madness – Scull, Mellett, Busfield, Skultans, Jones, Showalter and others

– differ, often quite sharply, in their interpretations. But they share a common scenario. In these and other recent accounts, the epic of English madness opens in the late eighteenth century; its main plot is the development of psychiatry, taken as a body of theory, a profession and a system of institutions, all within an overarching legislative framework. Brute figures lend weight to the view that psychiatric institutionalisation is the key to this history. Around 1800, no more than a few thousand 'lunatics' were confined in England in all kinds of institutions; by 1900 the total had skyrocketed to about 100,000. In human terms, this increase of perhaps twentyfold means that during the nineteenth century a disturbed person's fate was likely – indeed, ever more likely – to end up as the story of encounters with organised psychiatry; in fact, quite specifically, to be the tale of life and death within the asylum, caged in 'museums of madness'. Psychiatry established itself as a national institution, here to stay.

Recent interpretations have often cast these developments in a lurid light, presenting psychiatry as an agency of social control or as a professional ramp – though it is highly doubtful whether Britain should really be seen as a 'psychiatric society' or as a 'therapeutic state' as early as 1900. But however we interpret the rise of institutional psychiatry, it remains noteworthy that the most notorious lunatics of the nineteenth century, such as James Hadfield, Richard Dadd and Daniel MacNaughten, spent the great bulk of their lives 'inside'; and others, for instance John Perceval, are famous precisely because of their crusades against compulsory confinement. Moreover, Victorian psychiatrists were themselves preoccupied with the asylum as a thera-peutic institution; and similarly, when madness figures in fiction, from Tobias Smollett to Charles Reade, it is the madhouse which dominates, both physically and symbolically. Hence it is no surprise that scholars have concentrated on nineteenth-century developments, and that the keynote in such accounts has been tracing the irresistible rise – for better or worse – of organised psychiatry in its theoretical, legal-political and, above all, institutional dimensions. Indeed, the recent publication of

Anne Digby's exemplary history of the York Retreat, our first comprehensive, computerised asylum biography, will surely reinforce the tendency to write the history of English madness with Victorian institutional psychiatry stage-centre.

Yet what came before? Most histories pick up the story from the years around 1800, because the turn of the century seems a significant watershed, cutting off 'the world we have lost' from the modern era. Its landmarks include the 'madness' of George III; the opening of the York Retreat, with its 'moral therapy', in 1796, and of Ticehurst House in 1797; the trial of James Hadfield in 1800, and the subsequent Criminal Lunatics' Act of the same year; the first major parliamentary inquiries into madhouses in 1807 and 1815; and the passing of the Act first empowering the setting up of public lunatic asylums in 1808. If the years around 1800 thus mark what Scull has called a 'paradigm switch', the eighteenth century is thereby relegated to 'prehistory', a past severed by 'an epistemological rupture'. Probably for this reason, the earlier history of English madness has been neglected. The few books there are offer very bitty coverage. For instance, Volume I of Denis Leigh's *The Historical Development of British Psychiatry*, focusing on eighteenth-century England, hardly goes beyond a gallery of bio-bibliographical cameos. Admittedly, ampler coverage has been given to certain Georgian topics, such as the 'English malady', yet our ignorance remains great; not least, we know little of the history of public asylums, such as Bethlem. Above all, there has been no attempt to create an interpretative synthesis of English madness before institutionalisation became the dynamo of change in the nineteenth century.

Research on what I shall call the 'long eighteenth century' (roughly, from Restoration to Regency) thus remains patchy. Some bold shots have been made, however, to characterise the age. These have mainly been by way of polemical afterwords or preludes to books concentrating on earlier or later periods. Not surprisingly, perhaps, they create a confusing 'double vision'; in particular between those who – like MacDonald – see the eighteenth century as betraying a more humane past, and those who – like Sir Aubrey Lewis – regard psychiatry as altogether a later growth.

Yet on one matter historians, psychiatrists and anti-psychiatrists alike tend to agree: that the age of the Enlightenment was a 'dark age', both for psychiatry and for its charges. MacDonald leaves us in no doubt: 'the eighteenth century was a disaster for the insane.' It is easy to see, on the one hand, why Whiggish celebrators of psychiatric progress should look askance at the Georgians. After the strides made earlier by the first 'psychiatrist', Johannes Weyer (proving that 'demoniacs' and witches were not, after all, possessed but, rather, deluded), and by Robert Burton, much-sung father of English psychiatry, the eighteenth century provides no further precocious giants, at least until the Tukes at its very close – and even they must be unlikely heroes, being tea merchants, not doctors. On the other hand, for sympathisers with traditional spiritual therapies the eighteenth century, bedazzled by Descartes, seems the great treason. Thus MacDonald regards what he sees as the Georgian descent into 'cruel' medico-scientistic and mechanical treatments, accompanying the rise of the 'asylum system', as 'catastrophic'. The Georgian century, he argues, saw the rise of 'medical brutality', the 'abolition of family care' and the 'abandonment of therapeutic eclecticism'.

More particularly, Georgian developments have got a bad press from modern historians looking back from the 'age of reform'. Those who applaud the Victorians as promoters of psychiatric progress paint Georgian times, by contrast, as benighted and brutal. Take Woods and Car on the traditional asylum:

> Conditions were atrocious. There was no provision for cleanliness or comfort, much less for anything resembling therapy... Asylums were custodial institutions rather than therapeutic hospitals... Barbarity and ignorance were the rule.[2]

King-Hele drives it home:

> Lunatics were usually chained and brutally treated, in the hope of driving out the devils that possessed them... in 1794 [sic] the first humane lunatic asylum, the Retreat at York, was founded by the Quaker, William Tuke. But milder treatment did not become common until many years later.[3]

Allegedly preoccupied with punishment, therapies stagnated. 'The contribution of seventeenth- and eighteenth-century medicine to the problem of insanity', Galdston has judged, 'remained almost nil'; or, in Leigh's words, 'the English psychiatric writings of the eighteenth century were either tedious or second-hand'. Above all, Hanoverian madhouses are typically viewed as the ultimate disgrace, riddled with sadism and embezzlement, epitomised by those horrors of unreformed Bedlam which every schoolboy knows. As Patricia Allderidge has demonstrated, historians have given free rein to their Gothic imaginations in painting that notorious institution black.

In creating this 'demonology' historians have, of course, drawn freely on the anathemas of heroic nineteenth-century reformers. John Conolly, for example, concluded that the old 'restraint system' (in which attendants were 'frantic in cruelty', and 'torture' grew more 'ingenious') 'comprehended every possible evil of bad treatment, every fault of commission and omission', unlike the progressive non-restraint methods he had pioneered. And fellow non-restrainer Gardiner Hill decried the 'old era in psychiatry in which there was no humanity'. Luckily, concluded George Nesse Hill, the 'dawn of a more rational age' was at hand. Now it would be cavalier automatically to discredit such attacks as mere self-serving ideology. But neither should they be uncritically accepted. Reformers were, after all, moving minds rather than pursuing detached research into psychiatry's prehistory.

There is thus a Whiggish account of why the Georgian century was a 'dark age'. But in recent years this largely in-house history has found support from, at first sight, unlikely quarters. This comes, first and foremost, from the writings of the late Michel Foucault, although it is paralleled by the Frankfurt school-based interpretation of Klaus Doerner. Together Foucault, Doerner and their followers present a non-Whiggish conceptualisation of the eighteenth century as a disaster for the insane. It is important to evaluate this powerful and highly influential interpretation.

In his *Folie et Déraison*, Foucault advanced the challenging view that the epoch from about 1660 to around 1800 (he called it 'the classical period') constituted the 'great confinement' throughout Europe. During this era, madness – which had hitherto enjoyed a liberty and truth of its own, engaging in dialogue with reason – came to be disqualified, abominated and reduced to pure negation ('unreason'). There being 'no common language... any longer', Unreason was an affront, a threat to order, demanding 'reason's subjugation of unreason'. Hence, says Foucault, rationalism, backed up by the police powers of absolutism, initiated 'the great confinement', a movement of 'blind repression'. Within the *hôpitaux généraux* in France, the *Zuchthäuser* in Germany, and workhouses and bridewells in Britain, the mad were rounded up in an 'undifferentiated mass' with paupers, criminals, vagrants and beggars. In Doerner's phrase, 'the age of reason... put all forms of unreason... under lock and key'. Together all shared a generic deviancy which scandalised the bourgeois mind: they would not work. 'Madness was perceived', wrote Foucault, 'through the condemnation of idleness.' To remedy this, the mad were set to work, 'subject to the rule of forced labour'.

A key condition for this 'subjugation of unreason' (runs Foucault's argument) lay in the insane being perceived as animals rather than as human, hardly needing clothes, and being oblivious to climate and environment:

> In the classical period... the madman was not a sick man. Animality in fact protected the lunatic from whatever might be fragile, precarious or sickly in man... Unchained animality could be mastered only by discipline and brutalising.[4]

Hence savage treatment was not a dereliction but a duty: cages, whips and chains. There could not be a dialogue with the mad 'any longer', nor yet, however, any 'psychiatry', because (Foucault rather peculiarly claims) the Enlightenment possessed no 'psychology'.

Such a situation persisted for upward of a century till radically transformed in the 1790s by Pinel striking the chains off the inmates of the Bicêtre, and by the Tukes' moral therapy at the York Retreat (in that sense, Foucault endorsed the 'rupture' theory).Yet these events proved no red-letter days for the insane, according to Foucault. Despite pious eulogies, moral therapy was not 'unreason liberated' but rather 'madness mastered'. Physical constraint could finally be dispensed with, because the new 'moral imprisonment' proved so potent. This 'gigantic moral imprisonment', these 'mind forg'd manacles', were reinforced through infantilisation (the mad were as children), via the creation of surrogate families within the asylum, and by instilling guilt and self-control: at last 'thereby a psychology of madness became possible'.

Foucault's radical interpretation gives particular prominence to three points. First, during the 'great confinement', madness was 'reduced to silence', made a 'nothing', and penalised as never before; unreason's fate was to be 'shut up' in every sense. Second, the mad were newly locked up on a vastly greater scale during this period. The Paris *Hôpital Général*, founded in 1656, was already by the 1660s housing some 6,000 inmates, including lunatics and imbeciles. In France such institutions spread from the capital to the provinces, once an edict of 1676 had ordered cities to establish their own *hôpital général*. Third, the intermingling of the mad higgledy-piggledy with down-and-outs, petty criminals, idlers and tramps indicates that securing the mad was essentially the politics of custodialism, stockading rational bourgeois society against its enemies. The 'great confinement' was to discipline anarchy more than to heal the mentally sick.

There is bold insight here. For instance, the difficult, different, dangerous and distracted were indeed being shut up in increasing numbers during the Enlightenment, that glorious epoch of freedom and *sapere aude* ('dare to know'). And the authorities could clearly regard securing the mad as a police measure. Thus the English Vagrancy Act of 1714 linked lunatics with 'Rogues, Vagabonds, Sturdy Beggars and Vagrants', empowering Justices of the Peace to detain the 'furiously mad, and dangerous' in some 'secure place' – a lock-up, bridewell, or house of correction – where the disturbed in mind might be herded with other disturbers of the peace. This gloomy reading of emergent policy as essentially repressive certainly rings truer than those histories of psychiatry which salute the New Science and the Age of Reason as brave new dawns, freeing the mad from being mistakenly identified as demoniacs.

Foucault's revisionism cannot, however, be more than partially accepted, for it does not fit the facts, at least for England. This is true most strikingly for the scale of sequestration, which was hardly 'great'. Certainly the chief cities of France built receptacles for undesirables; but confinement was less concerted elsewhere. In England, for example, workhouses themselves developed unevenly – not surprisingly, for until 1834 the keystone of Poor Law policy remained not institutional confinement but outdoor relief, mixing care and coercion under the parish. Moreover, even in France the number of lunatics locked away remained small. Throughout the eighteenth century, there were never more than twenty mad people at any one time in the Montpellier Hôtel Dieu.

Indeed, outside France the very concept of a 'great confinement' – which Foucault claimed operated 'throughout Europe' – seems inappropriate for the 'long eighteenth century'. England provides an acid test. Under the Georges there was no co-ordinated drive by government, central or local, to sequester the mad poor. Provision of public asylums did not become mandatory until 1845. Unsurprisingly, therefore, the aggregate of confined lunatics remained small. Official figures compiled early in the nineteenth century and known at the time to be an underestimate, suggested that some 2,500 people were detained in licensed houses for lunatics, and approximately a further 2,200 pauper lunatics in houses of correction and similar places. These figures may be contrasted with the 3,000 patients housed in one single asylum, Colney Hatch, by 1900. Even at the close of the eighteenth century, the tally of the confined mad poor in Bristol, a town of some 30,000, was only twenty, and throughout the county of Oxfordshire there were just twenty-two. About 400 people a year were being admitted to private asylums. Foucault's notion that reason embarked upon a heroic 'exorcism of madness' is, for England at least, hyperbolic. Likewise, it is something of an exaggeration for MacDonald to state that in the eighteenth century the 'asylum system' spread 'throughout the nation'. Rather, something approaching fifty private receptacles, most housing fewer than a score, sprang up here and there – none at all existed in Wales or in Devon and Cornwall. Talk of 'system' is misleading. The age of the 'great confinement' in England was not the Georgian era but its successor.

Similarly, there is nothing to support Foucault's assertion, endorsed by Doerner, that confined lunatics, scandalising the bourgeois work ethos, were set to 'work as a moral duty'. Eye-witness reports suggest instead that what truly characterised asylum life was idleness. Some asylums provided token occupational therapy (gardening, needlework etc.), but this was offered as tonic, distraction and recreation, not to inure patients to the capitalist mill outside nor even to make the asylum cost-effective. The self-supporting colony-asylum was a dream of the future. Further, Foucault's claim that inmates were regarded as brutes and treated with exemplary cruelty, though it has some supporting evidence, seems positively perverse, since that is precisely the image of madness which leading Enlightenment writers on insanity were repudiating. For example, the madhouse-keeper Benjamin Faulkner asserted in the 1780s that lunatics should be treated as 'rational creatures... with attention and humanity'.

Overall, Foucault's characterisation of a 'great confinement' proves dubious for interpreting English developments during the 'long eighteenth century'. Indeed, his notion of reason chaining 'unreason' in new custodial institutions hardly applies anywhere (it seems to project French ideology onto the rest of the continent). Throughout peasant Europe – in Spain, Portugal, Russia, Scandinavia, Ireland, Poland etc. – little confinement of lunatics occurred. Where it was increasing, traditional institutions generally remained predominant, above all those under Christian auspices. Thus in Catholic nations, most confined lunatics were still tended by such healing orders as the Brothers and the Sisters of Charity. In Spain, Bohemia and Poland, these charities exercised almost a monopoly of care. Elsewhere initiatives typically came not from the absolutist state and its prefects, but from humanitarian impulses. Thus in England, philanthropic lunatic asylums were supported by private generosity in such towns as London, Manchester and York. And in the market-capitalist regions of north-west Europe, private madhouses run for profit became a feature.

This leads to a further point. It is a key contention of Foucault, and particularly Doerner, that the 'great confinement' was a drive by the powerful to police the poor: 'The bourgeoisie established psychiatry specifically for the poor insane.' Now, a numerical majority of the confined may well have been from the lower orders. But it would be a mistake to underestimate the numbers of the bourgeoisie, gentry and nobility who were also being confined. Without their well-heeled clientele, the 'trade in lunacy' would have foundered. Psychiatry was thus not just – probably not even primarily – a discipline for controlling the rabble.

REROUTING

These considerations have important bearings upon our images of eighteenth-century madhouses. Those horror stories of lunatics chained in underground dungeons in France, whipped in Germany, and jeered by ogling sightseers in London's Bedlam – all are true. Manacled, naked, foul, sleeping on straw in overcrowded and feculent conditions, the mad were dehumanised. The evils of certain madhouses, both public and private, beggar description. Inspecting the York Asylum, the JP Godfrey Higgins found cells whose stench made him instantly vomit, and discovered thirteen women cooped up for the day in a cell eight feet square.

Yet there are other sides to the story. Even some of the larger public asylums were kept in good repair. Take St Patrick's in Dublin, founded by Jonathan Swift: 'The whole clean and in good order', reported Henry Gray Bennet in 1815:

> There were but six straw patients in the whole establishment, two of whom were quite naked, having torn their clothes to pieces... the patients were remarkably quiet and orderly; there were only three persons in manacles, no one in a strait-waistcoat.[5]

And some asylums for paying patients were positively comfortable. The houses run by the Brothers of Charity in France had good amenities for the better-off, not least an enviable cuisine. Similar healthy and inspiriting conditions were not unknown in England, as for instance at the licensed house founded by the Revd Dr Francis Willis – George III's mad-doctor – at Greatford in Lincolnshire. Visiting it, Frederick Reynolds was taken aback:

> As the unprepared traveller approached the town, he was astonished to find almost all the surrounding ploughmen, gardeners, threshers, thatchers, and other labourers, attired in black coats, white waistcoats, black silk breeches and stockings, and the head of each *bien poudrée, frisée et arrangée*. These were the doctor's patients: and dress, neatness of person and exercise being the principal features of his admirable system, health and cheerfulness conjoined toward the recovery of every person attached to that most valuable asylum.[6]

Inside, the atmosphere was that of a Gothic house party:

> The Doctor kept an excellent table, and the day I dined with him I found a numerous company. Among others of his patients... there was a Mrs B., a lady of large fortune, who had lately

recovered under the Doctor's care, but declined returning into
the world from the dread of a relapse; and a young clergyman
who occasionally read service and preached for the Doctor.[7]

So what are we to make of this? There was no doubt a trend,
begun earlier but now accelerating, towards institutionalising the
mad. The totals, however, remained minuscule compared with
later developments. The great majority of the disturbed remained
within society, kept at home or boarded out. Incarceration was
not government policy. Most confined lunatics were handled
in the private sector by the 'trade in lunacy'. Asylums catered
for all social ranks. It would thus be a mistake automatically
to identify the unreformed madhouse with mere degradation,
punitiveness and social control. Moreover, attitudes towards
the mentally disturbed were more complex than Foucault or
Doerner have allowed. Georgian culture, both elite and popular,
became disposed to sympathise with and even to sentimentalise
the disordered, as well as to stigmatise them.

To voice these criticisms at the outset is not simply to beat
a retreat into minutiae or parochialism. It is merely to establish
that the early history of English madness lacks the uniformity
which centralised absolutism might have afforded, or which
public debate and parliamentary legislation were subsequently
to impart in the 'age of improvement'.

In sharp contrast, then, to the later consolidation of psychological medicine, buttressed with its journals, gatherings
and professional associations, pre-nineteenth-century practice
was characterised by diversity and individualism. This was both
good and bad. Eighteenth-century judicial arrangements for the
deranged were lax in contrast to the legalism, culminating in
the 1890 Act, which was later to straitjacket patients, doctors
and magistrates alike. It was extremely easy – as Defoe protested
– to put relatives away. Grossly improper confinement was made
more difficult in the Victorian age, though even public figures
such as Bulwer Lytton still managed to confine their wives under
dubious circumstances. But Georgian *ad hoc*-ery had its virtues.

When in 1796 Mary Lamb slew her mother in a mad fit, her fate was not to be put on trial and then either executed or found legally insane and secluded in Bethlem for the rest of her days, as would happen a generation later with the painter Richard Dadd. Rather, on a coroner's warrant, she was entrusted to her brother's safekeeping – surely for her, and possibly for her family, the best resolution of a hideous catastrophe. The poor of course could not expect such clemency.

Moreover, the pre-bureaucratic stage of mad-doctoring was favourable in many respects to innovation. Victorian asylum management may well have terminated the gross abuses and peculation poisoning eighteenth-century madhouses, but it was certainly stymied by the legalism of magistrates, the penny-pinching of Boards of Guardians, the centralising aspirations of the Lunacy Commissioners, and by blind faith in institutional discipline. By contrast, the previous century had showed prolific experiment. Jaundiced now by hindsight, it is easy to forget how novel early private asylums were. In a nation in which institutions typically meant workhouses for paupers and bridewells for malefactors, the appearance of opulent establishments such as Ticehurst and Brislington House marked an important break. Moreover, though the much-fêted 'moral therapy' has now been subjected to disenchanted revisionism, it remains true that radically new techniques of management were pioneered during the eighteenth century – most famously from the 1790s at the York Retreat, but before then at many other sites. Again, whether it appears an advance or an abomination, there was much experimentation with new therapeutic technology. Mechanical chairs, swings and, above all, medical electricity were not wholly new. But they did represent attempts to break free of the hidebound depletive therapeutics of bloodletting, vomits and purges.

Some historians have seen this new technology as essentially repressive, but hindsight can oversimplify. It is tempting, in the light of current anti-psychiatry, to denounce early psycho-technology simply as the harbinger of the evils of electro-convulsive therapy, highlighting the decline from Christian

thaumaturgy into the medical mechanism encouraged by the
Scientific Revolution. Such polarities beg many questions.
After all, the leading Georgian advocate of medical electricity
was none other than John Wesley, spiritual healer and exorcist
extraordinaire, a man who saw insanity largely in terms of the
Devil (Wesley also, it should be remembered, advocated putting
a maniac under a waterfall 'as long as his strength will bear').
And among others who treated mental and nervous afflictions with the new techniques of magneto-electricity were
Mesmerists, who fit equally badly into the tunnel-prehistory
of institutional psychological medicine and who, indeed, are
often lauded – using a different sort of hindsight – as the fathers
of psychotherapy and dynamic psychiatry. 'Saints and sinners'
history oversimplifies.

If the new machinery of madness has been criticised, so has
the scientific rationality apparently underpinning it. Critics such
as Berman and Capra have argued that the Scientific Revolution,
especially the Cartesian mind/body dualism (allegedly splitting
the whole person into a 'divided self'), was responsible for
psychic catastrophe. The new model of the self as an isolated
atom in an alien, dead cosmos allegedly produced existential
terror among disorientated moderns, compelled to live in the
deracinated, meaningless universe of the New Science. Moreover,
Cartesianism, by unsouling the flesh, may also have thereby sanctioned more rigorous treatments for the crazed. These issues
will be explored further in later chapters, but some preliminary
comments are worth making now.

First, we must be careful not to exaggerate or oversimplify
the impact of the New Science in reconceptualising the self
and its place in Nature. Despite Descartes and Newton, everyday medicine, for both mind and body, remained as routinely
psychosomatic as ever, presuming – as common experience suggested – a two-way traffic between mind and body within the
whole person as integral to both the cause and cure of afflictions.
Indeed, even traditional humoralism stayed deeply entrenched
through the eighteenth century – as is shown by the evidence

of sick people's diaries and also by novels such as *Tristram Shandy*, written 'against the spleen'.

Science did not have a blanket impact, and its influence amounted to much more than conjuring up a nightmare vision of mind adrift from the mechanised body, a ghost in the machine. The New Science could be put to many uses. Take, for example, the newly promoted physiology of the nervous system, with its attendant nervous illnesses. Medical men eagerly incorporated nerves into their aetiologies of disturbance, creating in the process the stereotype of the nervous, hysterical woman. Laypeople too enthusiastically embraced 'nerves' for their own purposes. Thus, when word got abroad that George III was delirious, he reassured the court of his sanity, insisting: 'I'm nervous, I'm not ill, but I'm nervous.' The jargon of 'nerves, spirits and fibres' was not simply foisted on to the public. Indeed, laymen were eager to exploit the resources of mental medicine to enhance individuality or shrug off responsibility. The auras of mental abnormality or creative malady readily conferred distinction, heightened sensibility, and hinted at originality and creativity. For every terrified Johnson, there was a tempted, titillated Boswell.

I have been stressing the sheer diversity of developments in the 'long eighteenth century'. Legally and institutionally there was no uniform 'great confinement', nor did new Rationalism simply invalidate unreason. This varied response indicates the fact that – both in reality and in the public imagination – lunatics were not such terrifying bogeys as witches earlier or as Jacobins later. The shires panicked over Papists and paupers more than over the mad. It was not until well into the nineteenth century that the insane – crack troops in the army of degenerates – were to precipitate 'moral panic'.

The situation of the mad in Georgian England was heterogeneous; they formed part of civil society, but they hardly fell under the state or under systematic medical *savoir-pouvoir*. Yet that is not to deny that they were visible. Certainly Victorian psychiatric reformers found a hidden iceberg of 'latent insanity', hitherto unsuspected. But the mad and the sad were extremely familiar figures in the early modern physical and mental landscapes. Indeed, precisely because so few disordered people were permanently locked away, the witless and the weird were bound to be on public view – in the lanes, loafing round taverns, or, like Margery Kempe some centuries earlier, shrieking away in church. They were sights. London crowds thronged to quiz Bethlem's 'scholars' – evidence that Pepys' or Dr Johnson's contemporaries did not, *pace* Foucault, feel that lunacy was something to quarantine but rather to experience. Johnson deemed that seeing the mad was as instructive as attending public executions: 'it is right that we should be kept in mind of madness'.

Being fascinated with madness was not condemned as ghoulish until the age of sensibility. Medieval drama had made sport with Folly; in their turn Jacobean playwrights filled the stage with maniacs and zanies, and mad-folk –Tom Fool, Crazy Jane, Mad Meg and the like – populate folklore and ballads; 'Mad Madge' was also the nickname of Margaret, Duchess of Newcastle. Not least, the disturbed were present in people's family experience. James Boswell, for example, had a brother, John, who became disordered and ended up confined. Boswell showed real concern for him.

Madness made its presence felt, from Hamlet, Ophelia and King Lear, through the mid-eighteenth-century graveyard poets, up to Keats' bittersweet melancholy, and the 'mad, bad, and dangerous to know' Lord Byron. Folly was the idiom of satirists, and Hogarth engraved mankind's madness in a crazy upside-down world in which London and Bedlam formed an ironic tale of two cities. The cunning of history had its say too, driving King George III mad, and turning him into a very presentable double of King Lear. Other public figures were also regarded as crackbrained, not least George's arch enemy Edmund Burke, who insisted on being buried in an unmarked grave so that his persecutors should not be able to pursue him beyond death.

THE REALITY OF MENTAL ILLNESS?

In thus setting up Georgian madness for discussion, I have necessarily made assumptions about its nature. Polonius' dilemma – precisely what is the objective status of insanity? – has obviously been raised by recent 'anti-psychiatries'. Should the historian view it as an organic disease, rather like smallpox or plague? Or should it be treated as a social label, akin to 'heretic', 'witch' or 'subversive'? For practical purposes, in my view, the history of madness stands between histories of subjects such as plague or death and (on the other hand) histories of witchcraft. It must treat insanity, like heart failure or buboes, as a physical fact; but it needs to interpret it, like witchcraft or possession, principally as a socially constructed fact.

Yet any hard-and-fast polarity we may draw between the 'objective' and the 'projective' will be constantly dissolving. For even such certain phenomena as death and disease are encrusted with language, culture and history, ranging from doubts in the particular case (is this person dead or merely deep in coma, or dead drunk, dead to the world?) to the cosmic, as in the Christian denial of death ('Death, thou shalt die'). Similarly, retrospective diagnosis of smallpox creates problems: can we match past symptoms against present epidemiology? Has smallpox itself changed down the ages? Even so, historical demographers studying mortality, and medical historians investigating epidemics, do not generally feel that they have to be essentially historians of *mentalité*, ideology and hegemony.

Not so, however, with study of demonic possession (except for the dedicated Satanist scholar). In his scholarly practice, today's typical historian is a Sadducee, denying the reality of the spirit world. He fundamentally regards witch-beliefs as false consciousness, true only in the sense that belief in them was once so intense as to induce the phenomena blamed on the Devil.

So, is the historian to treat the lunatic as akin more to the smallpox victim or to the witch? Neither of these extremes will serve our turn. Even the doughtiest champion of the organic aetiology of insanity will concede that madness has donned and doffed radically different masks down the ages, just as those who regard 'insanity' essentially as a social label will admit that the individual suffering is none the less intense. Some integrative position is required. Insanity is both a personal disorder (with a kaleidoscope of causes, ranging from the organic to the psychosocial), and is also articulated within a system of socio-linguistic signs and meanings. This complexity is made quite clear by the historical record. For pre- and early industrial English society had little difficulty in accepting that – generically speaking – lunacy existed, yet actually demarcating the insane often remained controversial in the particular case.

As with death, the real presence of madness formed part of the natural beliefs of the times. However in the century after the Civil War, witchcraft was increasingly discredited, or at least was regarded so that its reality became merely subjective. A witch, for opinion-makers such as Joseph Addison, turned out after all to be merely a woman who deluded herself into thinking she was one. No one 'proved' that madness was all an illusion, or believed a madman was nothing but a person who thought he was one. No new theory arose to explain away 'mad' behaviour, as it did to dissolve witchcraft; indeed witchcraft was itself denied partly by being incorporated into irrationality. Instead there remained the presence of the 'mad' themselves, or at least the mad clad in convention. Standard types, such as the Toms o' Bedlam who tramped the highways 'licentiated', as John Aubrey put it, 'to goe a-begging', the jilted lover gone demented or the ranting religious maniac, and standard actions – muttering gibberish, tearing off one's clothes – epitomised madness in the public mind.

Yet craziness was indeed situational, rather like possession or witchcraft. If madness was Protean, how then could one know its symptoms for certain? When the confinement of a Home Counties farmer was disputed in the early nineteenth century, the fact that he paid his labourers wages over the odds was adduced by his family to prove he had taken leave of his senses. Another time, another place, he would have been hailed as a true-blue paternalist. Similarly, the evangelical leader George Whitefield secured the release from Bethlem of a gospeller, Joseph Periam, whose faith had led him to hosanna at the top of his voice and to give his goods to the poor. To Georgian churchmen this was crazy; once it would have been holy. Because the meanings of madness were matters for continuous renegotiation, the history of insanity is more difficult (but also richer) than, say, that of smallpox or witchcraft.

This is so for further reasons. It was common in the centuries of court wits and jesters, of Burton and Hogarth, to personify madness itself as a rogue – two-faced, duplicitous, the supreme trickster. It impersonated civility, yet laughed behind its back. In the mad state, mind and body deceived each other, and John Ferriar had later to confess,

> We are ignorant by what laws the body possessed a power of representing the most hazardous disorders, without incurring danger; of counterfeiting the greatest derangement in the circulating system, without materially altering its movements; of producing madness, conscious of its extravagancies, and of increasing the acuteness of sensation, by oppressing the common sensorium... Nature, as if in ridicule of the attempts to unmask her, has in this class of diseases, reconciled contradictions, and realised improbabilities, with a mysterious versatility; which inspires the true philosopher with diffidence, and reduces the systematic to despair.[8]

What is more, as everyone knew, madness had its remissions and lucid intervals, and lunacy was as inconstant as the moon. So was one to think of lunatics having fits of sanity or sane people suffering bouts of madness? – a hare that James Carkesse started chasing in his provocative mad-verse manifesto *Lucida Intervalla* (1679). In other words, what was so maddening about madness was that it was simultaneously real, terrifying and catastrophic, yet also chimerical, duping both its victims and society at large.

Moreover, madness was Protean, in that the idea itself encompassed no end of meanings. It could assume all the solemnity of a clinical diagnosis, or be a street-corner insult; now a stigma, next an endearment. It could signify rage – *ira brevis furor* (anger is a brief madness) was an old saw – but also signal the comic and ludicrous. It could mark the passions, especially pride and vanity; indeed, it could be passion itself (a 'mad' person might simply, *par excellence*, be impassioned, like a mad bull); or be a synonym for illogicality, absurdity, reason in motley. 'Mad caps', 'mad rogues', 'mad devils' – all such idioms traded upon the mysteries of liminality, bursting the bounds of the workaday – notions which the Renaissance cult of the singular Saturnine genius replicated higher up the social scale.

In other words, with all its verbal kin from light-headedness to lycanthropy, lunacy was unbound, never confined exclusively to a charmed circle of meanings, never simply a slur or a nosological niche. It maintained its vernacular currency in tales of love madness, catchpenny ballads of Crazy Kate, and the slapstick wit of 'It's a Mad World My Masters'. In the world we have lost, the laity did not need expert psychiatric witnesses to tell them that the newly delivered mother, delirious with fever, who smothered her baby should be treated as mad and spared the noose, just as everyone recognised the 'madness' of *crime passionnel* when the jealous Revd James Hackman shot his inamorata Martha Ray, Lord Sandwich's mistress, but also saw why *he* must swing for his crime.

Yet this is not to argue, either, for some Olde Worlde folk-loric sagacity, super-sympathetic to the daft, the dim and the distracted. As doctors pointed out, toleration didn't spring up from the grass roots. Peasants ragged the village idiot no less than sightseers joshed the Bedlamites. Nor, indeed, were popular attitudes 'timeless'. In 1500 or 1600, jurymen would have found a man who did away with himself guilty of the felony of wilful self-murder; they were, it seems, content to sanction the escheat of his property and his burial in unhallowed ground at a crossroads, a stake through his heart. After all, such self-murderers had sinned against the Holy Ghost, and their troubled spirits might haunt the community. An eighteenth-century coroner's jury, however, would have found the equivalent suicide mad, and hence spared the law's rigours; that verdict allowed his family to inherit his property. Possibly this shift in attitude filtered down from above, though it is hard to be sure.

I have been highlighting two aspects. First, madness – with all its brood of melancholy, delirium, phrenzy, troubled spirits and the like – wore many faces. Second, talking about madness – even talking authoritatively about it – was not traditionally the preserve of any profession. There was no unique dictionary definition or moral response: it could be cosmic, comic, clinical or casual. Background beliefs about original sin and the senility of Creation (*mundus senescens*), as well as traditions of jesting and rites of inversion – all emphasised that craziness was indeed the way of the world, was even normal, and so sustained the double vision of the mad and the rational, and the potency of madness as a lampoon of the workaday world.

MADNESS AND THE PEOPLE

Documenting the social history of madness down the 'long eighteenth century' means starting from everyday perceptions, rather than taking our terms *ex cathedra* from legislators, text-books and psychiatrists. This is because, initially at least, the people talking most about madness were the people at large. As with witch-beliefs, ideas about madness were not merely implanted from above, but were entrenched within a common cultural consciousness, forming a social expression rather than a hegemonic construct.

Michael MacDonald has brilliantly mapped the linguistic resonances of insanity in the minds of the early seventeenth-century doctor Richard Napier and his clients. It would be of great value to extend this lexicon down throughout the 'long eighteenth century', to see what changed. I cannot do that here. But attention must be drawn to certain powerful traditions endowing madness with meaning in common discourse. Prominent among these was Christianity.

The Scriptures welcomed certain modes of madness. Of course the Bible pinpoints the ungodly, like Nebuchadnezzar, deranged by God by way of exemplary punishment just as Herod, Judas or, indeed, Lucifer had been maddened with pride. But – particularly in the New Testament and in Patristic theology – madness can also be holy, either as the innocent otherworldliness of the Pauline fool or as the ecstasy of the Old Testament prophet. If the temporal body cages the eternal soul, then to go out of one's senses – 'standing beyond' in ecstasy – spelt release from the carnal prison-house. Reformation piety was sympathetic to speaking prophetically or hearing voices from Beyond, as marks of a divine madness. Equally, of course, these might be Satan's wiles, symptoms of sickness or even of fraud. The problem was to distinguish and this, naturally, provoked bitter conflict. It was, for example, regarded as perfectly normal for a godly Protestant to hear spiritual voices; Richard Napier, treating the disturbed, consulted with the Archangel Raphael. However, as George Trosse was to find, Satan's voice mimicked God's, and when such diabolical ventriloquism happened, 'divine ecstasy' imploded into raving madness. Similarly, when God spoke to Lady Eleanor Davies prophesying the fall of Charles I, the divine message overstepped diplomacy and she was sent to Bethlem – an early example of 'psychiatric abuse'.

Of more widespread importance is the fact that Christianity provided, in the Fall, a compelling myth of the human condition itself as disordered. In God's sight, all were fallen as a result of Original Sin. If all are sunk in sin; if (as Luther saw it) reason is thus a 'whore', or at best a broken reed compared to essentials like faith and grace; or if, as Calvin contended, the will is bound, and souls predestined to their fates, their worldly qualities notwithstanding – in such theologies the divide between sanity and craziness would then, in the sight of God, signify little. At least it will count for less than the distinction between God's children and His foes, the saved and the damned, the faithful and the infidel, the orthodox and schismatic. As Erasmus' ironies implied, being worldly-wise was hardly cardinal to a faith that espoused the madness of the Cross, and taught that truth pours out of the mouths of babes and sucklings. If mankind was radically sinful, the gulf between *homo rationalis* and the fool was neither clear-cut nor crucial under God, for all are sinful, all mad. As Bishop Hall put it:

> He is a rare man, that hath not some kind of madness reigning in him: one a dull madness of melancholy; another, a conceited madness of pride [etc.] It is as hard, to reckon up all kinds of madness, as of dispositions.[9]

Only once belief in Original Sin became tempered – initially among the educated Anglican elite, in line first with Arminian liberal theology and then with Enlightenment naturalism – could this divide become primary.

Until then, however, the Church evinced a certain sympathy towards simpletons – though there is less evidence in England than, say, in Russia for any cult of 'holy fools', of 'fools for Christ's sake'. Although Christianity abounded in scapegoats – the infidel, witches, Jews, women even – there is little sign that lunatics were thought *ipso facto* God's enemies. In fact, their standing was as ambiguous as that formerly of lepers. Doubtless certain people whom we might diagnose clinically insane were accused as demoniacs or witches, but the courts energetically strove to differentiate between them, and Zilboorg and others were wrong to suppose that the magistracy systematically mistook the mad for the maleficent. It was never the policy of Christian churches to sequester the mad. Rather, within Christianity, it was precisely the convocation of the rational and the sane, of *dives* and *pauper*, the confusion of adults and children and even of humans and beasts – God's creatures all – that traditionally constituted the divine and human comedies.

Alongside specifically Christian theology, a wealth of assumptions about madness was also in circulation among secular culture, high and low, integrating erudition garnered from the Greeks with the kinds of colloquial lore fixed in such proverbs as 'mad as a hatter', 'mad as a weaver', 'mad as a March hare' and 'mad as May-butter' (tantalisingly echoed in 'but mad North North West').The Classical legacy encouraged the possibility of viewing madness as an essential, even a positive part of experience. For while ancient philosophy – filtered through Renaissance Humanism – assuredly championed reason, Greek culture had equally been riveted by the irrational. Tragedians in particular had portrayed the precariousness of the mind, resulting from man's dual and cruelly divided nature and from nemesis, the gods' vengeance against the hubris of rational pride.

And the Greeks and their successors grasped the potential – no less than the wretchedness – of man's dark and divided nature. For strangeness was also strength. Disequilibrium of the humours (those four key fluids – blood, phlegm, choler and black bile – whose harmony produced health) certainly endangered the mental and physical constitution; yet it could also confer distinctive energies. In particular, in Aristotle's formulation, the man superabundant in black bile was of course prey to fear, suspicion and misanthropy; yet such a melancholic would also characteristically be sharp of intellect, trenchant in criticism, acute in perception, pungent in expression – a genius no less. From black-clad Hamlet, through Jaques with his 'melancholy of mine own', to that self-consuming artefact which was Burton's *Anatomy of Melancholy*, Stuart England cultivated the melancholic as both the man of parts and the malcontent, whose fascination, if challenged by Montaigne, was celebrated by Burton in orgiastic Jacobean profusion.

Melancholy genius was a blood relation to another class of madness formulated by the Greeks and internationally endorsed by Renaissance Humanism: the poet as madman, possessed by transcendental fire (*furor*), a divine inspiration which thrust him out of himself. Above all, in the *Symposium* Plato had imagined the poet as a man filled with 'afflatus' (the divine breath) or 'divine fury', and such views were playfully echoed in Shakespeare's

sentiment that 'the lunatick, the lover and the poet are of imagination all compact', and his description of artistic creation:

> The poet's eye in a fine phrensy rolling
> Doth glance from heav'n to earth, from earth to heav'n
> And, as imagination bodies forth
> The forms of things unknown, the poet's pen
> Turns them to shape, and gives to aiery nothing
> A local habitation and a name.[10]

Within this cultural conceit – Dryden's 'Great Wits are sure
to Madness near ally'd' – to dub a poet mad was paying him a
compliment. As Michael Drayton praised Kit Marlowe:

> For that fine madness still he did retain
> Which rightly should possess a poet's brain.

And this cultural trope of the intermixing of wit and madness
mirrored the living realities of Tudor and Stuart England. Like
Shakespeare's motley fools, real jesters such as Will Somers and
Richard Tarlton were marked out by their zany improvisations,
ditties, jingles and barbs. As set on stage by Jacobean playwrights,
Bedlam always had its complement of Parnassians and wits who
had lost their wits. And herein life only mimicked art. Visiting
Bethlem (commonly called, in deference to Plato, the Academy
of Bedlam), John Evelyn found one inmate 'mad with making
verses', and a few years later he would have met there the eminent
dramatist Nathaniel Lee, crazed by claret. When ex-Bedlamites
tramped the highways, licensed to beg, their numbers swollen
by pretenders ('Abraham Men'), they were expected to busk,
singing Bedlamite ballads, for their bread.

Such mad music formed one of many links between learned
stereotypes and all the mundane manifestations of the mad.
Indeed, as MacDonald has emphasised, the rich and nuanced
early Stuart vocabulary for the abnormal was essentially shared
between the doctor and his patients and spanned the social

ranks, even if certain phrases (e.g. 'melancholic') were reserved for posher patients, and others (e.g. 'mopish', suggesting surly captiousness) for plebeians. Scores of epithets pepper Napier's casebooks – sad, sorry, distracted, furious, despairing, jabbering, and many more. And the fact that so many of them are adjectival may be revealing. Far more sufferers were identified as 'raving' than were actually labelled 'maniacs', probably indicating that madness was conceived more in terms of deeds and demeanour than of disease, or any permanent internal disposition.

In fact, insanity might be widely seen as a hazard of humanity, a fate which, under desperate circumstances, could seize anyone and everyone, for a galaxy of reasons, from the bite of a rabid dog to oppressive weather (especially during the 'Dog Days' of Midsummer Madness), to earwigs in the head (according to Cornish folklore) or overwhelming grief, pride, love or joy. So insanity was a blow afflicting by degrees, in fits, coming and going with remissions, oscillating in intensity. With such flux, governed by the inconstant moon, at what point did extreme passion or eccentricity pass over into madness? Or the vagabond mind return to lucidity? Presumably pondering the poet Kit Smart, but surely reflecting also on his own plight, Samuel Johnson was to assure Boswell,

> Many a man is mad in certain instances, and goes through life without having it perceived; – for example, a madness has seized a person, of supposing himself obliged literally to pray continually; had the madness turned the opposite way, and the person thought it a crime ever to pray, it might not improbably have continued unobserved.[11]

Johnson's insight – madness was not unequivocal but an existential hazard of living in the world of opinion – is confirmed at almost the same date in this interesting confidence by Horace Walpole to his friend, Horace Mann, about Walpole's nephew, Lord Orford. This fellow was clearly, in Walpole's eyes, somewhat disturbed, but Walpole saw it as part of the chances and changes of life:

I am debarrassed... of my nephew. He has resumed the entire
dominion of himself, and is gone into the country, and intends
to command the militia. Yet is he not ignorant of his situation.
He said the other day to his Dalilah, speaking of Dr. Monro [the
physician to Bethlem], 'Patty, I like this doctor! don't you? We will
have him next time.' What an amazing compost of sense, insen-
sibility, and frenzy! His recovery was as marvellous. He waked,
could scarce articulate, and thought himself paralytic. The keeper
gave him a common apothecary's draught. In a quarter of an hour
he said, 'What have you given me? It has removed a weight from
my head' – and thence talked rationally.[12]

Walpole guessed at organic reasons why Orford's condition
would intensify and remit:

It seems to me to indicate that frenzy is occasioned by a gathering
of matter or water that presses on the brain and disorders it, and
that what he felt as paralytic, was the crisis preceding an internal
discharge. It even looks in him as if it took the same time to come
to maturity. Last fit lasted under or about thirteen months; this
is not quite twelve – I hope the next will be as long gathering
as the last, three years![13]

Writing near the close of our period, the Bristol physician
Dr Thomas Beddoes was nettled over the pitfalls of reasoning
about madness: 'MAD is one of those words, which mean almost
everything and nothing'. Even physically, madness and sanity
were hard to tell apart:

The difficulty of a definition of madness... is evident from another
consideration. The insane have the same muscles with the sane.
In both, they perform the same general office.[14]

Beddoes grasped at rational – even anatomical – distinctions,
yet still could not overcome this slitheriness, frustrating to one
with his Edinburgh training. Yet the doctor's dilemma perfectly

captures the fact that terms like 'mad' revelled in linguistic licence, defying physicians' attempts to sterilise them for clinical use. But in one sense Beddoes seems almost wilfully wrong – in maintaining that madness means 'almost everything and nothing'. For vernacular use of such terms had discernible contours and these may be briefly mapped in here, backed by examples, to illuminate the topography of 'natural beliefs'.

In common parlance, people were typically called 'mad' when impassioned beyond moderation or 'reason'. 'A violent Vase madness broke out among the Irish', rejoiced the potter Josiah Wedgwood when his ceramic sales went through the roof. 'The people in London, Manchester and Birmingham are steam mill mad', reported his business crony, Matthew Boulton. 'The Town is Mad', deplored William Blake, à propos of the stampede to see the child actor, Master Betty. Sir Joseph Banks diagnosed his wife 'a little old china mad', considerately adding, however, 'but she wishes to mix as much reason with her madness as possible'.

Such enthusiasms were not thought uniquely English. The Dutch were said to suffer from tulip-mania. Horace Walpole, for example, exclaimed, à propos of France, 'a new madness reigns there... This is la fureur des cabriolets; Anglice, one-horse chairs' – and of course throughout the century, the French were supposed to be gripped by 'Anglomania'.

But mass frenzies were often seen as particularly English, from Bubble speculations ('I am almost South Sea mad', confessed the Hon. Mrs Molesworth in 1720), through the 1780s, when people were 'Balloon Mad', up to the 'Railway Manias' of the 1830s and 1840s. Personal enthusiasms qualified as well, as for example when the physician John Ferriar autodiagnostically coined the term 'bibliomania'.

Passions of all kinds could mushroom into madness. In the late seventeenth century, for example, Lady Granville was judged mad because she collected insects, and the naturalist John Ray had to testify on her behalf that entomology was a sane and sober science. Of course, it was the staple of satire to stigmatise whims and enthusiasms as crackbrained, yet the tone is generally indulgent. 'What mad freaks the mayds of Honour at Court have', recorded Pepys, pruriently agog 'that Mrs Jennings, one of the Duchess' maids, the other day dressed herself like an orange-wench and went up and down and cried oranges'. Indeed, it could even be delicious to confess *oneself* mad with enthusiasms. As the young Shelley insisted to Hogg, 'How can you fancy that I can think you mad; am I not the wildest, most delirious of enthusiasm's offspring', telling him later, 'I have wandered in the snow for I am cold wet and mad – Pardon me, pardon my delirious egotism.'

Madness was also synonymous with other turns of passion: pride, vanity and anger, viewed both as a blind, all-consuming fury, and as an emotion more positive and justified.

> While mad with foolish fame, or drunk with power
> Ambition slays his thousands in an hour[15]

rhymed Erasmus Darwin, associating madness and destructive fury – a tone informing Thomas Campbell's depiction of the London theatre audience ('the savages of the gallery') turned mob:

> The players were twice hissed off after this till a promise of Mrs Yates' appearance on Monday &c somewhat abated their madness.[16]

Countering this, of course, there was an animated moral and religious literature urging self-control which, like the *Treatise on the Dismal Effects of Low Spiritedness* (1750), identified madness as the vice of unbridled passions. Yet madness could equally be a point of pride, an expression of righteous indignation. Take Pepys' wrath on hearing his patron slandered:

> 'If my Lord had been a coward he had gone to sea no more it may be; then he might have been excused and made an Embassador' (meaning my Lord Sandwich); this made me mad, and I believe

she perceived my countenance change, and blushed herself very much.[17]

Pepys similarly got beside himself when he witnessed wanton cruelty:

> then to Kensington to the Grotto, and there we sat to my great content; only, vexed in going in to see a son of Sir Heneage Finch's beating of a poor little dog to death, letting it lie in so much pain that made me mad to see it...[18]

This finds an echo in his report of London's response to disaster:

> This day the great news is come of the French their taking the Island of St. Christopher from us... This makes the City mad.[19]

Madness could thus be raging passion. Everyone went wild from time to time with emotions good and bad, and all might be heartsick or lovesick or even, as the eighteenth century discovered, homesick. Ideas of raging passion highlighted the continuities between the common man and the mad, rather than setting the insane apart.

The language of madness also denoted, however, not just volcanic passions of the heart but also incongruity and error of the mind – all that defied norms or expectations, whatever lacked or transgressed good sense. The underlying emotional judgements could be neutral or positive, but were most frequently derogatory; the targets could be individual or collective. The astrologer Ebenezer Sibly, it was claimed, had written 'in the very language of Bedlam' – an attack echoed in the astronomer William Herschel's prediction that some would think him 'fit for Bedlam' for his stellar theories. Such equations of madness with intellectual eccentricity were bantering enough. Horace Walpole, however, was being less charitable when he attacked thundering evangelical preachers as wrong-headed slaves to error and consigning others to madness:

When Whitfield preaches, and when Whiston writes,
All cry, that madness dictates either's flights.
When Sherlock writes, or canting Secker preaches,
All think good sense inspires what either teaches,
Why, when all four for the same gospel fight,
Should two be crazy, two be in the right?
Plain is the reason – every son of Eve
Thinks the two madmen, what they teach, believe.[20]

Walpole's accusation was paralleled in tone by Mary Wortley
Montagu's sardonic digs against enthusiasts:

I am charmed with the account of the Moravians, who certainly
exceed all mankind in absurdity of principles and madness of
practice; yet these people walk erect, and are numbered among
rational beings[21]

but exceeded by her downright horror at a young lady's lunacy
in planning to elope with a seducer:

Any girl that runs away with a young fellow, without intending
to marry him, should be carried to Bridewell, or to Bedlam the
next day.[22]

And if individuals were liable to accusations of madness for
their morals or *mœurs*, whole groups – or indeed, the very times
hemselves – were often said to be running mad. The would-be intellectual Sylas Neville was so offended to hear a naval officer 'calling
all Philosophers Madmen', that he was stung to respond: 'On your
principles then... every man who endeavours to think justly and act
rightly is a madman'. Politicians for their part were commonly called
mad, and artists too. Robert Hunt pronged both on one fork:

If beside the stupid and mad-brained political projects of their
rulers, the sane part of the people of England required fresh proof
of the alarming increase of the effects of insanity, they will be

too well convinced from its having lately spread into the hitherto
sober region of Art.[23]

Defoe had also drawn on the same idiom, in his case seeing the
middle classes awash with madness:

> From mad statesmen, let us descend to mad Tradesmen,
> mad Creditors, and Companies, and all the Crowd of Shop-
> keeping Lunaticks, with which the world abounds – Some run
> in Debt to trust Lords, and are so mad, to think the other will
> be mad enough to pay them. Some are mad at the Diligence of
> Forreigners, and yet are idle themselves [and so forth].[24]

Such accusations knew no bounds. In the revanchist climate of
the Restoration, it became automatic to condemn the Civil War
and Cromwellian years as an era of lunacy; Bishop Sprat, for
example, referred to the 'madness of that dismal age'. The nation
itself was commonly deemed mad wholesale – an upside-down
world, wherein order, morals and authority had been usurped
by pride, presumption and extravagance; indeed, by the diabolical trinity of vice, vanity and folly. One solution, suggested the
Tatler, was that Bedlam itself be extended to house whole new
classes of lunatics: politicians, freethinkers and so forth. After all,
was Bedlam not already viewed as an 'Imperial College' or as
a fools' Parliament, whose senators and scholars had privileged
licence of expression? So Ned Ward went but one stage further
in his Hudibrastic inventory of contemporary evils by declaring
All Men Mad, Or England a Great Bedlam (1711), as did Thomas
Tryon, who insisted 'the world is just a great Bedlam, where those
that are more mad, lock up those that are less'. Yet it had all been
said long before, not least in Burton's *Anatomy of Melancholy*, that
omnium gatherum of anecdotes of insanity whose burden was that
mankind without exception – including the author himself – was
quite out of its mind: *nos insanavimus omnes*.

Burton's view of madness – early seventeenth-century opinion in a nutshell – was complex. At one level, that great lord of

misrule was out to tease; at another, however, he was painting a black and blue vision of human existence, taking cruel delight in racking mankind for its folly. You seek medicine for melancholy? he asks. Try intellectual diversions: why not 'calculate Spherical Triangles, square a circle... peruse subtle Scotus' and Suarez's Metaphysics... find the philosopher's stone?' How could we deserve better than such tortures? For after all, we are the wretches who

> insult, contemn, vex, torture, molest, and hold one another's noses to the grind-stone hard, provoke, rail, scoff, calumniate, challenge, hate, abuse, (hard-hearted, implacable, malicious, peevish, inexorable as we are) to satisfy our lust or private spleen, for toys, trifles, and impertinent occasions, spend ourselves, goods, friends, fortunes, to be revenged on our adversary, to ruin him... Monsters of men as we are, Dogs, Wolves, Tigers, Fiends, incarnate Devils, we do not only contend, oppress, and tyrannize ourselves, but, as so many firebrands, we set on, and animate others: our whole life is a perpetual combat, a conflict, a set battle, a snarling fit.[25]

Of course, Burton makes wheedling apologies for his outrageous authorial persona ('Democritus Junior had a merry kind of madness'); yet it was the real Democritus, he reminds us, who plucked out his own eyes because 'he could not bear to see wicked men prosper'. But the effect of Burton's stress on the universality of madness as a contagion, like sin, infecting all was actually to mitigate its specific terrors; to melancholise was human. When all are mad, none need rue it particularly; one could just say 'It's a mad world my masters', and laugh like Democritus or weep like Heraclitus. When 'all the world is melancholy... every member of it', lunatics do not get scapegoated in quite the ways in which Hans Mayer and Sander Gilman have seen racial outsiders such as Jews stigmatised in later ages.

Thus meanings of madness multiplied within lay culture, describing individuals, acts and situations out of the ordinary.

They did so in Burton's day without any automatic stigma or sense of a 'great divide' between 'two classes of men', the sane and the insane – was this likely when it was chummy to call someone to his face 'a mad fellow'?

In this situation, madness was familiarised by a rich explanatory lore. When Milton wrote in *Paradise Lost* of 'moon struck madness', he was evoking views about lunacy resonant among all walks of men (*Tristram Shandy*, it will be remembered, made the moon one of the dedicatees of his life and opinions). There were popular treatments galore for madness, ranging from herbal recipes to water-shock therapies, passed down orally and preserved in health-care publications. Burton recommended laurel, white hellebore, antimony and tobacco – 'divine, rare, super-excellent tobacco… a sovereign remedy to all diseases. A good vomit, I confess, if it be well qualified, opportunely taken and medicinally used.' In the mid-eighteenth century, in his *Primitive Physick*, John Wesley was to grant some remedies his personal *imprimatur*, along with new ones, for popular consumption:

> For Raving Madness:
> 1. It is a sure rule that all madmen are cowards, and may be conquered by binding only, without beating (Dr Mead). He also observes that blistering the head does more harm than good. Keep the head close shaved, and frequently wash it with vinegar.
> 2. Apply to the head clothes dipt in cold water.
> 3. Or, set the patient with his head under a great waterfall, as long as his strength will bear; or pour water on his head out of a tea-kettle.
> 4. Or, let him eat nothing but apples for a month.
> 5. Or, nothing but bread and milk. Tried.[26]

There was moreover a lively folklore which blamed madness on spells, or specifically on Satan and his henchmen. Yet this magico-spiritual element must not be misconstrued. It is all too easy to invent a linear progression from the Middle Ages when

– particularly among the ill-educated – madness was supposedly ascribed to supernatural (or rather infernal) forces, leading up towards a naturalistic present. But medievalists have amply demonstrated that madness was then no less commonly attributed to natural causes – to accidents, passions and personality – than to demons or curses; indeed, diagnostics were scrupulous about the distinctions. As with witchcraft in the sixteenth and seventeenth centuries, the learned quite possibly set more store by the divine and diabolic dimensions of madness than did common people.

Thus opinions, metaphors and maxims about madness proliferated within the 'natural beliefs' of early modern times. It could be fearsome; but it could also be familiar. There was even a relaxed quality in vernacular references to madness: how else could Shakespeare get away with his classic joke in Hamlet about the mad English (''tis no great matter there')? All this was to change, eventually generating that complex superstructure of theories, institutions and stereotypes encompassing insanity which I noted at the opening of this chapter; and the rest of this book will chart and interpret these changes. I shall emphasise that the developing discipline of 'psychiatry' was shaped 'from below'. By this I do not exclusively mean from the lower social ranks, but from within society, rather than from autonomous state and professional apparatuses. Lay and medical outlooks diverged only very slowly. We are not dealing – at least before the nineteenth century – with the management of madness primarily as medical policing, hegemonic social control, or as an agency for drilling the masses for industrialism. Any such crude functionalist or conspiratorial renderings do scant justice to the complexity of the processes or the equivocal role of their promoters.

LOOKING FORWARD

I have drawn attention to vernacular meanings of madness, proliferating and jostling against each other. One aim of the following chapters will be to show how these clusters of ideas fared – some waning, some strengthening, most being transformed, in the struggles of post-Restoration mixed monarchy and market capitalism. Moreover, attitudes towards madness were never an island; they complemented wider images of self, rationality and social health, and they interacted with changing evaluations of such comparable groups of threateningly marginal individuals as slaves, witches and foreigners.

Moreover, tradition was all the time being confronted with novelty, especially what the doctors said. There had always of course been a medicine of madness, stretching back to the Greeks. It is important to remember this when scholars write as if the 'medicalisation of madness' was new to the eighteenth century. Alongside such models of madness as possession and ecstasy, a medical corpus had flourished through the Middle Ages interpreting insanity via theories of the humours, the passions, the inner senses, and so forth.

Nevertheless, the seventeenth and eighteenth centuries saw particularly lively developments in the medical renderings of madness. In part, this involved the decline and fall of old humoralism, challenged by iatrochemistry and a mechanical physiology of nervous hydraulics and then of nervous electricity. Scepticism challenged old wisdom, for example the association of the moon with lunacy. In some ways all this enhanced medical superiority; in others it created new roles for doctors as popularisers of expertise – witness for example the influential writings of George Cheyne. Furthermore, there was a marked increase in the overall quantity of writing on insanity and depressive disorders. This was true of course of all facets of contemporary culture. But nervous complaints formed a quite remarkable growing point of eighteenth-century medical culture, articulated in the writings of Cheyne, Blackmore, Mandeville and others, and then through later popularisers such as William Rowley and Thomas Beddoes.

Concurrently, new forms of treating the mad were emerging, generating new claims to expert authority. Therapeutics remained relatively stagnant before the mid-eighteenth century. The tiny clique of medical men with extensive first-hand experience of treating the mad had traditionally kept their knowledge to themselves. But that began to change. Authors – some medically qualified, others 'empirics' – went into print discussing mental management. Their experiences began to pinpoint new problems and opportunities. One involved the personal powers of the mad-doctor himself. Another was the site of healing. Increasingly the mad were to be treated institutionally in madhouses or asylums. Of course, it was not until the nineteenth century that a full-scale technology developed of asylum architecture, internal classification, and madhouse management; nor did extensive public debate arise till then on asylum reform. Yet, whereas for Burton in 1621 the madhouse was essentially a metaphor, by the time of the 1815 House of Commons Committee it had become a literal matter of nuts and bolts.

Probing how far such developments before 1800 should be styled 'the discovery of the asylum' or the 'rise of psychiatry' – the problems with which I opened this chapter – will form the marrow of this book. The York Retreat, opened in 1796, was founded by absolute beginners; one of the most prestigious asylum-keepers in the early nineteenth century, Thomas Bakewell, was a self-styled 'empiric'. The formal public 'coming-out' of psychiatry was still a long way off. Yet by 1800 public discussion on madness was becoming better focused, stirred up fortuitously by the king's derangement. Debate grew between the public and a new cadre of experts. The uneasy relations between these would form the nodal points of future change.

2

Cultures of Madness

POPULAR VIEWS

In the context of debates about the 'manufacture of madness', I have been suggesting that mental disturbance was a fact of life to English people throughout the early modern period. Particular specifications of madness were, of course, 'socially constructed'. Yet they were constructed out of grassroots experiences and community tensions, rather than being essentially medical codifications serving the interests of a 'psy profession' or a 'therapeutic state', as arguably they eventually became. Insanity was a real presence in the popular mind long before psychiatry spelt independent professional expertise. Indeed, psychiatry later emerged on the basis of 'natural beliefs' about madness already well entrenched within the common culture. When, in 1810, the London physician William Black tabulated the causes of insanity among admissions to Bethlem, the aetiological categories he used – Bethlem's own – were all common parlance. They would have been familiar to Robert

Burton or Richard Napier two centuries earlier, or to any man in the street:

> A Table of the Causes of Insanity of about one third of the patients admitted into Bedlam:[1]

> Misfortunes, Troubles, Disappointments, Grief 206
> Religion and Methodism 90
> Love 74
> Jealousy 9
> Pride 8
> Study 15
> Fright 51
> Drink and Intoxication 58
> Fevers 110
> Childbed 79
> Obstruction 10
> Family and Heredity 115
> Contusions and Fractures of the Skull 12
> Venereal 14
> Small pox 7
> Ulcers and Scabs dried up 5

As Black's table suggests, explanations of insanity were quite eclectic. It could arise from moral and character defects ('pride'), from emotional difficulties ('troubles'), from organic diseases ('fevers'), from head wounds ('fractures of the skull'), from the brain or belly ('drink'), from heredity ('family').

Bethlem's official tabulation of disturbance presumably reflects a widespread belief that it was a dangerous world, in which almost any flaw or misfortune could precipitate insanity. But caution is needed. Our evidence is fragmentary, and we must pause before ascribing perceptions to the people at large. Shakespeare and his fellow dramatists were surely familiar, at first or second hand, with the psychological doctrines of Renaissance Humanism; their plays offer abundant proof. But how far were their audiences attuned to them? Presumably all ranks of play-goers recognised the Bedlamites jabbering on stage: but did the groundlings pick up that Jaques (with his scholar's melancholy) was a classic melancholic as defined by humoralism? How many understood Hamlet being mad 'North North West', or knew – as Victorian psychiatrists thought *they* did – whether he was truly mad or just acting crazy?

Our difficulty is acute because access to popular beliefs is typically via the literati who wrote them down, often – as, for example, with attributing lunacy to the moon – only to scoff at or refute them. Texts such as Burton's *Anatomy of Melancholy* are compendia of what Sir Thomas Browne dubbed 'vulgar errors'; but can we be sure whether a servant at Christ Church would have recognised, still more endorsed, Burton's 'tapings' of oral lore about madness? Or take Richard Napier's case notes. We may be disposed to believe that the parson-physician's humane accounts of his light-headed, low-spirited, or lovesick patients accurately record what they themselves told him; surely his success stemmed from being a sympathetic listener. Yet the fact remains that we possess only one side – Napier's – of the consultations.

Interpreting sources thus poses ticklish problems. Nevertheless, weighty evidence indicates that certain attitudes towards madness were genuinely widespread across early modern English society. Two of these problems are particularly fundamental.

The first concerns how madness was recognised. All agreed that it was of the essence of lunacy to be visible, and known by its appearance. Indeed, Thomas Tryon sourly noted that because men of reason were such hypocrites, it was only the mad whose nature could be read in their face. Madness advertised itself in a proliferation of symptoms, in gait, in physiognomy, in weird demeanour and habits. It was synonymous with behaving crazy, looking crazy, talking crazy. Villagers, churchwardens and doctors alike – all could spot 'antic dispositions'.

This public transparency of madmen and fools is worth emphasising, for it was a situation later to become contested.

For one tenet of the professional psychiatry developing in the nineteenth century was the conviction that insanity could be fearsomely latent, biding its time, and visible only to the expert diagnostic gaze of the alienist. Eventually this view was to infiltrate the public mythology of madness, popularised, for example, in Robert Louis Stevenson's *Dr Jekyll and Mr Hyde*, through the notion of double personality: one self seemingly normal and rational; the other subterranean, hideously perverted. Within such theorisings, what counted were not visible traits – 'madness is as madness does' – but defects of the inner self, variously called 'personality', 'ego', or later the Freudian unconscious. By analogy with tertiary syphilis, madness was the 'poison within'.

But Burton's or Boswell's contemporaries had reckoned otherwise. Both alehouse wisdom and Humanist erudition inhabited a world of signs, made sense of experience through analogies and emblems, and trusted to Nature's legibility. There were indeed inner as well as outer truths, but outward signs encoded inner realities. Hence madness gave itself away. The mad looked quite peculiar. They went near-naked, tore their clothes or dressed fantastical, their hair festooned with straw. They acted oddly: now motionless, withdrawn; now praeternaturally violent. They gobbled strange foods, such as vermin and dung, or refused to eat. They moved and gesticulated incessantly, apparently never sleeping, racked by tics and convulsions. Some bayed at the moon, or howled like dogs. Others tried to kill themselves. Altogether, they were sub- or anti-human.

Not least, the mad stood out because of their silences or bizarre or foul speech. Thus in the mid-seventeenth century, Nicholas Culpeper reassured readers that they could easily tell the mad apart, as they were 'sometimes laughing, sighing... doting, crying out, threatening, and so forth'. And, as MacDonald has shown, lunatics were commonly described with words such as 'babbling', pointing to their jabbering, dislocated din, their nonsensical word-play, their riddling, or being possessed by voices from Beyond, like the woman who cried out 'Christ Jesus have mercy on me' day and night for a whole year.

The visibility of madness was, of course, inscribed by art. As Gilman and Kromm have shown, paintings of the mad, at least up to Van Gogh, worked within powerful stereotypes which identified and passed moral verdicts on them. The fool is typically sketched with his cap and bells, bladder, pinwheel and streamers; motley clad, he leads the foolish world a dance. The melancholic, by contrast, appears listless, hands hidden as a token of lethargy, signalling the deadly sin of acedia (sloth): the Devil will find work for these idle hands. For his part, the maniac is near naked, leonine in countenance, rippling with a brute strength which only fetters can contain. The common message of such stereotypes – expressed in ballads, on the stage and in pictures – is that madness, far from being the silent enemy within, is a moral warning (against pride, sloth, rage or vanity) blazoned forth for all to heed.

Precisely what relation did such literary and artistic images bear, however, to popular perceptions of lunacy? It is hard to be sure. From the 1680s visitors to the newly rebuilt Bethlem Hospital at Moorfields passed through a portico, flanking either side of which stood statues by Cajus Gabriel Cibber, the one of Melancholy, the other of Maniacal Madness. These conventional images ('Brainless Brothers') were aimed to key in the eye to the anatomy of madness. Cibber's sculptures were to become almost definitive icons. William Hogarth was personally familiar with Bethlem's interior. But when he depicted it in the final tableau (VIII) of 'The Rake's Progress', he sketched a cast of crazy caricatures (the mad king or 'pretender', the papist fanatic, the unrequited lover etc.) in the centre of whom lay the fallen anti-hero, Tom Rakewell, frozen in the posture of Cibber's maniac. Behind him a mad artist, scratching on the walls, resembles Hogarth himself. Working in types rather than individuals suited Hogarth's purpose, which was not documentary but didactic. He was inviting the public to superimpose Bedlam and Britain: were not Britons crazier than Bedlamites? How far Georgian Bethlem and its inmates actually resembled Hogarth's engraving we have no means of knowing, since subsequent pictures of Bedlam then mirrored Hogarth, and art commented on art, not life.

The same problem of authentication applies to the written word. Soon after 1700, Ned Ward described a visit to Bedlam which traded on all the ready-made literary clichés:

> We turned in thro' another iron barricade where we heard such a rattling of chains, drumming of doors, ranting, hollaing, singing and rattling, that I could think of nothing but Don Quevedo's vision, where the damned broke loose, and put Hell in an uproar.[2]

Thus Ward's Bedlam was both a jail and hell: the mad, with their 'frantic humours and rambling ejaculations', were lost souls; but all this spectacle was filtered through a Spanish satirist's vision of Pandemonium. Perhaps the ranting and hollaing were real. But are Ward's lunatics, who perform like a circus troupe of zanies, credible? Can we really believe him when he depicts one of the Bedlamites

> holding forth with much vehemence against Kingly government. I told him he deserv'd to be hang'd for talking of treason. 'Now', says he, 'you're a fool, for we madmen have as much privilege of speaking our minds as an ignorant dictator when he spews out his nonsense to a whole parish... you may talk what you will, and nobody will call you in question for it. Truth is persecuted everywhere abroad, and flies hither for sanctuary, where she sits as safe as a knave in a church, or a whore in a nunnery. I can use her as I please and that's more than you dare do.'[3]

This witty fool – is he not merely a mouthpiece for Ward's upside-down-world jibe that in a crazy nation only lunatics are sane, and that under oppression only the confined are free? So we dismiss his figures as fictions. Yet things may have been more complicated. For in *ancien régime* Bedlam, where until 1770 almost unlimited sightseeing was allowed, surely the Bedlamites themselves played to the gallery, putting on a 'show' in return for attention, ha'pence and food, turning the tables and mocking the voyeurs at the same time.

A parallel case of 'acting mad' may be the 'Abraham men', genuine or bogus Bedlamite vagrants licensed to beg and singing Bedlamite ballads, thus 'presenting' madness, to wheedle charity. One thinks then of dramatic performances at Charenton and, later still, those prize hysterics at the Salpêtrière in Paris, who had clearly been 'trained' by Charcot – or had 'trained' themselves – to present textbook enactments of hysteria. So lunatics may well have 'acted crazy' to establish a mocking rapport with the sane, turning all into a gallery of distorting mirrors. The fact that madness thereby became a show merely confirms how, to contemporary minds, what counted was its face.

Such beliefs were reflected in public policy and the law. The Crown and the courts took no interest in madness as such: it was no crime to be mad. Harmless lunatics and 'natural' fools were traditionally left alone. Authority intervened only when insanity's public presence broke the bounds of acceptability by threatening property or creating danger or scandal: when the maniac burned down barns, stoned passers-by, smashed windows, brawled, blasphemed, cursed, went naked, or made attempts on his own life.

The same applies to the courts. Might the accused be unsound of mind? Before the nineteenth century, medical experts were rarely summoned to pronounce. What counted was the community perception – witnesses, friends, family, magistrate and jury. And here the key question was: did the accused habitually behave like a lunatic? His fate hung on his ensemble of actions. When, in the nineteenth century, psychiatric doctors such as Forbes Winslow increasingly put themselves forward as expert forensic witnesses, they caused raised eyebrows when they claimed unique insight into the 'secret' springs of insanity beyond what everyone could see from the accused's disposition and deeds. Michael Hay has studied courtroom practice in eighteenth-century Scotland. He concluded that for the proper-tied classes, magistrates typically set the behavioural hurdle high before they would judge a party to be of unsound mind. So long as a person was not a gross public menace or scandal, judges might turn a blind eye even to notorious private eccentricity. The court was concerned with due process of the law, not with psychiatric diagnoses.

Common culture thus had views on how madness was *known*. These hinged on ideas about what insanity was: the second fundamental problem. Here the belief was that madness was also *tangible*, in other words something physically defective, briefly or permanently, in the sufferer's constitution. Insanity typically was – or at least included – a distemper of the body, arising from constitutional malfunctioning and producing organic symptoms. In low and high culture alike, disturbance was not regarded as purely 'mental', stemming from or confined to an 'occult', or hidden, faculty such as the psyche, mind, soul or will, though it was clearly symptomatically marked by bizarre feelings, ideas and urges.

'Madness is as much a corporeal distemper as the gout or asthma.' Attuned to debates in the psycho-politics of today, we readily identify such somaticism with aggressively 'medically materialist' strands of psychological medicine and neuro-psychiatry. But this was actually the opinion of Lady Mary Wortley Montagu, the mid-eighteenth-century *belle lettriste*. And she was simply giving voice to what – in various forms – was a commonplace of high and low, lay and medical opinion alike, throughout the early modern centuries.

Precisely how such disorders were essentially corporeal was hotly disputed (Lady Mary argued that they were 'lodged in the blood'). But all such views traded heavily upon the physi-ological theory of the humours, first formalised by the Greeks, passed down through the Middle Ages, and then standard within educated society after the Renaissance. Humoralism proposed to explain mortal man within a holistic philosophy of an ordered cosmos, whose earthly ('sublunary') dimension was regarded as harmoniously functioning, yet also liable to mutability. All things terrestrial comprised a balance (temporarily in equilibrium, yet

ultimately corruptible and unstable) of four basic elements
– Earth, Air, Fire and Water – embodying in differing degrees
the basic qualities of hotness and coldness, wetness and dryness.
Man – a microcosm crystallising the macrocosm – was also
constituted of a balance of four basic vital fluids: blood, phlegm,
yellow bile (or choler) and black bile. These were replenished
through digesting food ('coction'), and duly discharged from
the body when in excess, stale or noxious ('peccant'). A proper
economy of the humours – the right mix of heat and cold,
dryness and moisture – was the state of good health. Gross imbalance produced sickness. Too much heat, for example, resulting
perhaps from surplus blood, the hot and moist humour, spelt
fever. Such imbalances could be rectified by purging excesses
or making up deficiencies. Hence bloodletting ('venesection')
could be a suitable therapeutic procedure for fevers.

Each person, however, had a constitution distinguished by his
own unique humoral balance. Factors such as parentage, diet,
gender, climate, environment or – some believed – the astrological influence of the planets disposed individuals to somewhat
disproportionate quantities of blood, phlegm and bile. This
stamped on them a visible physical type, their complexion. Thus
a constitution which manufactured a plethora of blood would
present a florid or ruddy complexion. Physical distinctiveness
would in turn colour character. Hence such a person would be
sanguine in temperament, manifesting high spirits, lively parts, and
a generally 'full-blooded' disposition. There was a broad gender
distinction too. Women were thought to be cooler and moister
than men, thus accounting for their being generally weaker.

Humoralism offered ways of seeing the person as a unity, in
sickness and in health, keying the body's physical operations to
tokens of appearance and behaviour (or disease symptoms) and
to more permanent character traits. It thereby explained the
whole person. Furthermore, not the least of its strengths was that
it chimed with everyday perceptions, as expressed in such 'body
language' descriptions – then not merely metaphors – as one's
'blood boiling' or being 'hot-blooded' or 'bilious'. Humoralism's

language of the self combined medical credit with a graphic common appeal.

Humours thus provided a blueprint for understanding the human economy. Their distribution would explain the power of the appetites, those fundamental instincts mankind shared with the brutes. Thus anger registered a surfeit of choler. Humoral disposition would also interact with the flow of 'animal spirits'. Such spirits were commonly regarded as superfine 'messengers' connecting the vital bodily structures (such as the blood system) to the higher faculties. Generated out of the stomach's digestive processes, animal or vital spirits coursed through the blood and along the nerves, stimulating the brain and the distinct 'soul'. Their tone would render a person high- or low-spirited.

Sustained by – yet also governing – the humours and spirits were the nobler parts. All living creatures were believed to be animated by souls, regarded as the most aethereal organs. The vegetative soul directed growth and generation; the sensitive soul – common to man and brute alike – determined the passions and the five 'outward' senses and instincts, controlling actions and passions. But man alone was dignified by a rational soul. This had various offices and faculties. It supervised the 'inward senses' of imagination, memory and common sense. It governed speech. But above all it was the seat of the will and understanding, mind and consciousness, of reason itself. 'Reason is the noblest gift bestowed by the Creator on man', judged the eighteenth-century madhouse-keeper Benjamin Faulkner, putting in a nutshell the Humanist or Stoic creed down the ages.

This traditional vision of man crowning the Great Chain of Being as the uniquely rational animal – a view fundamental to metaphysics, theorised by classical medicine, congruent with common observation, and not least hallowed by Christianity – saw him as an incarnate whole, subdivided into a multitude of distinct offices within a hierarchical unity, whose proper running depended upon due subordination of parts. Keeping reason on top was a duty requiring tireless vigilance. As Samuel Johnson was to stress, 'to have the management of the mind is a great art' – adding 'it may be attained in a considerable degree by experience and habitual exercise'.

In guidelines for producing *mens sana in corpore sano*, a healthy mind in a healthy body, analogies between the body natural and the body politic of course carried weight. As in the nation, the mind's government must necessarily be hierarchical, for the passions were a low, blind and rude rabble lacking self-control, unlike Reason, 'the sovereign power of the soul'. Just as the mob threatened the breakdown of law and order, so madness would shatter the individual when inflamed appetites, fanned by imagination, rebelled, usurped Reason's office, and became ruling passions. '*Madness* and *Phrensie*', noted the late seventeenth-century Dissenter Thomas Tryon, 'arise and proceed from various passions and extream Inclinations, as *Love, Hate, Grief, Covetousness, Dispair*, and the like', which 'stir up the *Central Fires*', leading to 'Hurley-burley, Confusion, Strife and Inequality', an 'intestine Civil War', all of which 'subverts the government of the inward Senses and Spirit of Wisdom, and puts Reason under Hatches'. Appetites were commonly pictured as animal, a bucking mount, threatening to unseat its rider. As the aptly named John Brydall put it, 'Reason being thus laid aside, Fancy gets the ascendant, and Phaeton-like, drives on furiously'; or in Swift's image, mental anarchy sets in 'when a Man's Fancy gets astride his Reason, when Imagination is at Cuffs with the Senses, and Common Understanding, as well as common sense, is Kickt out of Door'.

Thus human nature, ideally harmonious, was in fact poised on a knife-edge. So long as Reason held the reins, life would be orderly and sane. But if its grip were relaxed, chaos followed. Most exceptionally, of course, someone could go out of his mind, not by sinking but by rising above his corporeal self. This was the Christian beatific vision of divine madness, in which the soul broke loose from the Augustinian prison-house of the flesh, winning transcendence through faith or grace. But much more typically and tragically, the loss of reason was a descent into delirium and destruction. Moralists, medical men and preachers alike could agree that the archetype of madness was the overthrow of mind by carnal appetite. 'Madnesse', emphasised Hobbes, 'is nothing else but too much appearing passion.'

Reason thus usurped, what remained was a mere travesty of humanity. This was a view often depicted. Take for instance the portrayal by the minor Augustan poet Thomas Fitzgerald of the wild Bedlamites, who, lacking self-control, are restrained within society's cage of reason – a vision trading on systematic antitheses between reason and passion, art and animality, the civilised and the savage mind:

> Where proud Augusta, blest with long Repose,
> Her ancient Wall and ruin'd Bulwark shows;
> Close by a verdant Plain, with graceful Height,
> A stately Fabric rises to the Sight.
> Yet, though its Parts all elegantly shine,
> And sweet proportion crowns the whole Design;
> Though Art, in strong expressive Sculpture shown,
> Consummate Art informs the breathing Stone;
> Far other Views than these within appear,
> And Woe and Horror dwell for ever here.
> For ever from the echoing Roofs rebounds,
> A dreadful Din of heterogeneous Sounds;
> From this, from that, from ev'ry Quarter rise,
> Loud Shouts, and sullen Groans, and doleful Cries;
> Heart-soft'ning Plaints demand the pitying Tear,
> And Peals of hideous Laughter shock the Ear.[4]

Fitzgerald hymns civilisation, yet his stilted antitheses pointed their moral ultimately to the sane: know thyself, control thyself:

> Mean time, on These reflect with kind Concern,
> And hence this just, this useful Lesson learn;
> If strong Desires thy reasoning pow'rs control:
> If arbitrary Passions sway thy Soul,

If Pride, if Envy, if the Lust of Gain,
If wild ambition in thy Bosom reign,
Alas! thou vaunt'st thy sober Sense in vain.
In these poor Bedlamites thy Self survey,
Thy Self, less innocently mad than they.[5]

Preachers and poets alike identified base passions and carnal lusts with madness. Remove Reason's just rule, and man is left prey to the ragings of the flesh. The late eighteenth-century psychiatric doctor William Pargeter painted just such a portrait of the inner and outer man:

a fellow creature destitute of the guidance of that governing prin-ciple, reason – which chiefly distinguishes us from the inferior animals around us, and gives us a striking superiority over the beasts that perish. View man deprived of that noble endowment, and see in how melancholy a posture he appears. He retains indeed the outward figure of the human species, but like the ruins of a once magnificent edifice, it only serves to remind us of his former dignity, and fills us with gloomy reflections for the loss of it. Within, all is confused and deranged, every look and expression testifies internal anarchy and disorder.[6]

Thus moralists stressed that madness was typically self-destruction, the wages of vice or sin. He who falls passion's slave wilfully, culpa-bly plunges into madness or animality. Contemplating the Dublin asylum he was founding in his will, Jonathan Swift reflected:

What a mixed multitude of ballad-writers, ode-makers, translators, farce-compounders, opera-mongers, biographers, pamphleteers, and journalists, would appear crowding to the hospital; not unlike the brutes resorting to the ark before the deluge.[7]

All such puny sciolists, disgraces to civilisation, had brutalised themselves, Swift thought, through vanity and pride. This was, of

course, a satirical fling (was it also self-mocking?). But the analogy
with beasts ran deep. Semi-naked, filthy, hirsute, often chained or
caged and tamed with whips – lunatics in Swift's age were handled
very much like animals. It was often assumed, for example, that
madhouses would not need heating, nor their windows glazing,
because madmen, like brutes, were insensitive to cold. Treated in
this way, the mad conspicuously lacked those attributes which gave
mankind dignity: clothing, language, conscience. As Keith Thomas
has insisted, establishing proper distance from the brutes became a
matter of high anxiety in seventeenth-century religion. By trans-
gressing that boundary, the lunatic betrayed mankind. Thus the
degradation and depravity of madness were underlined by its contiguity to animality. Perhaps all truly possessed a 'wild man within',
and Swift could satirically suggest that horses were more rational;
but not until Blake did anyone urge that the tigers of wrath should
be let loose, or suggest that they possessed a truer wisdom.

Reason thus had to reign. But it ruled through a mixed
constitution, because man was so complex, so heterogeneous a
being. Passions, humours, appetites, the 'outer senses', and the
'inward wits' (memory, judgement, common sense, imagination),
the animal spirits and the different souls – all had their several offices, sympathetically interacting in a delicate symbiosis.
Not surprisingly, then, early modern views of human nature, as
advanced by doctors and laymen alike, were somatopsychic and
psychosomatic through and through. On the one hand, the body
clearly impinged upon the mind. As Benjamin Faulkner put it,

> The influence which bodily disorder has on the mind, every
> one knows is various, and exhibits itself in innumerable forms.
> Frequent convulsions, habitual intoxication, violent fevers, &c.
> &c. often affect the mental faculty so as to produce the appear-
> ance, *pro tempore*, of actual mania.[8]

But consciousness reciprocally impacted on the body – something strikingly visible in blushing, in the erection of the penis,
in pounding hearts, racing pulses and many similar responses as

discussed, for example, in Joseph Parrish's *An Inaugural Dissertation on the influence of the passions upon the body, in the production and cure of diseases* (1805). Thus the influences were reciprocal. As the Dissenting minister Richard Baxter was to insist, 'The Soul and Body are wonderful Copartners in their Diseases and Cure.' This holistic view of man as a dynamic interplay of differentiated powers provided, of course, abundant explanations for the galaxy of behavioural and perceptual disturbances, mild and severe, manifest in endless permutations of symptoms. Someone was low-spirited, moody, suspicious, pained, 'humorous'. What was his complaint? Perhaps his vital spirits were disordered; his fancy might have distempered his brain-pan; ill-digested food might be giving off foul vapours and causing 'crudities'; the nerves linking body to brain might be 'relaxed'. Aetiological possibilities proliferated. Yet in the common range of explanations, some corporeal malfunctioning was typically regarded either as the root cause of the affliction, or at least as the prime medium of sickness symptoms. That body and mind formed a continuum was axiomatic, but the emphasis in traditional medicine, both lay and professional, was upon the ontological primacy of mind over body. The corollary of this was that the body bore responsibility for alienation of mind.

In particular, in both humoral medicine and its successors, disordered senses were generally traced to the abdomen, which in turn might disturb the brain. Thus early in the eighteenth century George Cheyne concluded on the basis of his experiences, clinical and personal:

> I never saw a person labour under severe, obstinate, and strong nervous complaints, but I always found at last, the stomach, guts, liver, spleen, mesentery or some of the great and necessary organs or glands of the belly were obstructed, knotted, schirrous, spoiled or perhaps all these together.[9]

Two humours were thought chiefly responsible for such disturbances. One was yellow bile or choler. Excessive secretion of this hot and dry fluid would create irritation and inflammation, or in extreme cases mania and frenzy. This was reckoned a relatively rare affliction, at least in England (things were different in the tropics, or where spicy foods and ardent spirits were habitually consumed). The other was black bile, 'cold and dry, thick, black, and sour, begotten of the more feculent part of nourishment, and purged from the spleen', according to Burton. Melancholy humour created ticklish problems for the anatomist, however, since it was rarely found neat but rather blended with other humours, as when blood or excrements were found blackened. Often its presence was merely inferred from dark skin, hair or eyes, or from 'black looks'. Traditional physiology taught that it was the function of the spleen to absorb surplus black bile. The failure of that operation created the condition known as the 'spleen', though this whole process remained rather mysterious. Even so, its power to torment the system was all too clear. Anxiety, panic, trembling, lassitude and self-loathing – these were the commonest symptoms of melancholy; but its manifestations were innumerable. Burton called it a Proteus, incorporating every facet of the human comedy. A century later Richard Blackmore agreed:

> As a melancholy Constitution of the Spirits is fruitful of a surprising and copious Diversity of odd and ridiculous phantasms, and fills the Imagination with a thousand uncouth Figures, monstrous Appearances, and troublesome Illusions; so it is no less fertile in producing disquieting and restless passions, inseparable and distinguishing Concomitants of this Distemper.[10]

Melancholy's empire was awesome. This was partly because disorders of the spirits did not possess an invariant symptomatology of their own but mimicked other diseases (by the close of the eighteenth century, John Ferriar was speaking of 'the fallacy of symptoms' and 'the conversion of disease'). But it was partly also because the two prime types of disorder, mania and melancholy, were as Blackmore saw it doubles, intermingling and merging with each other:

Indeed the Limits and Partitions that bound and discriminate the highest Hypocondriack and Hysterick Disorders, and Melancholy, Lunacy, and Phrenzy are so nice, that it is not easy to distinguish them, and set the Boundaries where one Ends, and the other Begins.[11]

Thomas Willis had likewise seen mania and melancholy as essentially of a piece:

...three things are almost common to all: viz. First, That their Phantasies or Imaginations are perpetually busied with a storm of impetuous thoughts... Secondly, That their Notions or conceptions are either incongruous, or represented to them under a false or erroneous image. Thirdly, To their Delirium is most often joyned Audaciousness and Fury.[12]

Of course, raging mania and low melancholy *prima facie* looked like polar opposites. But, argued Dr Nicholas Robinson, they were truly two sides of the same coin:

I call that kind of melancholy Madness, where Men rave in an extravagant Manner, Lunacy; because it is only the same Disease, improved in a hot biliose Constitution:[13]

Such a gradient of symptoms was of course to be expected within humoralism, which regarded diseases as essentially individual constitutional distempers. But in addition, melancholy had a uniquely dual nature as a result of a special oddity – the fact that it was not fixedly due to one single humour, black bile. For it could also be choler's child, or, more precisely, the product of *choler adust*, burnt choler, producing the brittle, edgy, acrimonious temper of the malcontent or tetchy ('humorous') genius. Unpredictability and reversals were of its essence. The melancholic man was contrary, all contradiction, proudly self-deprecating and self-hatingly vain.

In the course of time, traditional humoralism (which stressed how biliousness soured the spirits) yielded to new medical theories, in particular to the chemical and mechanistic physiologies promoted by the Scientific Revolution. The process was slow, one of evolution rather than revolution, and the politics of this shift in allegiances is still obscure. In medicine, it clearly involved infiltration rather than radical revolution, as a new vocabulary – of particles, fibres, pressure etc. – became invoked to replace the old language of humours. Consider Dr John Purcell's iatrochemical elucidation of mania:

> Raving is produc'd by a Mixture of Heterogeneous Particles with the Spirits, which fermenting with them, make their Motion violent and irregular in the Emporium of the Brain, where they do at once irritate a great many little Nervous Fibres, and renew many confus'd Ideas of things past... [14]

– what was this but pouring old wine into new linguistic bottles?

The decline of humoralism, initially among doctors and later with the public, was not, however, merely a semantic smokescreen. From the mid-seventeenth century onwards, new developments in anatomy made their mark. In particular, highly influential researches by Thomas Willis focused attention on the nervous system. Though iatrochemical in his general physiology, Willis explored how nervous organisation channelled sensations, coordinated reflexes and directed actions, anchoring his theories in case studies of convulsives, epileptics and defectives. His emphasis upon the key role of the spinal column in neurogeography, tracing the nerve trunk-routes between brain and spine, tended to demote the heart and abdomen from their traditional key positions in explanations of mood and behaviour. Thenceforth the salient axis would be the cerebrospinal, somatising the break, but also the bridge, between mind and body.

Responding to such anatomical investigations, theories of melancholy and madness became preoccupied, from late Stuart times, with the role of the nerves as mediators between distempered bodies and troubled minds. The old somatopsychic explanations were thereby reinvigorated. Best theory came to regard body disorders as funnelled through nerve fibres to the brain, where they were experienced as pains and disturbance. The new centrality of the nerves will become evident through sampling discussions of different sorts of melancholy disorders as ventured by leading early Georgian medical authors.

Take hysteria. Traditional medicine had gathered under this head a mishmash of distressing symptoms – sudden pain, constrictions, breathlessness, chokings – all supposedly arising, as etymology suggested, from gynaecological irregularities. Hence hysteria was, strictly speaking, a female malaise, classical medicine specifically attributing it to the 'wandering womb'. The idea of uterine mobility was not bizarre – physicians were familiar with prolapsed wombs – and the linked idea of the womb as an 'animal within an animal' – i.e. a sinister, autonomous organ with powers of its own – chimed with an ingrained misogyny. Attacks of acute distress, palpitations and suffocation had traditionally been attributed to the diseased womb worming its way up through the body and rising ultimately into the throat, producing the strangulating *globus hystericus* effect.

Blaming hysteria on the womb could form part of an attractive strategy – as in the early Jacobean writings of Edward Jorden – for denying that such symptoms were marks of witchcraft or demonic possession. But they had become discredited by the latter part of the century. Thomas Willis dismissed them as rank anatomical absurdities:

> for that the body of the womb is of so small bulk,... and is so strictly tyed by the neighbouring parts round about, that it cannot of itself be moved, or ascend from its place.[15]

On the contrary, Willis argued, hysterical symptoms must arise from quite a different dysfunction, a defect of the nerves:

> the distemper named from the womb, is chiefly and primarily convulsive, and chiefly depends on the brain and the nervous stock being affected.[16]

If, as he contended, echoing other leading physicians, notably Thomas Sydenham, hysteria was not due to the womb but rather to a chemopathology of the spirits and nerves, there was no reason why it should be exclusively a female malady. Yet women clearly became more hysterical than men. Why? Because the animal spirits and nerves of the 'weaker vessels' were notoriously weaker. As Blackmore put it:

> the convulsive Disorders and Agitations in the various parts of the Body... are more conspicuous and violent in the Female Sex, than in Men; the Reason of which is, a more volatile, dissipable, and weak Constitution of the Spirits, and a more soft, tender, and delicate Texture of the Nerves.[17]

Traditionally the male analogue of hysteria was hypochondria, a disorder (as its Greek etymology also shows) of the cavity beneath the ribs. Though attended by agonising anxieties about health – not surprisingly, since its outbreaks were both erratic and chronic – it must be stressed that hypochondriasis was medically classified as a *bona fide* organic disorder rather than (as in modern usage) merely the foible of the *malade imaginaire*. There had, of course, been a traditional humoral aetiology for it in terms of black bile. As Blackmore noted, Greek doctors

> imagined that all Hypocondriacal Symptoms were derived from a Collection of black Dregs and Lees separated from the Blood, and lodged in the Spleen: whence, as they supposed, noxious Reeks and Cloudy Evaporations were always ascending to the superior Regions (the Chest, the Heart, and Head, Which by turns were made the Seat of Hypocondriacal War, turbulent Conflicts, and seditious Insurrections) to the great Distraction and Confusion of the animal State.[18]

In line with his colleagues, Blackmore argued that anatomy had now scotched such a hypothesis. For as there are no passages, or proper Conveyances, by which these Steams and Exhalations may mount from the inferior to the superior parts... it is now exploded by learned Men, though retained, at least in Name, among the people...[19]

The new anatomy, by contrast, could explain it in terms of the mechanical faults of tiny fibres:

The Spasms, Twitches, jumping of the Tendons, and convulsive Motions, with which these patients are often afflicted, being occasioned by the acrimonious and acid Fluids separated from the Blood in a disproportionate Measure, irritating and urging the Extremities of the Nerves and the animal Spirits, must be owing to the too wide and enlarged Orifices of the Strainers, that suffered an exorbitant Quantity of Humours to pass through.[20]

Here the terminological dregs of humoralism survived but were made to serve new iatrochemical and physical explanatory paradigms.

A further disorder was the 'spleen', traditionally attributed within Galenic medicine to the non-absorption of surplus black bile. Splenetic people displayed symptoms similar to hypochondriacs. These were, according to Dr John Arbuthnot,

obstinate watchfulness, or short sleeps, troublesome and terrible dreams, great solicitude and anxiety of mind, with sighing, sudden fits of anger without any occasion given, love of solitude, obstinacy in defending trifling opinions and contempt for such as are about them, suppression of usual evacuations, as of the menses in women and haemorrhoids in men: great heat, eyes hollow and fixed, immoderate laughter or crying without occasion; too great loquacity, and too great taciturnity, by fits; great attention to one object, all these symptoms without a fever.[21]

The most respected anatomical researches, such as those summarised by Dr William Stukeley, failed, however, to find direct links between the spleen, black bile and the symptoms. Some new seat had to be found, and the 'spleen' too was now ascribed to disordered nerves and spirits.

Finally, the same applies to the 'vapours'. Within humoral medicine, poor digestion ('coction') was believed to belch black fumes up from the abdomen towards the head, creating dizziness and even befogging the understanding. The ensuing foul symptoms knew no bounds. Dr John Purcell conjured up a nightmare:

> Those who are troubled with Vapours, generally perceive them approach in the following manner; first, they feel a Heaviness upon their Breast, a Grumbling in their Belly; they belch up, and sometimes vomit sower, sharp, insipid, or bitter Humours: They have a Difficulty in Breathing; and think they feel something that comes up into their Throat, which is ready to choak them; they struggle; cry out; make odd and inarticulate Sounds, or Mutterings: they perceive a Swimming in their Heads: a Dimness comes over their Eyes, they turn pale; are scarce able to stand: their Pulse is weak; they shut their Eyes; fall down; and remain senseless for some time.[22]

Even worse could ensue. Some sufferers struggled, foamed at the mouth, or beat their breasts:

> [They] suffer such violent and long continu'd Contractions of the Diaphragm and Intercostal Muscles, that their Breast and lower Belly remain elevated for a long time together, so that they cannot draw their breath all that while; nay, some have layn for three whole days without the least Sign of breathing that could be perceived by those that were about them.[23]

So the vapours were real enough, but Purcell denied that they were due to fumes literally wafting up from the guts and smoking out the brain. Instead they signified a sickness located

in the Stomach and Guts, whereof the Grumblings of the one,
and the Heaviness and Uneasiness of the other generally preceding the Paroxysm, are no small proofs.[24]

Noting that one of Hippocrates' immortal contributions to
medicine was his recognition that epilepsy was not after all a
divine affliction ('the sacred disease') but natural and organic,
Purcell deemed the vapours akin to epilepsy; indeed, essentially
identical:

and if there be any difference to be made between them, it only
consists in this, that an Epilepsy, is Vapours arriv'd to a more
violent degree; that the Convulsions are more general and more
apparent over all the Body, and they foam at the Mouth much
more than in Hysterick Fits.[25]

Thus, as all these discussions suggest, from the late seventeenth
century best medical opinion was sketching a revised geography
of disturbance. Humoralism was vacuous and question-begging.
Thus for Willis, depression was no longer due to black bile in
the epigastrium, but

is a complicated Distemper of the Brain and Heart: For as
Melancholick people talk idly, it proceeds from the vice or fault
of the Brain, and the inordination of the Animal Spirits dwelling
in it;... we cannot here yield to what some Physicians affirm, that
Melancholy doth arise from a Melancholick humor.[26]

But in unseating humoralism, these physicians had no strategy of setting less organic theories in its place. Far from it.
Humoralism had been exposed as mere verbal hocus-pocus.
Verba must yield to *res* – to real, substantial, mechanical explanations. As the Newtonian Dr Nicholas Robinson insisted, lunacy
was not a matter of mere 'imaginary Whims and Fancies, but
real Affections of the Mind, arising from the real, mechanical
Affections of Matter and Motion, whenever the Constitution

of the Brain warps from its natural Standard'. Pain must have a real material cause. Some said melancholy was all in the mind. If so, Robinson challenged,

> I hope these Gentlemen will be so candid as to inform us, from whence that wrong Turn of the Fancy it self arises, that is suppos'd to give Being to all those Symptoms: For I deny, that all the Thoughts themselves can ever start from a regular Way of Thinking without... a Change in the Motions of the Animal Fibres;[27]

Only physical explanations could satisfy physicians:

> Every Change of the Mind, therefore, indicates a Change in the bodily Organs; nor is it possible for the Wit of Man to conceive how the Mind can from a chearful, gay Disposition, fall into a sad and disconsolate State, without some Alterations in the fibres, at the same time; Lowness of the Spirits, is no otherwise increas'd upon these Changes, but as the Body weighs heavier to the Mind:[28]

Above all, the nervous system now held the key. As Cheyne insisted, warped nerves – those 'Bundles of solid, springy and elastick Threads or Filaments (Like Twisted Catguts or Hairs)' – explained warped thought:

> I could never find a natural and philosophical Cause for, or Account of, Ideotism, Stupidity, Loss of Senses, Memory, or Judgement, for Lunacy or Madness, or of any of these Distempers that are called Cephalic or Nervous, or which is attended with a Deviation from what is called common Sense, or just Thinking, but an Obstruction, Extinction, Relaxation, or Malformation of the proper Organs which are commonly reckon'd the Nerves.[29]

In turn, nervous disorder stemmed from the intestines:

> I never saw any person labour under severe obstinate, and strong
> Nervous Complaints, but I always found at last, the Stomach,
> Guts, Liver, Spleen, Mesentery, or some of the great and necessary
> Organs or Glands of the lower Belly were obstructed, knotted,
> schirrous, or spoil't.[30]

And so, for Cheyne, mastering melancholy boiled down to the
maxim that man is what he eats:

> True Mania's, real Lunacy, Madness, and a disorder'd Brain,...
> can possibly be accounted for from no other natural Cause, but
> a Malregimen of Diet.[31]

Not everyone agreed with Cheyne that the cure lay in milk
and seeds. Yet heavy eating was commonly blamed for heavy
spirits. Bernard Mandeville's *Treatise of the Hypochondriack and
Hysterick Passions* – that fascinating dialogue of distress – pictured a physician treating a nuclear family of depressives, whose
maladies were traced to overindulgence in rich food and strong
liquor (which not only rotted the stomach but also proved habit-
forming) and to self-drugging. Fearful for the stomach,
Mandeville was sceptical about medicines.

He was exceptional. For physick was widely recommended,
as one would expect, given that disordered senses were regarded
as a physical ailment. Burton had offered hundreds of purges,
vomits and restoratives, many fierce, including laurel, white hellebore and antimony. A century later, and despite his delicacy
about the digestion, Cheyne enthused over mercurials and antimoniacs; Blackmore, like so many of his contemporaries, waxed
lyrical over opium as a specific against hysteria and hypochondriasis, waving aside objections that it made takers 'sottish' or
would prove addictive; while, for his part, Robinson advocated
positively heroic drugging:

> It is Cruelty in the highest Degree, not to be bold in the
> Administration of Medicines, when the Nature of the Disease

absolutely demands the Assistance of a powerful Remedy, and more especially in Cases where there can be no Relief without it... the most violent Vomits, the strongest purging Medicines, and large Bleedings, are to be often repeated.[32]

For the sufferer fearful of regular medicines, however, popular or quackish remedies were also available aplenty, but most of these were also drug-based. Purchasers of the Receipts of the famous John Moncrief (1716) were recommended venesection, leeches, vinegar, hellebore and the cold wet cloth therapy, while hysterical misses might have taken comfort from the Ladies Dispensatory's recipe for home-made Splenetic Pills:

Take Ens Veneris, four Scruples, Saffron, Long Pepper, Virginia Snake-Root, and Spikenard, of each a Scruple; Galbanum, four Scruples; Tincture of Myrrh, a sufficient Quantity to make Pills.

This was excellent in:

all hysterical and hypochondriacal Disorders... and by continuing for some Time to take three or four at a Dose, twice at least in a Day, they will prevail against the most obstinate and inveterate Complaints of this kind.[33]

This thoroughgoing somatic grounding of disorders of thought, feeling and behaviour provided guidelines for both diagnosis and treatment. Medical practice bears this out. When winning his spurs as a young Oxford physician in the mid-seventeenth century, Thomas Willis had sundry patients suffering from melancholy-madness. He treated them as for standard organic complaints. Mrs Bolt of Eaton languished under chronic melancholy which flared into mania. Willis had her bound with chains and tied to her bed. He then bled her, gave laudanum, and administered an enema. Eventually, finding her ranting, weeping and singing, he

prescribed a liniment of Vigo's ointment... smeared on a rose
cake to be applied to her forehead and temples and a poultice
of gently cooked water-hemlock to be put on the region of the
spleen; and also repeated draughts of a cardiac julep. The next
night she died.[34]

Willis gives not the slightest indication of regarding either her
melancholy or her mania as afflictions essentially distinct from
any other illness, such as fever.

There was thus a deep-seated disposition to view abnormalities as body-based. Nowadays many sufferers from comparable
conditions would commonly be said – by their doctors and
by themselves – to be suffering from psychosomatic, psychosocial, functional disorders or other 'neuroses', without known
independent organic pathology. In other words, during the
intervening centuries there has been a massive shift – whether
'progressive' or 'retrograde' – ushering in the new cognitive
realms of 'psychology' and 'psychiatry'. Explanation of both
mental sets, and the emergence of the latter, is required.

EXPLAINING DISTURBANCE

It might, *prima facie*, be tempting to assume that somatic explanations of mental afflictions were promoted by physicians as part
of an imperialistic 'medical model'; but that would be a mistake.
Medical materialism was not foisted on to the public willy-nilly
by the doctors. For one thing, in the prevailing medical balance
of power, doctors hardly carried the clout to impose their systems
onto unwilling clients. But in any case, all the signs are that sufferers were just as eager as the doctors to see what we might today
call 'mental' disorders somatised and incorporated in the body.
Indeed, physicians record sufferers' resistance to the possibility
that their disorders might stem primarily from, and be indications
of, diseased minds. As Cheyne bewailed, he was often put on the
spot when presented with personal disorders, because they could
be callously belittled – by those in rude health! – as marks of

'peevishness', 'whim', 'ill humour', or, in the case of women, of 'fantasticalness' or 'coquetry'. Even worse, such complaints might be regarded as halfway to outright lunacy. Hence great diagnostic delicacy was needed, lest terms like 'vapourish' should seem to cast aspersions. Above all it was vital to the patient's peace of mind to assign a real disease, since although it was extremely easy to banter about these conditions as 'nothing but the effect of Fancy, and a delusive Imagination, yet it must be allowed... the consequent Sufferings are without doubt real and unfeigned'. Cheyne's solution – widely shared – was to emphasise the organic substrate, although even this required diplomacy:

> Often when I have been consulted in a Case, before I was acquainted with the Character and Temper of the Patient, and found it to be what is commonly call'd Nervous, I have been in the utmost Difficulty, when desir'd to define or name the Distemper, for fear of affronting them or fixing a Reproach on a Family or person. If I call'd the Case Glandular with nervous Symptoms, they concluded I thought them pox'd, or had the King's Evil... Notwithstanding all this, the Disease is as much a bodily Distemper (as I have demonstrated) as the Smallpox or a Fever.[35]

Dr Richard Blackmore grappled with the same predicament. Those constantly 'bellyaching' about strange discomforts could easily be maligned as malingerers or as incipient lunatics. The doctor's dilemma was acute, for he

> cannot ordinarily make his Court worse, than by suggesting to such patients the true Nature and Name of their Distemper... One great Reason why these Patients are unwilling their Disease should go by its right Name is, I imagine, this, that the Spleen and Vapours are, by those that never felt their Symptoms, looked upon as an imaginary and fantastick Sickness of the Brain, filled with odd and irregular Ideas.[36]

Faced with patients ashamed 'to own a Disease that will expose them to Dishonour and Reproach', the only solution was to designate the complaint organic.

But the somatisation of such disorders involved far more than the tactful stratagems of fashionable physicians. Sufferers themselves strove to attribute their own palpitations, tetchiness, morbid delusions or mood swings to organic malady. A tortuous striving for such an explanation, at once morally, spiritually and medically acceptable, occupies the autobiographical writings of the superannuated Puritan Dissenting minister Richard Baxter. Baxter experienced chronic internal pain and morbid health anxieties. He personally ascribed his troubles to kidney stones, though his physicians were unable to locate them. He tried many remedies, some from the doctors, some home-brews; and consulted up to thirty-six practitioners without relief or remedy. The real blow came when 'divers eminent physicians agreed that my disease was the hypochondriack melancholy'. What exactly the (by now surely exasperated) practitioners intended by that, we cannot be sure. For Baxter, however, the term carried shattering connotations of morbid delusion and even of real madness, which his *amour propre* and religious mission had to deny:

> I was never overwhelm'd with real melancholy. My distemper never went to so far as to possess me with any inordinate fancies, or damp me with sinking sadness, although the physicians call'd it the hypochondriack melancholy.[37]

Thus outmanoeuvring the doctors, Baxter legitimated his malaise by rendering it organic:

> I thought myself, that my disease was almost all from debility of the stomach, and extream acrimony of blood by some fault of the liver.[38]

Baxter's experiences suggest that the mere *malade imaginaire* could expect no more sympathy from ordinary people than

Molière's fictional hero: he too, in fact, would be a figure of sport – indeed, Baxter reports, being rumoured to be merely hypochondriacal, 'I became the common talk of the city, especially the women.' The case also shows how a staunch Puritan, who saw Providence and spiritual forces behind so many events, felt most comfortable in laying his own mysterious malaises at the door of regular organic causes.

In such circumstances, sympathetic doctors and patients tended to concur in a diagnosis which made such conditions 'real' by basing them in the body, and 'natural' so as to minimise personal responsibility, guilt and shame. As Bishop John Moore stated in a sermon in 1692, depressed spirits were better regarded as truly 'Distempers of the Body, rather than Faults of the Mind'; Timothy Rogers, instructing readers how to cope with melancholy, agreed, emphasising, 'it does generally indeed first begin at the Body, and then conveys its Venom to the Mind'. Nevertheless, a tightrope had to be walked. When Dr John Radcliffe told Queen Anne she was suffering from the 'vapours', his patient took umbrage and sacked him; evidently that particular term was too double-edged for royalty.

There were, moreover, even more compelling reasons why contemporary medical culture was very wary of judging disordered senses 'in the mind' rather than 'in the body'. For on top of aspersions of malingering, there could arise imputations of a capital disturbance of the Reason, and all that that entailed for man's soul and life eternal. This shows in fears of the tyranny of imagination.

Minds steeped in Humanism paid fearful tribute to the extraordinary cosmic powers of 'imagination'. It had been the sustaining force of sympathy, astrology and magic; it had underlain witchcraft fascination. Physicians were, of course, aware that imagination might be potent in curing diseases – witness the successes of faith healers and other irregulars, from Valentine Greatrakes through to Mesmer – though the faculty considered it scandalous that maladies immune to the best medicine proved susceptible to mere suggestion. More commonly, however, doctors dreaded the power of imagination to wreak havoc. As Nehemiah Grew warned:

> Phancy... operates... in the Production of Diseases. Consumptions often come with Grief. From Venereal Love, Madness, and Hysterick Fits.[39]

A commonly cited example of this harm was the reputed power of imagination in women, either at the instant of conception or when pregnant, to 'impress' whatever preoccupied their mind upon the embryo of their unborn child. A woman who imagined ('conceived') a monster would indeed give birth to a deformed child.

Imagination was thus at best a very mixed blessing. Once permitted to slip the reins of reason, it would readily imperil health. Awareness of this fuelled the profound anxieties about dreaming so frequently expressed during the 'long eighteenth century'. To the superstitious or suggestible mind, nightmares too readily turned into self-fulfilling prophecies, as well as exhausting the body. If then, as Goya was to put it, the sleep of Reason produced monsters, small wonder medical theorists were so eager to break the hold of such monstrous imaginings by proffering simple somatic explanations for bad dreams. Nightmare, physicians commonly argued, was not a literal case of possession or of being hag-ridden, nor a true vision, but was the outcome of heavy suppers and bad sleeping postures.

It was hardly surprising then, that the dramatic potential of imagination – in dreams in particular but more generally too – should be anxiously associated with the slippery slope into madness; or, as Thomas Tryon epitomised the connection towards the end of the seventeenth century, 'Madness seems to be a Watching or Waking Dream.' Dread that unbridled imagination might engender peculiarly terrifying forms of madness was widely expressed, but by none more powerfully than Samuel Johnson, classically in Chapter XLIV of his moral fable, *Rasselas*, entitled 'The Dangerous Prevalence of Imagination', which opens with Imlac's chill assessment:

> Disorders of intellect... happen much more often than superficial observers will easily admit... There is no man whose imagination does not sometimes predominate over his reason, who can regulate his attention wholly by his will, and whose ideas will come and go at his command.[40]

What gives Johnson's fictional insight that madness is bred by imagination its special poignancy is the fact that it was clearly autobiographical. A middle-aged widower, with his *Dictionary* behind him, Johnson developed a phobia about idleness. Recoiling from toil, his conscience began corrosive solitary self-accusations, arraigning himself of wasting his life and sinking into vacuity. As he confessed to his diary on 21 April 1764:

> My indolence, since my last reception of the Sacrament, has sunk into grosser sluggishness,... my appetites have predominated over my reason. A kind of strange oblivion has overspread me, so that I know not what has become of the last year.[41]

This strain became the signature of long tracts of his life. His diary for 7 April 1776 thus reads:

> My reigning sin, to which perhaps many others are appendent, is waste of time... Melancholy has had in me its paroxysm and remissions.[42]

Johnson, who confessed he had been 'mad all my life, at least, not sober', clearly believed that idleness paved the way to insanity. Why so? Surely because it handed a blank cheque to the fiends of imagination, filling his head with torments. Soon after his wife's death he refers to being 'depraved with vain imaginations' – evidently sexual fantasies. After beseeching God to 'purify my thoughts from pollutions', he was relieved to find at Easter 1758 that he was not 'once distracted by the thoughts of any other woman'. His mind brooded wistfully on the past, and wishfully about the future. He writes in *Rasselas*, 'no mind is much employed upon the present; recollections and anticipation fill up almost all our moments'.

Johnson's melancholy did not, however, stem simply from what he imagined, but from the very surrender of finding himself enslaved to fantasies. Driven by the 'hunger of imagination', he craved his daydreams, but dreaded succumbing to a never-never-land of wishes, as all self-control caved in:

> I had formerly great command of my attention [he wrote in 1772] and what I did not like could forbear to think. But of this power which is of the highest importance to the tranquillity of life, I have for some time past been so much exhausted.[43]

The mad astronomer episode in *Rasselas* is Johnson's ('imaginative') exploration of this doom. The sage's solitary fantasisings about the heavens have turned monstrous, and his laudable craving for knowledge has warped into the *idée fixe* that command over the elements lies at his nod:

> By degrees the reign of fancy is confirmed; she grows first imperious, and in time despotic. Then fictions begin to operate as realities, false opinions fasten upon the mind, and life passes in dreams of rapture or of anguish.[44]

Johnson thus dreaded that, with his 'mind corrupted with an inveterate disease of wishing', he would eventually pay the price: he would go mad.

This diagnosis was not, of course, uniquely Johnsonian – far from it. For he was introspecting within a paradigm of mental collapse full of Classical suspicion of the flames of fancy, and reinforced by Locke's linking of madness with the association of ideas. The sleep of Reason left imagination free to spawn monsters. Such prognostications of the imagination's despotism preyed upon Johnson; indeed, they became self-fulfilling. Fleeing to dissipation to escape melancholy was a leap out of the frying pan into the fire. Impressed by the *Anatomy of Melancholy*, he knew the wisdom of Burton's adage, 'Be not solitary, be not idle'. For otherwise there was the descent:

> Idleness produces necessity, necessity incites to wickedness, and wickedness again supplies the means of living in idleness.[45]

The end of the road was clearly madness.

In expressing these personal fears, Johnson was thus giving voice to an extremely widespread tradition of associating imagination and melancholy. 'A great Fancy is one kind of Madnesse' was Hobbes' view. Johnson concurred. 'Madness', he told Fanny Burney, 'is occasioned by too much indulgence of imagination.' No wonder the possibility that morbid distempers were monsters of disordered minds could strike such terror. Blaming symptoms on bodily disease was far more reassuring.

Even worse, however, might be the prospect of being 'possessed' not merely by tumultuous imagination but by outside forces, infernal powers. As I shall explore more fully below, seventeenth-century scriptural Protestantism treated the drama of salvation as a literal psychomachy, in which individual souls were fought over by the warring spiritual forces of the Lord and, on the other hand, by His Satanic Majesty, backed by the armies of the night. If God and the Devil battled for every soul, the danger of diabolical invasion was always acute. Scores of spiritual autobiographies – typically, of course, the memoirs of survivors – tell of infiltration by emissaries of the Tempter, provoking terror and despair, particularly at times of tribulation or of sickness, when resistance would in any case be low (illness was the 'Devil's bath', commented Burton).

Divinity saw temptation as every Christian's cross. Satan might be repulsed through faith or grace, and some Puritan saints might relish the struggle. Yet, faced with the prospects of hell and damnation, believers stricken by pains, anguish and despondency would rarely wish to think that these were symptomatic of diabolical invasion or witches' maleficium. As the sober late seventeenth-century Archbishop Tillotson put it:

> I chuse rather to ascribe as much of these to a bodily distemper as may be, because it is a very uncomfortable consideration, to think that the devil hath such an immediate power upon the hearts of men.[46]

Rather, like Tillotson, sufferers would seek refuge in more comforting physical explanations, tracing such troubles to the diaphragm not to devils, the stomach not Satan. During the seventeenth century, a stream of medical practitioners such as Edward Jorden reattributed putative possession phenomena to disease, locating it in the body; and all the signs suggest that the educated elite increasingly concurred in rejecting the Pandora's box which diabolism opened.

It was similar fears which could make the Cartesian mind-body dualism an attractive option to some. Strict Cartesianism had few English followers and, as Brown has argued, even pro-Cartesian physicians did not deny those integrative mind-body interactions which traditional physic and common experience alike attested: instead what Cartesianism did was to provide exclusively mechanical explanations for them in place of humoral ones. The attraction of Descartes' strategy in designating reason as disembodied consciousness, however, was that it removed the risk that inquiry into the brain and its links with the senses would implicate the transcendental soul itself in disorder or disease. Henceforth, mechanical analysis of brain malfunctions and behavioural peculiarities could proceed without any hint of diabolical possession, or of the subversion of the rational Soul itself. Thus for Cartesian sufferers or physicians, such conditions as delusional melancholy could be frankly accepted as really organic, without fear that they were the suggestions of the Devil.

I have been painting a broad picture of attitudes towards mental disorder shared by many patients and physicians alike through the 'long eighteenth century', suggesting why it made sense to them to regard disorders ranging from melancholy to mania as fundamentally similar to fevers, scrofula, or other organic complaints. Of course, 'superstitious' causes and 'magical' cures for mental disorders still had their popular currency, and distempers were regularly attributed to the passions and to personal peculiarities – often in a tone of blame or reproach, or by way of abdicating responsibility. Equally, a very few highly distinctive souls might claim to be divinely mad, and certain others were deemed captivated by evil thoughts or diabolically possessed. Such derangement of the soul itself was, however, overwhelmingly terrifying. In such circumstances, the great majority of the disordered and the depressed were agreed to have organic afflictions, to be treated with drugs and medical care. Thus Richard Napier's responses to his disordered patients were discriminating, very occasionally including exorcism, but universally involving medication, purges and bloodletting, together with good counsel.

In the remainder of this chapter, I shall shift from these broad matters of *mentalité* and examine particular foci of controversy, seeing how new meanings of madness came about. Such changes were most profound in the interface between religion and madness, so I shall address this area first.

RELIGIOUS MELANCHOLY

Within Christianity, the divine, the numinous and the transcendental dwarf the paltry earthly city where the drama of human salvation is played out. Both Protestantism and Counter-Reformation Catholicism deemed mankind numerically overwhelmed by the spiritual squadrons of Good and Evil doing Miltonic battle in the heavens overhead, haunting the forest (the seventeenth century was the great age of witchcraft and witch-craze) and penetrating every nook and cranny of minds waking and asleep. Miracles, providences, prophecies, prodigies – all testified to an eschatology in which human actors lay under direction of the Divine. For the educated, this theology was buttressed by the astrological, occult, magical and hermetic lore of the Renaissance, all attesting to the empire of powers unseen.

Yet the spirit-drenched cosmos was also a cockpit of appalling conflict. As the grip of millennialism shows, Antichrist seemed terrifyingly ascendant in that great age of melancholy, the first half of the seventeenth century. Pious Protestants saw the Beast extending his kingdom still further, through captivating the foolish and the wicked. One mark of possession by the Devil was insanity. Understanding precisely how madness was commonly the Devil's work was thematic to Burton's *Anatomy of Melancholy* (1621), though it is a feature of his text often neglected, constituting as it does the final section of that inordinately discursive work and representing a darkening of tone from the playful folly of the human comedy in the first two Partitions.

Burton unfolds a vision of the little world of man, the *atrium mundi* where all mankind plays the fool as an 'antic or personate actor'. Through the *Anatomy*, mankind is oft-times convicted of melancholy madness. It is, however, a suspended sentence, tempered with mercy, because in the human comedy all suffer, yet also relish the role of 'melancholising', creating a 'charming illusion', under the direction of 'Mistress Melancholy'. In any case, Burton also devotes hundreds of pages to remedies; mundane melancholy is a malady we live with, rather than die of.

But Burton's text darkens abruptly when he turns to religious melancholy; all is blacker, in deadly earnest. Burton doffs his motley and mounts the pulpit. And as a divine, he was not an irenic Erasmian, a tolerant Latitudinarian, a Cambridge Platonist *avant la lettre*, or a prophet of the Lockian reasonableness of Christianity.

Religious melancholy was no joke; towards its victims, confides Burton, he could not play *Democritus ridens* but only *Heraclitus fleans*, for it spelt disease, death and damnation. Religious melancholy had its own particular aetiology. It was, first, the stain of Original Sin. Thus in broaching religious melancholy, Burton's subject was not mere mankind but mankind fallen. Lapsarian man's 'will' and 'love of God' are 'corrupt': he is a 'monster'. For the Fall spelt death, a 'punishment for our sins'; and 'melancholy is the character of mortality'. Unlike the Revd Laurence Sterne in the following century, Burton would not stay to break a jest with Death. The Fall meant Hell: 'naught so damned as melancholy'.

More particularly, religious melancholy cut so much deeper than other modes of folly because it was, for Burton, quite literally, ensnarement by the Devil. His disquisition on religious melancholy is, in effect, the history of Satan's statecraft. 'The Devil reigns', Burton explains, aiming to 'captivate souls', being 'the principal agent and procurer of this mischief', with a little help from the fifth column of black choler which is Satan's 'shoeing horn' or 'bath'. Burton signals the diabolical pedigree of religious melancholy even in his subject headings – e.g. 'Subsection 8, Causes of Despair, the Devil [etc.]'.

What is remarkable here is not that Burton had a lurid vision of religious madness as a Satanic pandemic – holding such a view was impeccably orthodox. Its pedigree derived from Augustine, and extended down through Protestant theologians such as Melanchthon and humanists such as Bodin. Burton's literalism over religious melancholy was typical of his times. Rather, it is the fact that Burton's demonology has been so utterly ignored or explained away by scholars, presumably appalled at his benightedness (Babb, for example, has argued that 'the religious intolerance of Burton the parson was considerably qualified by the understanding and sympathy of Burton the psychiatrist'). Many whittle away his demonomania. So Blaine Evans contends that Burton's references to the Devil are best read not literally, as implying physical diabolical possession, but rather metaphorically as symbolising an inner state, to which Satan is merely a 'contributory factor'. Taking a similar tack, Paul Kocher glosses the *Anatomy* as if for Burton the Devil 'seldom entered the body', and then only 'through the mediation of the bodily humours' – a view which distorts Burton's argument.

Now, it is true that a few voices during Burton's lifetime were questioning diabolic intervention in the little world of man – these opinion-changers included divines such as Samuel Harsnet and Timothy Bright, some medical men such as Johannes Weyer, André du Laurens and Edward Jorden, and scholar-gentlemen such as Reginald Scot. Thus, in his *Suffocation of the Mother* (1603), Jorden contested the popular but, he thought, pernicious view that hysteria betokened diabolical possession: it was, rather, an organic disease; Reginald Scot denied that witches were truly in league with the Devil, and Weyer deemed that Satan had no sway over material bodies. Certain up-to-date treatises which Burton quarried – those of Bright, Thomas Wright and du Laurens – hardly glanced at the Devil in their analysis of melancholy.

But Burton – like his king and the majority of his subjects – was not of their party. Indeed he specifically repudiated Sadduceeism, holding it as a cardinal tenet that 'the Devil reigns'. On this Burton is insistent and unambiguous. 'Where God hath a temple, the Devil will have a chapel'; 'the air is not so full of flies in summer, as it is at all times of invisible devils'. Thus melancholy is the 'Devil's instigation', and 'the first mover of all superstition is the Devil'. But the Devil is above all Protean, a master of disguise. Melancholy's terror was a 'personating disease', and the Devil is the arch-impersonator. Sometimes he acts directly, mobilising his invisible army of witches, demons, hobgoblins, incubi and succubi, *ignes fatui*, evil spirits, and witches who could 'hurt plants, make women abortive, not to conceive, barren, men and women unapt and unable'. The Beast also recruits subordinates to his purposes, above all the 'bull-bellowing Pope', and his underling priests and Jesuits, who co-operate 'to keep it [the world] in subjection', 'to stupify, to besot', and 'gull the commons', implanting captivating beliefs like purgatory, limbo, transsubstantiation, and other 'superstitions'. The Devil fascinates, co-opting 'imagination' to conjure the 'Devil's

illusions', ensnaring men in theological paradoxes about predestination and salvation, and exploiting fears, obsessions, and the
lust for domination.

In other words, because it could well be the Devil's work,
religious melancholy – unlike other forms – was unfit for merry
satire. Indeed Burton was notably pessimistic about its cure
– contrast, say, Erasmus, who had concluded the *Praise of Folly*
with a festive celebration of Christian madness. Burton viewed
man's soul not, as did Thomas Browne, as a globe to revolve for
pleasure, but as the trophy in a duel between God and Satan.
Hence creeds were critical, not 'matters indifferent', and heresy
so dangerous it had to be extirpated, if necessary by the sword,
or even by fire, for 'fire cures what the sword cannot': 'a wound
that cannot be cured must be cut away'.

So what help was there for individual melancholics, trapped
by Satan's wiles? Burton believed that medicine would mend
most forms of melancholy, but with religious melancholy, 'physick can do no good':

> There is no sickness, almost, but will provide a salve: friend-
> ship helps poverty: hope of liberty easeth imprisonment:...
> authority and time wear away reproach: but what Physick, what
> Chirurgery... can relieve... a troubled conscience?[47]

Neither did he trust to the traditional religious instruments for
casting out devils. As a good Protestant, of course, he utterly
deprecated charms, spells, and other 'unlawful cures': superstitious and magical, all were, in fact, further insidious diabolical
snares. Moreover, following the Canons of 1604, he did not look
to exorcism or healing fasts. And he was peculiarly pessimistic
about self-help or collective support attempts to conquer religious melancholy, for too often the cure was worse than the
disease. He who sought to quell his terrors by scrupulous self-
scrutiny or Bible-reading, wrote Burton – surely with a swipe at
the Puritans – would plunge into deeper despond, for 'medita-
tion mars all'. Hellfire preachers were even worse. Conjuring

up ghastly images of perdition, their overheated imaginations merely added fuel to the flames. Polluted consciences were too heavy to bear – and rightly, for God was indeed vengeful, and His vengeance terrible.

In short, therapy lay not in man's hands but in the Divine Physician's. The sinner must repent, 'call on God', and 'ask forgiveness'. Faith was necessary; but faith was sufficient. Burton's solution was thus not Stoic self-knowledge, nor Montaigne's self-acceptance, nor the gentle supportive dialogue of comfort composed by Timothy Bright for 'M', his fictive sufferer, nor a manual of holy living and holy dying. Denying Humanism, Burton looked to Lutheran justification by faith alone in all its grandeur.

What this extended exposition has been concerned to show is that for Burton the human race was mad and the Devil mostly possessed it. Religious melancholy was in reality excruciating diabolical possession. Burton's contemporaries would mostly have agreed. Over 600 of Richard Napier's patients believed themselves bewitched or possessed. Yet this culture of terror, marking the 'age of melancholy' spanning the 'general crisis' of the Baroque, was to be comprehensively repudiated by cosmopolitan elites from the close of the Thirty Years' War and the ending of the English Civil War onwards. The new ideology expressed a resolve to replace the kingdom of darkness with Enlightenment, and build new intellectual, social and political worlds as free of clerical or demonic as of demotic power, safe from sin, damnation and the grim terrors from Beyond. This campaign to render everything natural and rational, including religion – Max Weber termed it the 'demystification of the world' – had crucial implications for the construal of religious madness.

By no means all believers, of course, gave their blessing to the new temper of rational religion. Indeed, fundamentalist resistance was what gave the Enlightenment's *ecrasez l'infâme* sloganising its edge. Antinomian sectaries throughout Stuart England continued wholeheartedly to endorse traditional types of divine and ecstatic madness. Ranters, Fifth Monarchists and the first Quakers engaged in such 'mad' behaviour as 'going naked for a sign'. George Fox, founder Quaker, practised faith healing, laid on hands, and expected to raise the dead. Trances, fits, speaking in tongues and ranting marked the ecstatic conversions of many a gathered flock; these continued into the eighteenth century, not least in the transports of the 'French prophets', a group of convulsionary Huguenot exiles who settled, under fashionable protection, in Queen Anne's England.

Interpreting madness as psychomachy remained integral to the religion of salvation. Consider the case of George Trosse, a 'born-again' Presbyterian of the late seventeenth century, who records that as a debauched young Cavalier, engaged 'in a Course of Sin and Folly', he began to hear the commands of the Devil (whom he mistook for God), tempting him to sin, and culminating in calls for self-destruction. Disabused, tormented by fear and loathing and convinced that he was damned, Trosse fell into raving and was confined in a pious physician's household. In time, he records, by reading the Scriptures with the minister who was caring for him, committing St Matthew's Gospel to heart, praying with the 'Gentlewoman and her family', attending public worship, and sitting 'constantly under the Instructions of a minister of Christ of the Presbyterian persuasion', he grasped that Christ's blood had been shed for him, was released from his conviction of damnation, and recovered. What Trosse depicts is a not uncommon religious crisis, as recorded in spiritual autobiographies: Timothy Rogers offers a similar account 'from the Author's own Experience'. The wiles of the Devil induce a raving self-destructiveness; this is finally resolved, if not by exorcism at least by religious persuasives.

Conversion experience, revelation and the *imitatio Christi* continued – despite the Enlightenment – to induce the faithful to behave in ways which appeared stark mad to the worldly-wise. Take for instance, one Joseph Periam. The revivalist George Whitefield recorded:

> Had the pleasure of being an instrument under God, with Mr
> Seward, of bringing a young man out of Bethlehem, who was
> lately put into that place for being, as they term it, Methodically
> mad.[48]

Periam had begged Whitefield's aid:

> According to his request, I paid him a visit, and found him in
> perfect health both in body and mind. A day or two after, I and
> Mr Seward went and talked with his sister, who gave me the three
> following symptoms of his being mad. 1. That he fasted for near
> a fortnight. 2. That he prayed so as to be heard four stories high.
> 3. That he had sold his clothes, and given them to the poor. This
> the young man himself explained to me before, and ingeniously
> confessed, that under his first awakenings, he was one day reading
> the story of the young man whom our Lord commanded to sell
> all, and to give to the poor: and thinking it must be taken in the
> literal sense, out of love to Jesus Christ he sold his clothes, and
> gave the money to the poor.[49]

Whitefield's spellbinding preaching caused many converts to lose
their senses in divine ecstasy; and he himself explicitly embraced
the Pauline ideal of holy madness, asking 'who would but be
accounted a fool for Christ's sake?... we must be despised before
we can be vessels fit for God's use'.

Yet the most energetic apostle of divine madness was John
Wesley. Wesley staunchly denied that madness was merely reduc-
ible to physical illness – though his self-help health manual,
Primitive Physick, recommended drugs and medical treatments
for lunatics. He was alert all his life to interpreting all manner
of mystery illnesses as symptoms of diabolical possession, as for
example the case of this gentlewoman,

> whose distemper had puzzled the most eminent physicians for
> many years; it being such as they could neither give any rational
> account of, nor find any remedy for. The plain case is, she is

tormented by an evil spirit following her day and night. Yea, try
all your drugs over and over, but at length it will plainly appear,
that this kind goeth not out but by prayer and fasting.[50]

Mad fits were the surest symptoms. 'I rode to Stratford Upon
Avon', he wrote,

> I had scarce sat down, before I was informed Mrs K_, a middle
> aged woman, of Shattery, half a mile from Stratford, had been for
> many weeks last past in a way which nobody could understand;
> that she had sent for a Minister, but almost as soon as he came,
> began roaring in so strange a manner, (her tongue at the same
> time hanging out of her mouth, and her face being distorted
> into the most terrifying form,) that he cried Out, 'It is the Devil,
> doubtless! It is the Devil!' and immediately went away.[51]

(Wesley interjects sardonically, 'I suppose this was some unphi-
losophical Minister; else he would have said, "Stark mad! send
her to Bedlam."'):

> I asked 'What good do you think I can do?' One answered, 'We
> cannot tell; but Mrs. K_... earnestly desired you might come...
> saying She had seen you in a dream, and should know you imme-
> diately. But the Devil said (those were her own expressions), I will
> tear thy throat out before he comes.' But afterwards, (she said), his
> words were, 'If he does come, I will let thee be quiet; and thou
> shalt be as if nothing ailed thee till he is gone away.'

> A very odd kind of madness this!... One showing me the way, I
> went up straight to her room. As soon as I came to the bedside,
> she fixed her eyes, and said 'You are Mr. Wesley; I am very weak
> now I thank God: nothing ails me; only I am weak.' I called them
> up, and we began to sing,

> 'Jesu thou hast bid us pray,
> Pray always and not faint;

With the word, a power convey
To utter our complaint.'

After singing a verse or two, we kneeled down to prayer. I had
but just begun, (my eyes being shut,) when I felt as if I had been
plunged into cold water: and immediately there was such a roar,
that my voice was quite drowned. [52]

This episode and many others suggest a powerful rapport between
Wesley as evangelist and a strand at least of popular piety in linking together diabolism, madness, and spiritual physic. The actual
parson is relegated to the sidelines, while a straw-man bogey
parson (a 'philosophical minister') stands quite beyond the pale.

Wesley rejected medicalising such fits ('A very odd kind of
madness this!'). Thus in 1759 he was called

to a young woman, who was some days since suddenly struck
with what they called madness; and so it was, but a diabolical madness, as plainly appeared from numerous circumstances:
however, after she had been at prayer, she fell asleep, and never
raged or blasphemed after.[53]

The Devil had many ways of driving people mad. Some sur-
rendered themselves to Satan in despair, as with this demented
woman:

Sat. 20. I saw a melancholy sight. A gentlewoman of an unspotted
character, sitting at home, on May the 4th, 1771, cried out, that
'Something seized her by the side.' Then she said it was in her
mouth. Quickly after she complained of her head. From that
time she wept continually for four months, and afterwards grew
outrageous: but always insisted, 'That God had forsaken her, and
that the Devil possessed her, body and soul.'
I found it availed nothing to reason with her: she only blasphemed the more, cursing God, and vehemently desiring, yet
fearing to die.[54]

Here, Wesley discovered, despair ran in the family:

> Her brother gave me almost as strange account of himself. Some
> years since, as he was in the full career of sin, in a moment he
> felt the wrath of God upon him, and was in the deepest horror
> and agony of soul. He had no rest, day or night, feeling he was
> under the full power of the Devil... Thus he wandered up and
> down, in exquisite torture, for just eighteen months; and then in
> a moment the pressure was removed: he believed God had not
> forsaken him. His understanding was clear as ever. He resumed
> his employ, and followed it in the fear of God.[55]

In other cases, vice or sin created chinks which Satan, ever
vigilant, could enter; as with this further 'amazing instance of
distress':

> A sensible young woman (no Methodist,) constantly attending
> her church, had all her life long believed herself to be a right good
> Christian; and in this persuasion she continued during a violent
> fever, till the physician told her brother she must die; on which
> she cried out, 'So my brother and you are going to heaven, and
> I am going to hell.' Her brother said, 'From that hour she was in
> hell already; she felt the flames; the Devil had her soul and body,
> and was now tearing her in pieces. If she swallowed any thing,
> she cried out she was swallowing fire and brimstone; and for
> twelve days she took nothing at all, – for above twenty, nothing
> but water. She had no sleep day or night'... [56]

In other instances religious madness, Wesley discerned, was not
diabolical possession but a divine judgement or trial. Take the
tortured case of J.H., who had 'fallen raving mad':

> It seems he had sat down to dinner, but had a mind first to end a
> sermon he had borrowed on 'Salvation by Faith.' In reading the last
> page, he changed colour, fell off his chair, and began screaming ter-
> ribly, and beating himself against the ground. The neighbours were

alarmed, and flocked together to the house. Between one and two I
came in, and found him on the floor, the room being full of people,
whom his wife would have kept without; but he cried aloud, 'No;
let them all come; let all the world see the just judgement of God.'
Two or three men were holding him as well as they could.[57]

Here the sufferer himself supplied the explanation:

'God has overtaken me. I said it was all a delusion. But this is no
delusion.' He then roared out, 'O thou devil! thou cursed devil!
yea, thou legion of devils! thou canst not stay. Christ will cast
thee out. I know his work is begun. Tear me to pieces, if thou
wilt; but thou canst not hurt me.' He then beat himself against
the ground again: his breast heaving at the same time, as in the
pangs of death, and great drops of sweat trickling down his face.
We all betook ourselves to prayer. His pangs ceased, and both his
body and soul were set at liberty.[58]

Wesley battled against the eagerness of people to treat such cast-
iron cases of divine or demonic seizure as mere physical disease.
What was the true source of low spirits?

The plain truth is, they wanted God, they wanted Christ, they
wanted faith; and God convinced them of their want in a way their
physicians no more understood than themselves. Accordingly
nothing availed till the Great Physician came; for in spite of all
natural means, He who made them for himself would not suffer
them to rest till they rested in Him.[59]

Observing the ecstatic convulsions frequently suffered by his congre-
gations further clarified his thoughts as to the theology of madness.
Such people had no organic distemper. Rather, he concluded,

1. That all of them (I think not one excepted) were persons in
perfect health, and had not been subject to fits of any kind, till
they were thus affected.

2. That this had come upon every one of them in a moment, without any previous notice, while they were either hearing the word of God, or thinking on what they had heard.

3. That, in that moment, they dropped down, lost all their strength, and were seized with violent pain... Some said, 'They were quite choked, so that they could not breathe:' others, 'That it was as if their heart, as if their inside, as if their whole body, was tearing all to pieces.'[60]

To Wesley all this proved demonic possession:

These symptoms I can no more impute to any natural cause, than to the Spirit of God... it was Satan tearing them as they were coming to Christ:... The word of God pierced their souls... And here the accuser came with great power, telling them, 'There was no hope: they were lost for ever.'[61]

If such madness was thus from Beyond, what use physic? Spiritual physic alone would prove effective. Thaumaturgy worked:

Mon. 27. We reached Osmotherley. After preaching in the eve-ning, I was desired to visit a person who had been an eminent scoffer at all religion, but was now they said, 'in a strange way.' I found her in a strange way indeed: either raving mad or pos-sessed by the Devil. The woman herself affirmed, 'That the Devil had appeared to her the day before, and after talking some time, leaped upon, and grievously tormented her ever since.' We prayed with her: her agonies ceased: she fell asleep, and awoke in the morning calm and easy.[62]

Thus Wesley championed belief in a demonomania, and the practice of spiritual healing, as had many churchmen of the previous century. But by the mid-eighteenth century, how many were there like him? Unfortunately, we lack the full-scale research which would map how demonological allegiances shifted. It seems clear, however, that pietistic brethren, many

ministers and believers within New Dissent (though decreas-
ingly so among old Nonconformists such as the Presbyterians),
and above all, Methodist leaders continued to espouse the pri-
macy of spiritual madness throughout the eighteenth century.
For other Christians, however – pious as well as lukewarm
Latitudinarians, outright Rationalists, Unitarians etc. – the
Miltonic spirit-drenched world no longer commanded assent.
Optimistic Enlightenment minds treated God's creation basically as a regular machine. Order reigned in the economy of
Nature, and reason and humanitarianism made literal belief in
Satan, witches, demons and particular providences seem silly,
superstitious, or even sick. If Christianity were reasonable, could
there be any positive religious madness?

Indeed, the manifestations themselves seem to have been on
the wane. Unlike Catholic Europe, England had no pilgrimage
shrines, no cloisters, no apparitions of saints to kindle collective
religious transports. Convulsionist epidemics became confined to
revivalist and evangelical groups, particularly among pietists and
Wesleyans. Mass ecstasies ceased to accompany even Wesley's field
preachings after the first decade, and Old Dissent withdrew from
its earlier commitments to thoroughgoing spiritualism. Indeed
one of the most influential critics of the traditional (Burtonian)
endorsement of demoniacal madness, Hugh Farmer, was himself
a Dissenting minister. Most spectacularly, even Quakers retreated
from their original free-spirit Antinomianism, becoming quiet-
istic and respectable. Indeed, the Quaker founders of the York
Retreat did not look upon 'religious madness' as a positive religious experience, treating it rather as a morbid condition (the
seriously disturbed were barred from religious services).

Some lamented the decay of transcendentalism; 'ghosts are not
lawful' was William Blake's angry comment on the times. Others
congratulated enlightened minds for sparing the grandchildren
of tormented Calvinists needless suffering. Humane physicians, moralists and clergymen denounced the irresponsibility
of Wesleyan 'fanatics' for playing with fire, with their rant and
cant about possession, and expressed pity or contempt for their

victims. Prominent among these was Erasmus Darwin, sworn foe to the Wesleyan firebrands. In his *Zoonomia*, he squarely listed fundamentalism as a disease:

> Orcitimor: The fear of Hell. Many theatric preachers among the Methodists successfully inspire this terror, and live comfortably upon the folly of their hearers. In this kind of madness the poor patients frequently commit suicide; although they believe they run headlong into the Hell which they dread! Such is the power of oratory, and such the debility of the human understanding![63]

Common folk, Darwin believed, were ultra-susceptible to this contagion:

> Those who suffer under this insanity are generally the most innocent and harmless people... The maniacal hallucination at length becomes so painful that the poor insane flies from life to become free of it.[64]

Darwin adduced numerous case histories of desperate sufferers whose 'scruples' had plunged them into religious madness, and often thence to despair and death:

> Mr_, a clergyman, formerly of this neighbourhood, began to bruise and wound himself for the sake of religious mortification... As he had a wife and family of small children, I believed the case to be incurable; as otherwise the affection and employment in his family connections would have opposed the beginning of this insanity. He was taken to a madhouse without effect, and after he returned home, continued to beat and bruise himself, and by this kind of mortification, and by sometimes long fasting, he at length became emaciated and died... When these works of supererogation have been of a public nature, what cruelties, murders, massacres, has not this insanity introduced into the world.[65]

Taking a rather more sympathetic tone, Richard Blackmore had pondered the melancholy dilemma that strict devotion posed for the pious:

> When the Imaginations of religious persons receive a melancholy Turn,... Scruples and Fears concerning the Sincerity of their Faith and Repentance, and their everlasting State, are by their Distemper increased, even sometimes to so deep a Despondence and Self-condemnation as borders on Despair.[66]

Do not scoff at such troubled souls, Blackmore warned the smart set. Do not despair, he advised sufferers: you are not really possessed, but just ill, in the grip of somatic disease which could be managed by medicine.

So the more liberal outlooks of the Enlightenment deprecated those dogmas, in particular literal belief in Original Sin, Predestination, Hell and the Devil, for fermenting the deadly medley of credulity, superstition and fanaticism. Possibly this reduced its occurrence. Ironically, however, it may have rendered the condition all the more appalling for individual sufferers, who in that dry, coolly secular climate were often left dramatically isolated and bereft. For, with many latter-day religious melancholics, the old clear-cut battle against the Devil ceased to apply. instead they suffered against the backdrop of the demystified clockwork universe and polite society, doubly cut off from saving grace. A further glance at the anguish of Samuel Johnson will illustrate this dilemma.

Johnson presents an apt case, for he was a devourer of Burton's *Anatomy of Melancholy*, the only book that ever got him out of bed 'two hours sooner than he wished to rise'. Hence the mental chasm between Burton's world and his becomes all the more striking. Burton and Johnson shared many melancholy traits. Both viewed themselves as 'nobodies' (Johnson told Fanny Burney that he had begun as 'nothing and nobody'), perhaps because both had denying mothers, impossible to please. In distinctive ways, both were solitaries, looking to authorship for rescue from oblivion. Both suffered want of emotional and sexual fulfilment, envying those to whom fortune, fame, and happiness came easily. 'Mad all my life, at least not sober', Johnson's melancholy was certainly fanned, and probably even initiated, by holy dread – above all, a conviction of sinfulness and a terror of death and damnation, all magnified by self-reproach for dereliction of sacred obligations. As discussed above, Johnson blamed indolence for allowing his mind to be captivated by imagination, thus opening the floodgates to madness. Yet this great Anglican, who imagined himself teetering towards insanity, had – unlike Burton – no inkling that this might be due to *diabolical possession*. He underwent religious agonies but did so entirely in terms of personal pollution, devotional lapses and self-lacerating guilt.

Christianity held out to Johnson indispensable prospects of triumph over mortality, of life eternal. But only at a terrible price, that of obeying the evangelical William Law's injunction to keep one's mind so 'possessed with such a sense of [death's] nearness that you may have it always in your thoughts'. Enforcing this suspended death sentence, Johnson's God was indeed wrathful and arbitrary:

> The quiver of Omnipotence is stored with arrows, against which the shield of human virtue, however adamantine it has been boasted, is held up in vain.[67]

God racked mankind with superhuman duties, meting out justice to sinners by damning them (which meant, Johnson explained, being 'sent to hell and punished everlastingly'). Heeding the rule of Law, Johnson buckled under the burden of God's call, that *via crucis* of duties – prayers, fasting, church-going, Bible reading, soul-searching – at which he bridled, conscious that it brought him inescapably face to face with his own worthlessness. Not least, he felt sentenced to mental hard labour. His morbid anxieties about wasting time make sense only under the ultimate threat of cosmic terror (that time wastes us), beneath the divine taskmaster. He abased himself with prayer upon prayer:

> O Lord, enable me by thy Grace to use all Diligence in
> redeeming the Time which I have spent in Sloth, Vanity, and
> Wickedness.[68]

Successive promises of reformation confirmed his inability to
reform, and broken promises induced only more guilt, further
confessions of 'manifold sins and negligences', spawning yet
more 'oppressive terrors'.

Johnson's religion proved a torment. Perhaps he never found
religious peace. Even as he neared his deathbed, he confessed,

> he had himself lived in great negligence of Religion and Worship
> for forty years, that he had neglected greatly to read his Bible
> and that he had since often reflected what he could hereafter say
> when he should be asked why he had not read it.[69]

His friend, Hester Thrale, understood it only too well. As she
perceived, it was pre-eminently Johnson's religion which fanned
his fears of madness:

> daily terror lest he had not done enough originated in piety, but
> ended in little less than disease... He... filled his imagination with
> fears that he should ever obtain forgiveness for omission of duty
> and criminal waste of time.[70]

Johnson himself was helplessly aware how he made rods for his
own back by his 'scruples'. To assuage guilt, strengthen his resolve
and placate God, he habitually bound himself by vows and
resolutions. These 'scruples' deferred crises and acted as charms
against further backslidings. But they too had their revenges. For
making them created guilt, aware as he was of their superstitious
nature ('a vow is a horrible thing... a snare for sin'); and he felt
still guiltier about breaking them: 'I have resolved... till I am
afraid to resolve again', he confessed, despairingly, in 1761.

There was no escape. Johnson's religious fears tormented his
reason yet, unlike William Cowper, he could not let go and

exculpate himself in madness, for his Arminian faith forbade such euthanasia of the spirit, believing that it was his cardinal responsibility to 'render up my soul to God unclouded'. Characteristically, Johnson gave up his medically prescribed opiates on his deathbed, to pass over with his mind clear. Religion thus made Reason a jewel of infinite price, confirming Johnson's intuition that whatever he was, he was through his intellect. But he also knew only too well that 'of the uncertainties of our present state, the most dreadful is the uncertain continuance of reason'. It was religious terrors precisely which raised those tempests in Johnson's mind that jeopardised his reason.

Other cases parallel Johnson's, for instance the torments of the 'castaway', William Cowper, cowering under an implacable and distant God and bereft of spiritual comfort; these will be examined in Chapter 5. Religious madness thus commonly triggered existential terror rather than liberation. And some 'inspired prophets' were by any standards dangerous, such as the Pentecostal Bannister Truelock, whose voices persuaded James Hadfield to shoot George III, or later Jonathan Martin, the divine arsonist of York Minster. Small wonder, then, that the leaders of Georgian opinion were so perturbed. Its chief advocates, evangelical preachers such as George Whitefield and John Wesley, came in for volleys of satire, abuse and fury. A witty touch is audible, perhaps, in William Warburton's conceit that Wesley had invented a new trade, that of 'turning fools into madmen', or when Pope argued tongue in cheek that 'the only means of advancing Christianity was by the New-birth of religious madness'. In a similar vein, Horace Walpole traded on the sort of sexual innuendo that was on the tip of every critic's tongue, summing up Whitefield's evangelicalism:

> His largest crop of proselytes lay among servant maids: and his warmest devotees went to Bedlam without going to war.[71]

But Methodistical madness struck real fear into the polite and propertied, alarmed lest a popular religion of the heart should

foment civil disorders, as in the bad old times of the Civil War;
a dread, ironically, provoking riots against Methodist neophytes,
leading Wesley to comment sardonically:

> Sat. 30. We rode to Stallbridge, long the seat of war by a senseless,
> insolent mob, encouraged by their betters, so called, to outrage
> their quiet neighbours. For what? 'Why they were mad; they
> would beat their brains out.'[72]

The evil, as perceived by the orthodox, was that those experiencing religious transports were claiming privileged access to divine
'truths'. This was dangerous nonsense. In Puritanism's heyday,
many had abandoned the *via media* of the once-born in favour
of a hotline to God through the inner voices, bypassing carnal
reason. Divine communication had been part of legitimate piety.
But in the disabused atmosphere of post-Restoration England,
leaders of elite opinion – philosophers such as Hobbes and
Henry More, Whigs such as Shaftesbury, High Tories such as
Sacheverell and Swift, and freethinkers such as Anthony Collins
– converged to discredit the 'saints'' claims to divine illumination
as mere credulity, superstition and enthusiasm.

Reason and ridicule were powerful weapons; but the sting of
the zealots' challenge to Church and state could be drawn, not
least by 'medicalisation'. 'Religious madness' was indeed real; but
it was not, after all, Burtonian literal possession by otherworldly
powers, higher or lower. Rather, it was now reinterpreted as a
symptom of common-or-garden madness, as essentially organic.
Enthusiasm – so detractors argued – was pathological. It was a
mark of appetites – the hunger for salvation, dread of damnation,
the vanity of believing oneself of the elect – out of control, and
poisoning the imagination. And – mad-doctors alleged – religious transports, like epileptic seizures, had their own physical
geography. Thus Dr Nicholas Robinson deemed that the French
prophets were victims merely of 'strong convulsive fits', arguing
that the visions of sectaries such as James Nayler, George Fox
and Lodowick Muggleton had been 'nothing but the effect of

mere madness, and arose from the stronger impulses of a warm brain'.

Thus, by delving to the organic roots of these bogus revelations, critics and medical men hoped to eradicate them. In the process, the Pauline idea of positive religious ecstasy, sanctioned from the Bible to Bunyan, lost credit, at least among churchmen and the coffee-house sets. No longer a blessing, it had been turned into a symptom. In George Man Burrows' verdict, early in the nineteenth century,

> Enthusiasm and insanity bear such close affinity that the shades are often too indistinct to define which is one and which the other. Exuberance of zeal on any subject, in some constitutions, soon ripens into madness: but excess of religious enthusiasm... usually and readily degenerates into fanaticism;... and permanent delirium too often closes the scene.[73]

Undoubtedly, as MacDonald and others have argued, the Augustan stigmatisation of religious rapture as disease involved a reactionary strategy, linked to Whig notions of progress. It was one of many ways in which elite culture – both experiencing threat, but also aggressively expansionist – was distancing itself from, defining itself against, and aiming to control traditional popular beliefs. Psychiatrising religious deviance thus served the Anglican ruling order as a technique of social policing. But it is important to remember as well that branding religious 'prophets' as sick had a longer and wider history, for it had been a common label in Britain and on the Continent, at least as far back as the French Wars of Religion. The formula was only in part a strategic response to the hardening and widening of social divides in the wake of the Civil War.

Moreover, the medicalisation of divine madness was not crudely manipulative or conspiratorial. The waning of the spirit-drenched cosmos involved more than an opportunist tactic by the powerful; rather, it marks a sea-change of consciousness synchronous with such fundamental developments as the rise of mechanical science, the progress of material civilisation, and the extension of man's dominion over Nature. In any case, it would be an oversimplification to conjure up a vision of popular culture's 'spiritual' notions of illumination and madness being suppressed by elite culture's medical materialism. For, as discussed above, common culture itself embraced highly organic theories of, and remedies for, insanity.

Two conclusions emerge. First, during the Enlightenment, the spirit kingdom was losing its status as a cosmological reality, and was being aetherealised or turned to metaphor, as part of what Abrams has called 'natural supernaturalism'. Such sublimation jeopardised authentic religious witness. Many in the Georgian era who experienced themselves as going out of their senses or who were so labelled, were simply living through what would once have been seen as a standard *Pilgrim's Progress*. The quest for religious identity could become acutely agonising for men like Alexander Cruden or Kit Smart, because, immersed in fundamentalism, they now had to walk out of step with a secularising society. When the Aberdonian Cruden tried to uphold the Sabbath by force, using a shovel, in the East End of London, he was regarded not as a saint but as a cranky nuisance. Yesterday's visionaries were now more likely to be stigmatised as mad and even confined; and once confined, their 'experimental faith' was ignored or negated. And those wrestling with spiritual crisis were increasingly likely to be placed in the care not of ministers but of physicians. Trosse had had his sympathetic Presbyterian lady. But, after him, Cruden, Periam, Richard Brothers and others had Bethlem or private asylums, under mad-doctors who regarded transports as disease symptoms. No asylums as yet had chapels. In the Georgian age, the free spirit came under observation for treatment.

Thus spiritual immanence fell under suspicion. But it was rarely actually suppressed. 'Methodism mocked' was a common tale, but very few prominent enthusiasts were actually silenced in madhouses. Indeed, as mentioned above, George Whitefield was even successful in getting the release from Bethlem of one such believer. Joanna Southcott, the great Regency prophetess, was often called crazy, not least for her blasphemy in proclaiming that she was about to give birth to Shiloh: yet she was never locked away.

Some light is perhaps shed on this by medical discussions, for from the beginning of the eighteenth century, texts on insanity simply ceased to give priority to religious melancholy. Certainly the diagnosis continued to do doughty service in polemics against fanaticism, as the furore over the 'French prophets' shows. Yet Burtonian melancholy stopped being held up as the fatal disease of fallen man. Major early Georgian texts on melancholy, such as George Cheyne's *The English Malady* (1733), hardly touch on religious melancholy. In his *Treatise of the Hypochondriack and Hysterick Passions* (1711), Mandeville explored at great length, from the sufferer's viewpoint, the varieties of depression the physician encountered (and Mandeville's self-interest surely lay in widening the condition as much as possible); yet religious melancholy was not so much as mentioned.

In Cheyne's case the silence is almost deafening. For Cheyne himself was a depressive, suffering religious crises and personally proselytising a chiliastic, quasi-mystical faith. Yet no discussion of souls in crisis appears in his medical work. Religious melancholy had no place – as blessing or as stigma – within the 'English malady'. Richard Blackmore at least addressed the subject, demolishing the scoffers' case that religion was itself pathological, while indicting pagans and Papists of sickly enthusiasm. Yet his *via media* merely underlines how far troubled souls had been secularised since Napier or Burton, for Blackmore treats religious melancholy not with Democritean laughter, nor Heraclitean tears, nor indeed Burtonian abominations, but with a cosy sympathy reminiscent of Addison's explanations of how once-terrifying witches were in reality merely pitiable old crones. Thus true religion as divine madness, and derangement as demonic possession, had both been displaced from enlightened minds. The praise of folly bowed out before Chesterfieldian politeness, and demonomania yielded to that most Georgian horror, Dullness.

THE ENGLISH MALADY

The decline and fall of Burtonian religious melancholy transformed the anatomy of abnormality. In a climate of well-tempered
religion and heady worldliness, personal crises were experienced
and expressed in ways less specifically Christian. The damned soul
of the Stuart age mutated into the Georgian hypochondriac, and
Satanic possession was superseded by the 'blue devils' (dyspepsia).
Ironically, the very term 'demoniac' could be appropriated in
mid-Georgian England by a clique of rakes, the Hellfire Club.
When Addison called *le spleen anglais* 'a kind of demon that haunts
the nation', he silently acknowledged the metaphorisation of the
Devil. Likewise, it is apt that the very first volume of that great
epitome of Georgian polite culture, the *Gentleman's Magazine*,
should announce that 'Apparitions, Genii, Demons, Hobgoblins,
Sorcerers, and Magicians, are now reckon'd idle Stories'.

This 'secularisation' in turn released other changes. Once
abnormal states could be viewed independently of diabolism
but rather as integral to the self, it became easier to stop regarding disordered people as dupes of Satan, or as wild beasts akin
to Gadarene swine. Alternative models emerged for constru-
ing madness naturalistically, historically and socially, within the
Aristotelian vision of man as a *zôon politikon*. The theology of
insanity made way for its sociology, and ultimately its psychology,
and disturbance became reconceived as a social function, indeed
as a disease of civilisation, and most particularly as the 'English
malady'. For reasons largely obscure – but somehow connected
with Hippocratic medical environmentalism – England had a
reputation, at least from the sixteenth century, as a hotbed of
wrongheads, crack-brains and suicides, and it was a national
joke which continental writers – Anglophiles and Anglophobes
alike – chose to chorus throughout the Enlightenment. What
is remarkable, however, is the alacrity with which the English
themselves accepted the crown of thorns conferred by *le spleen
anglais*. By 1807, Dr Thomas Trotter could thus cast his eye back
and assure his readers:

Sydenham at the conclusion of the seventeenth century computed fevers to constitute two thirds of the diseases of mankind. But, at the beginning of the nineteenth century, we do not hesitate to affirm, that nervous disorders have now taken the place of fevers, and may be justly reckoned two thirds of the whole, with which civilised society is afflicted.[74]

Doubtless this auto-diagnosis was an expression of authentic English self-laceration – a guilty fear, stimulated by Civic Humanist ideology, that Albion's opportunity society and boom economy spelt corruption and were sure to take their toll. Thus in his best-selling mid-century diatribe, John Brown stated it for a fact that

our effeminate and unmanly Life, working along with our Island Climate, hath notoriously produced an Increase of low Spirits and nervous Disorders.[75]

As if to clinch his case, Brown was soon to commit suicide.

But the moralists' Jeremiad was shared by medical men as well. According to the madhouse-keeper Dr Thomas Arnold, mental instability was out of hand in England thanks to its 'excess of wealth and luxury', a view on which his contemporary, Dr William Rowley, expatiated:

In proportion as the arts, sciences, and luxury increase, so do vices and madness... in those kingdoms where the greatest luxuries, refinements, wealth, and unrestrained liberty abound, are the most numerous instances of madness. England, according to its size and number of inhabitants, produces and contains more insane than any other country in Europe, and suicide is more common.[76]

It was liberty, thought Rowley, which was England's mixed blessing:

in Britain everyone thinks and acts as he pleases; this produces all
that variety and originality in the English character, and causes
arts, sciences, and inventions to flourish.[77]

It also, however, meant the liberty to pursue individualism into
insanity.

These were critiques of corruption. But they also involved
complex cross-currents, as is made clearest in their *locus classicus*, Dr George Cheyne's *The English Malady* (1733). Cheyne
confirmed that England was suffering an epidemic of 'nervous
disorders'. Such maladies must be brought into the open, treated
as objects neither of shame nor of satire but of sympathy, almost
even of pride. As Blackmore stated, 'the temper of the Natives
of Britain is most various, which proceeds from the Spleen, an
Ingredient of their Constitution, which is almost Peculiar, at least
in the Degree of it, to this Island.' So why did the spleen blossom
in England? 'The moisture of our air', Cheyne explained,

the Variableness of our Weather, (from our situation amidst the
Ocean), the Rankness and Fertility of our Soil, the Richness and
Heaviness of our Food, the Wealth and Abundance of Inhabitants
(from their universal Trade), the Inactivity and Sedentary
Occupations of the better Sort (among whom this Evil mostly
rages) and the Humour of living in great, populous and con-
sequently unhealthy Towns, have brought forth a Class and Set
of Distempers, with atrocious and frightful Symptoms, scarce
known to our Ancestors and never rising to such fatal Heights,
nor afflicting such Numbers in any other known Nation.[78]

This diagnosis was double-edged. Nervous disorders constituted
authentic physical diseases, causing profound suffering. Yet they
were the price of progress as much as the wages of sin. Attacking
the prosperous, they were marks of distinction, a success tax on a
busy hive buzzing as never before – urban, affluent, aspiring and
ambitious. When Cheyne explained, 'We have more nervous diseases since the present Age has made Efforts to go beyond former

Times, in all the Arts of Ingenuity, Invention, Study, Learning, and all the Contemplative and Sedentary Professions', he was boasting more than bewailing. Being ill could be symptomatic of well-being.

In this new theodicy, stress was the by-product of civilisation – a toll exacted not because (as later for Freud) society entailed repression and repression bred neurosis, but because the strains of the good life enervated the system. Wealth corroded health by encouraging the high life, gourmandising, lounging, artificial stimulants, exemption from manual labour. Property granted leisure, but maintaining investments bred anxieties, and sedentary idleness left time weighing heavily on vacant minds. For, as Mandeville stressed, the spleen leeched on to the comfortable, those free to indulge their imaginations, sparing

people of lower Fortunes, who have seldom higher Ends, than... the getting of their Daily Bread;[79]

Nervous diseases were thus class-specific, affecting the cream, refined and delicate spirits, high-flyers, those, explained Cheyne, 'who have a great deal of sensibility, are quick thinkers, feel pleasure and pain the most readily, and are of most lively imagination' – the distemper displaying (thought Dr Purcell) a particular 'gusto for the tender sex'. Such disorders, Cheyne asserted, 'I think never happen, or can happen to any but those of the liveliest and quickest natural parts whose Faculties are the brightest and most spiritual, and whose Genius is most keen and penetrating, and particularly when there is the most delicate Sensation and Taste, both of pleasure and pain'. His case histories bore this out, detailing patients exclusively from the *beau monde*, such as a 'lady of great fortune', one 'eminent for fine breeding', a 'knight baronet of ancient family', and so forth.

Similarly, the spleen and gout specialist William Stukeley thought melancholy afflicted 'men that have been most famous for wars, for art, philosophy, legislature, poetry'. 'For it is evident by common experience', agreed Blackmore, 'that Men of a splenetic Complexion... are usually endowed with refined and elevated parts, quick Apprehension, distinguishing Judgement, clear Reason, and great Vivacity of Imagination; and in these Perfections they are superior to the common Level of Mankind.' So the spleen was a silver spoon or a passport to high places. All this proved that the social order had a real physiological legitimacy, showing that Nature herself had divided mankind into 'quick thinkers', 'slow thinkers', and 'no thinkers'. The quick were prone to nervous disorders, such sickness being almost a litmus of leadership:

> There are those who govern and those who are govern'd, originally form'd and mark'd out by Nature, in their original Frame and indelible Signatures: The last may safely, at least for some Time, wallow in sensual Pleasure... having generally very blunt and obtuse intellectual Organs... The first have more delicate and elastic Organs of Thinking and Sensibility... they are like fine Lancets or Razors, that coarse Usage will soon ruffle and spoil; and therefore must forego gross and rank sensual Pleasures... otherwise their Sufferings will be intollerable, which is the Case of all nervous Hypochondriacal and Hysterical persons; most of which were created Genii, Philosophers and Lawgivers. [80]

Such theories about the 'hyp' and the 'spleen' stimulated rethinking about abnormality. They called for fresh tolerance, created social excuses and, not least, were optimistic because they also held out hopes for improvement. Being a real somatic disease, hypochondria had its remedies. Mediating between body and mind, the nerves of fine-spirited people needed to be highly elastic and vibrant (yokels, by contrast, had leathery, dull fibres, and so 'scarce any passion at all... so they enjoy the finest health, and are subject to the fewest diseases; such are ideots, peasants and mechanicks'). Among the fine-spirited, however, the danger was that high living would clog the nerves; these therefore needed periodic cleaning or retuning. A health-farm regimen, or a simple diet, recreation, exercise, and attention to the other 'non-naturals', was prescribed by Cheyne. Because 'study of difficult and intricate matters will infallibly do hurt', diversions were in order (think of Hume, philosophising in 'forlorn solitude', taking a break at the billiard table).

Cheyne denied, of course, that he was advocating low lifestyles to counter low spirits, protesting that his 'low diet' did not mean he was 'at bottom a mere Leveller, and for destroying Order, Rank and Property'. Unlike Rousseau, he did not think civilisation was itself pathological: it bred diseases but these could be remedied (for civilisation also bred physicians).

This socio-psycho-pathology of progress, a Georgian precursor of Civilisation and its Discontents, was a remarkable ideological coup, every bit comparable to Freud's later *tour de force*. Nor was it merely a slice of smart sales talk spun by fashionable physicians, out to expand medical demand. For a glance through contemporary letters and diaries reveals how such disorders – biliousness, prostration, lethargy, depression, mood swings – infected polite culture; having nerves was almost as much a status symbol as having taste. Indeed, the two were anatomically linked. The endless references in Georgian plays and novels to hysterical Misses and hyppish fathers evidently rang a bell. In 1728 a doctor commented upon how such disorders and fashion had become utterly whirled up together:

> When I first dabbled in this art, the old distemper call'd Melancholy was exchanged for Vapours, and afterwards for the Hypp, and at last took up the now current appelation of the Spleen, which it still retains, tho' a learned doctor of the west, in a little tract he hath written, divides the Spleen and Vapours, not only into the Hypp, the Hyppos, and the Hyppocons; but subdivides these divisions into the Markambles, the Moonpalls, the Strong Fiacs, and the Hockogrogles.[81]

Clearly, a momentous step has been taken when abnormalities are becoming not just acceptable but smart. In that acceptance, a key role was played by the emphasis among the proponents of the 'English malady' that it was exclusively a top people's disease. The vapours were eligible because, unlike colds and coughs, they were not caught from the poor. Within the traditional hierarchical metaphors of psychic health (reason-passions, master-slave), the elite had been seen as sane and the masses raged; in the new model, by contrast, bumpkins wallowing in the idiocy of rural life remained 'naturals', lacking the wit or sensibility to share the English malady. 'Fools, weak or stupid persons, heavy and dull souls', condescended Cheyne, 'are seldom much troubled with Vapours or lowness of Spirits.' Thus, by a Mandevillian sleight of hand, fashionable physicians flattered melancholy, making the corruption of the oligarchy's brains as acceptable as the corruption of their politics. In Chatham, Clive or Burke such malady became the fibre of empire-builders.

In the elevation of 'nerves' above vulgar disorders, Locke's new analysis of human understanding (discussed at greater length in Chapter 4 below) proved influential. Locke discriminated between the vacancy of village idiotism and true thought-disturbance, to vindicate hectic minds. For Locke, madness was no longer the overthrow of noble reason by base passions, but rather (mis)association of ideas, false consciousness. Madmen, he wrote, 'do not appear to have lost the faculty of reasoning but having joined together some ideas very wrongly, they mistake them for truths, and they err as men do that argue right from wrong principles'. Thus wrong-thinkers could be re-educated, for, as 'custom settles habits of thinking in the understanding', false associations could be corrected. Hence crazy ideas carried no congenital taint; they could be a temporary aberration, rather like sowing one's wild oats.

Furthermore, the formulation of the 'English malady' was all the more acceptable because it was founded on the somatic bedrock discussed above. Far from being the prelude to a lost soul, it was instead a distemper sited in the guts, and transmitted through slack nerves. Cheyne blamed diet. Too much food, its excessive richness, piquancy, or rancidity, and over-fondness for the bottle all congested the nerves. High living lowered the spirits. Dr Cheyne's own 'case' bore this out, for a surfeit of high life during his early years in London, when he was trying to carouse himself into a good medical practice, blew him up to thirty-two stone but reduced him to death-obsessed anxiety. Cheyne came out as the evangelist for vegetarianism, his ideal diet being light and low, consisting mainly of grain and vegetables. For this he was thought cranky, but his advocacy of moderation was widely accepted as the best corrective for the periodical depressions, flatulencies, nauseas and lethargies racking the bright and beautiful. Health cures rose high on the Quality's agenda. Taking the waters in Bath, Scarborough or Harrogate or at the multitude of lesser spas and mushrooming seaside resorts ('Sanditons') was to treat the 'blue devils' as much as for gout or rheumatism.

Being thus basically organic, 'lifestyle conditions' and nervous complaints could be owned without overtones of perversions of the will or of dabbling with the Devil. They were occupational hazards. Moreover, the formulation of the 'English malady' transformed the image of the melancholy man. The traditional melancholic has presented an equivocal face. On the favourable side, he paraded an awesome, aristocratic aloofness:

> The melancholy outsider was thought of as a noble gentleman in every sense of those words. He was well regarded among his own kind, just as artists, born under Saturn, and erotic outsiders were treated with regard – by their own kind.[82]

On the debit side, he was typically a malcontent, scoffer, or a solitary misanthrope. The formulation of the 'English malady' however, gave the morose melancholic a facelift. Gone was black Jaques fretting through the Forest of Arden, or the railing Democritus Junior of Burton's *Anatomy*, types tormented by an evil genius or a dominant humour: envy, jealousy, ambition, or despair. Such was traditionally the undersocialised man or the moody, broody, distrait *penseroso*. The Augustans continued to warn, with Burton, 'be not solitary', but the melancholic type was undergoing resocialisation – indeed, as innatist humoral psychology declined, the anatomy of melancholy yielded to its sociology, reflecting Enlightenment interest in social progress rather than in the pilgrimage of the soul. The Georgians came to regard melancholy as a social malaise, an *anomie* produced by the demands of city, court and crowd (almost, in due course, requiring the Romantic reinstatement of solitude). Whereas Burton thought melancholy was dangerous – it caused enmity, bloodshed, wars – the Georgians made it an object of sympathy.

Having the blues became safe and eligible, and melancholy's sting was drawn. Its allure for James Boswell makes this clear. Boswell was subject to periodic fits of depression, which he sometimes blamed on his guilt-inducing Scottish Calvinist upbringing. His family may have been a source of the problem, for his brother John grew so disturbed as to be confined to an asylum. Even so, Boswell enjoyed flirting with morbid introspection. Indeed, he wrote a newspaper column under the pseudonym of 'Hypochondriack', penning numerous pieces on that very subject, and was clearly enamoured of the melancholic's persona as an exceptional fellow, with marked profound feelings and superior insight: 'we *Hypochondriacks* may console ourselves in the hour of gloomy distress, by thinking that our sufferings make our superiority'.

What made Boswell's bravura feel safe for him was the consoling escape clause that nervous weaknesses such as his were poles apart from madness proper. One could thus indulge 'pleasing anxieties' without risking dire insanity. Samuel Johnson judged that this was courting disaster. Herein they differed fundamentally:

> Dr Johnson and I had a serious conversation by ourselves on melancholy and madness: which he was, I always thought, enormously inclined to confound together. Melancholy, like 'great wit' may be near allied to madness; but there is, in my opinion, a distinct separation between them.[83]

Johnson, however, distrusted Boswell's modish self-indulgence:

> You are always complaining of melancholy, and I conclude from those complaints that you are fond of it. No man talks of that which he is desirous to conceal, and every man desires to conceal that of which he is ashamed... make it an invariable and obligatory law to yourself, never to mention your own mental diseases: if you are never to speak of them you will think on them but little, and if you think little of them, they will molest you rarely.[84]

Hypochondria was indeed for Boswell a self-dramatisation which pandered to his desire to be a man of 'soul'. Johnson, by contrast, feared melancholy as the slippery slope to madness proper. Though Boswell enjoyed its frisson, did it, in the long term, speed the pathetic collapse of his final years?

SYMPATHISING WITH INSANITY

Nerves became *à la mode*, and 'madness appears to be fatally common in Great Britain, and among the higher ranks'. Admittedly, melancholy had enjoyed cachet before, especially in the Jacobean fantasy-world. But the tone changed in the high-pressure, high-visibility salons, boudoirs and coffee-houses of the Georgians. The Abbé Le Blanc was startled to find that what was traditionally called vice was now being excused as oddity, and Dr Thomas Beddoes was later to ponder whether any previous age would have been so foolish as to talk itself into elevating *ennui* and apathy into style. Top people were now willing to confess themselves less than perfectly normal. And this 'modernism' threatened traditional values.

For, as shown already, loss of reason had always been seen as perilous and stigmatising (one reason why sufferers and doctors took pains to somatise disorder). In the eyes of strict moralists, preachers and satirists, the madman had been equivalent to the sinner or the ne'er-do-well – indeed, his condition was the penalty of vice and sin. In Hogarth's 'Rake's Progress' series, fecklessness, folly and greed plunged Tom Rakewell headlong into his Bedlam chains. These classical condemnations were vociferously upheld in Augustan England by a troop of mainly Tory satirists, spearheaded by Swift, Gay, Arbuthnot and Pope. For them, the lunatic's symbolic function was to stand as the negation of rational order. He was an object lesson, a warning, exemplifying *homo rationalis* by his opposite, proving how flimsy and vulnerable reason was.

Satires such as *Gulliver's Travels* and the *Dunciad* drove home such fears about the madness of the 'divided society'. Critics thought it was not just a handful of false prophets who were crazed. Instead, they dreaded that the whole society was 'running mad after innovation', dissolving into a chaotic cacophony of prating, posturing individuals. Scribleran satire parades before the eyes a nightmare hubbub of would-be inventors and *soi-disant* geniuses, Dunce poetasters filled with *afflatus* (*recte* flatulence), windbag political saviours, crackbrained projectors, madcap philosophers like 'Monsieur Descartes' and the other inmates of the 'Academy of Modern Bedlam', buttonholing freethinkers and puffed-up atheists, speculators in economic bubbles, faiths and cosmologies, frenzied, fantastical egoists and their gulls like Lemuel Gulliver – all told, the vain, the proud, the opinionated, the fixated. Solvents of society, they all lacked humility, judgement and self-knowledge; self-obsessed, they were excrescences (traditionalists argued), prophets of a new, anything-goes regime where, as masquerades, paper money and South Sea Bubble speculations proved, illusion was eclipsing reality. It was a world peopled by Laputans and Yahoos.

Championing traditional views of madness regarded as a curse, Tory moralists anathematised these cranks as evil, stupid and sick. Radical preachers did not possess true divine madness; rather, the divines were possessed by madness and the 'inspired' were just full of wind, arising in the case of the Aeolists (Swift's term in the *Tale of a Tub* for the Puritans) from rotting guts: 'the corruption of the senses is the creation of the spirit'. Enemies of truth, order and civilisation, the mad were a scandal: endemic, incurable, deserving not pity but pills or the pillory. The sane needed to be protected from that madness which had been the 'Parent of all those mighty Revolutions that have happened in Empire, in Philosophy and in Religion'.

Thus critics of the brave new world of the Whig hegemony, with its mad scramble for wealth, place and fashion, hurled anathemas against 'the dull, the proud, the wicked and the mad', as Pope phrased it in his *Epistle to Dr Arbuthnot*. Healthy minds and healthy societies must stand together. Swift thus piqued himself on being 'a perfect stranger to the spleen', rather as Pope asserted, 'I was never hippish in my life'. By contrast, new currents of 'progressive' thought in the eighteenth century were to generate sympathies towards – even affinities for – the mawkish, the melancholy and the mad, as part of a new espousal of permissive liberal individualism. Attitudes towards the disturbed changed by degrees and never in straight lines, but it is easy to see straws in the wind.

For all his crusty Toryism, Dr Johnson was, for instance, according to his biographer Sir John Hawkins, 'a great enemy to the present fashionable way of supposing worthless and infamous persons mad'. Rather than endorse Pope's yoking of 'the wicked and the mad', which cruelly incriminated lunatics in vice and sin, Johnson regarded them as the supreme instance of unfortunates. He would have no truck, however, with the new humbug which sentimentalised their plight. Hence his indignation when the whingeing apologist Soame Jenyns, espousing a Panglossian optimism, fatuously paraded the happy moron as his prize exhibit: 'I doubt not but there is some truth in that rant of a mad poet, that there is a pleasure in being mad, which none but madmen know', Johnson answered back, with all his gravity:

I never knew disorders of mind encrease felicity; every madman is either arrogant and irascible, or gloomy and suspicious, or possessed by some passion or notion destructive to his quiet. He has always discontent in his look, and malignity in his bosom. [85]

William Cowper's reminiscences of a mid-century youthful visit to Bethlem convey a similar sense of attitudes in transition. He had gone anticipating sport; his recollection, however, was of shame:

> Though a boy, I was not altogether insensible of the misery of the poor captives, nor destitute of feeling for them. But the madness of some of them had such a humorous air, and displayed itself in so many whimsical freaks, that it was impossible not to be entertained, and at the same time that I was angry with myself for being so.[86]

Indeed, responses towards Bedlam became a touchstone of progressive attitudes. Before mid-century there is little sign that visitors treated Bethlem other than as a sideshow: good, clean fun. But reactions changed dramatically. Take, for example, this anonymous correspondent in *The World* magazine in 1753, stressing the horror of the experience for 'feeling minds', for whom

> there is nothing so affecting as sights like these; nor can a better lesson be taught us in any part of the globe than in this school of misery. Here we may see the mighty reasoners of the earth, below even the insects that crawl upon it; and from so humbling a sight we may learn to moderate our pride.[87]

Not surprisingly, fiction too nurtured this new pathos. In his influential sentimental novel *The Man of Feeling*, Henry Mackenzie's morbidly sensitive hero, Harley, is roused to pity by a procession of sentimental characters – prostitutes, the poor, the homeless – but by none more so than the sad, mad women in Bedlam. He encounters bitter tears:

> 'My Billy is no more! said she, 'do you weep for my Billy? Blessings on your tears! I would weep too, but my brain is dry; and it burns, it burns, it burns!' She drew nearer to Harley, – 'Be comforted, young Lady,' said he, 'your Billy is in heaven.' 'Is he, indeed? and shall we meet again?… when I can, I pray: and some-

times I sing: when I am saddest, I sing: – You shall hear me, hush! "Light be the earth on Billy's breast, And green the sod that wraps his grave!"[88]

The account is of course grossly maudlin, and Ophelia fills Mackenzie's imagination more than any real Bedlamite; yet the break with Ned Ward's thick-skinned roisterings half a century earlier is total.

Madhouses such as Bethlem play a significant, if minor, part in the emergent emotional landscape of the novel. Typically, they symbolise instruments of unlawful confinement, incarcerating the sane protagonists of Tobias Smollett's *Sir Launcelot Greaves* and the heroine in Mary Wollstonecraft's *Maria or the Wrongs of Woman*. In both, the wronged subject is prey to persecution by warped and wicked enemies. Smollett makes his hero Quixotic, so that the unworldliness of his own folly may underline the vicious madness of the world. While with *Maria*, it is crucial that the eponymous heroine is female, indicating the identification critics were by then commonly making between the mad, newly exonerated as victims of oppression, and women's plight under the heartless tyranny of their masters. For Swift or Pope, the mad were villains: by the late eighteenth century they have become victims. Once the lunatic threatened society; now society is a threat to him. Instead of the sane needing to be protected ('Shut, shut the door, good John', Pope had pleaded, to stave off Bedlamite scribblers), the mad, we are told, now need security against society.

This emergent sympathy towards the mad – some of it authentic, some smacking of affectation – matched a growing preoccupation among the literati with the relations of self and society, the private and the public, the individual and the normal, the mazy motions of the mind. Just how to account for this introspective turn obviously raises tangled issues of modulations in *mentalité*. How should we interpret that flow of individualism, subjectivity, and sentiment which becomes so powerful a current through the eighteenth century? In material terms, unparalleled political stability and prosperity probably permitted relaxation of the old stern familial, moral and religious behaviour codes, thus permitting new freedoms of expression and choice (such as a greater say for the young in marriage partners). Changing lifestyles and domestic architecture encouraged greater privacy. Silent individual reading, letter-writing and diary-keeping nurtured reflection.

Moreover, in the theatre of the mind, old certainties were eroded. In pedagogics, in taste, opinion, and piety, public dogma made way for pluralism and personal judgement, sanctioned by the ultra-influential Lockian model of personal culture, the mind and emotions popularised in middlebrow Spectatorism. Thus encouraged, the rising generations may well have experienced rising expectations of greater opportunities for personal development and self-realisation. They explored their selves and sampled 'sensibility' (for Burke, 'the *mania* of the day'). Yet such freedoms brought their own anxieties and pressures. And, apparently paradoxically, polite society simultaneously set more intense store upon decorum and conformity, regarded as the price to be paid for ensuring the smooth-running of a civil society which depended, as Hume noted, upon opinion not force. A gauche man-about-town in London, young Boswell had to keep reminding himself about *retenu* and playing his prescribed part upon the stage of life.

As Boswell's own journals record so well, the permissive mid-century generations commonly felt themselves tugged apart, enticed by dizzy yet dangerous freedoms while leaning heavily upon the traditional social pillars, or entangled in the pleasures yet also pressures of solitude. For many, the inevitable subterranean tensions surfaced in unease, ennui and melancholy, as symptoms of indecision and indirection, yet also as indulgent expressions of release. Georgian solipsistic melancholy could thus form a condition perilous neither to society (it was not revolution) nor to the self (it was not mania), both gratifying, yet also 'punitive'. Spleen was sometimes gross affectation or a literary pose; yet many articulate men and women, struggling to make sense of self in an increasingly secular and unfamiliar world, truly hovered uneasily between pleasurable absorption in an enhanced, narcissistic state of self-awareness, and black, uncontrollable depression. The lonely, rudderless life of the scholar poet Thomas Gray affords a good instance. In his lighter, more fanciful melancholy vein he could write to his friend West:

> Mine, you are to know, is a white Melancholy, or rather Leucocholy for the most part: which though it seldom laughs or dances, nor ever amounts to what one calls Joy or Pleasure, yet is a good easy sort of a state, and *sa* [*sic*] *ne laisse que de s'amuser.* The only fault of it is insipidity; which is apt now and then to give a sort of Ennui, which makes one form certain little wishes that signify nothing.[89]

Gray did not always, however, feel in command of his moods:

> But there is another sort, black indeed, which I have now and then felt... [This] excludes and shuts its eyes to the most possible hopes, and every thing that is pleasurable: from this the Lord deliver us! for none but he and sunshiny weather can do it.[90]

For all the Good Lord and the sunshine, many years of Gray's life lie deep in elegiac shadow, suggesting a depression ('black indeed') which genuinely created oblivion. Or take Gray's fellow poet, William Collins. Some of his best verse – for example, the 'Ode to Fear' – dwelt on the mystery of the mind. Yet, for reasons which remain unclear – though probably connected with neglect and alcohol – Collins dried up as a poet, lapsing into hopeless depression, and being confined for a time in an asylum. Solitude, sentimentality and self-absorption marked the literary temper from mid-century.

One risk run by such temptations to daydreaming, introspection, and close self-analysis was the dissolution of an assured sense of identity, particularly among those lacking robust religious vocation. Locke's sensationalist epistemology, especially as filtered through Hume's solipsistic scepticism, could involve radical disorientation. After all, according to a plausible reading of Locke, what was the self but the sum of all the sensations passing through the windows of the five senses? Yet the outside world, in turn, was known only as 'refracted through the senses'. Where then was the Petrine rock, the Archimedean point, the clear and distinct Cartesian *cogito* beyond the vertigo? Indeed, as Yolton has shown, contemporary philosophers of mind characteristically found it almost impossible to give satisfactory mechanisms of the mystery of consciousness. Hume's scepticism about one's assurance of self-identity was extreme (had he been Johnson, he would have kicked himself and pronounced that an end on't), yet similar doubts were much in the air, being played up for example throughout Sterne's *Tristram Shandy*, and encapsulated in the exchange:

> And who are you? said he.
> Don't puzzle me, said I.[91]

In his journals Boswell repeatedly instructed himself 'Be Johnson', 'Be Paoli', but never dared urge: Be Yourself; though it is worth noting that that phrase – being oneself – was in common contemporary use to describe a state of normalcy.

Enlightenment self-searching could be heady stuff, and plenty of eighteenth-century minds launched themselves on voyages of self-understanding, flying the flag of philosophical doubt. Suggestive of the novel delights of this quest for the New Found Lands of inner space is a reflection made by Boswell in his 'Hypochondriack' column: 'There is too general a propensity to consider Hypochondria as altogether a bodily disorder.' Here he was expressing a willingness – rare earlier – to risk the equivocations of free-floating mental and imaginative experiments. For Richard Baxter and many others a couple of generations before, hypochondriasis had been too terrible to toy with as a mental mystery tour. For Boswell, it promised a bewitching adventure into the interior.

One possible outcome of self-discovery was, of course, self-loathing and self-destructiveness. It remains unclear whether the Georgians were as suicide-prone as *Schadenfreude*-filled alarmists made out; certainly many contemporaries were deeply perturbed. What is relevant is the startling reversal in attitudes towards those who made away with themselves. In pre-Restoration times, both civil and ecclesiastical authorities concurred that self-murder was no less a crime and sin than murder. In committing *felo de se*, the criminal had wilfully broken God's commandments by entering into a 'suicide pact' with the Devil.

This constellation of attitudes changed drastically and, MacDonald has proved, quite decisively between the Restoration and the dawn of the eighteenth century. Increasingly – and by Georgian times almost universally – coroners and juries concurred in finding the suicide insane; his act had been committed while his mind was disturbed. Traditionalists condemned the condoning of vice seemingly involved in the new verdict, and it remains unclear how far it was merely conventional and convenient or how far sincere: and if sincere, did it register real pity (there but for the grace of God...)? If so, it would suggest that suicide forms another instance in which affinities between the mentality of people at large and the insane were being underlined.

Mainstream Christian morality prized self-knowledge, but had always condemned egotistic self-absorption as vain and presumptuous. I have been arguing, however, that the burgeoning cult of sensibility came to regard minute exploration of one's own feelings and failings and the cultivation of introspection, as challenges worth embarking upon in the name of experience and personal development even at the risk of angst. The 'perilous balance' of this quest, the paradox of the senses, where pleasure and pain intermingled – almost changed places – in the hunger for heightened experience, and self-consciousness readily became burdensome, are all registered in the oceans of melancholy poetry published in the age of sensibility. Exemplary within this genre – and how different from Milton's 'Hence

Loathed Melancholy!' – was Thomas Warton's 'The Pleasures
of Melancholy', with its overt partnership between melancholy
and the muse:

> O lead me, queen sublime, to solemn glooms
> Congenial with my soul: to cheerless shades,
> To ruin'd seats, to twilight cells and bow'rs,
> Where thoughtful Melancholy loves to muse,
> Her fav'rite midnight haunts.[92]

Comparable to this is Elizabeth Carter's 'Ode to Melancholy',
which apostrophised melancholy as a companion for the authentic, solitary self:

> COME, Melancholy! silent power,
> Companion of my lonely hour,
> To sober thought confin'd;
> Thou sweetly sad ideal guest,
> In all thy soothing charms confest,
> Indulge my pensive mind.

MADNESS AND IMAGINATION

Melancholy writing above all marks a 'privatisation' of the poet's
office and of the processes of invention, paying homage to inner
creative powers. Where was fancy bred? Which the organ of the
muse? Standard accounts of inspiration of course drew upon the
formulations of poetic furor, established by Plato and endorsed
by Renaissance Neo-Platonism. Yet old stereotypes of the mad
poet were being called into question during the course of the
seventeenth century, as part of the blanket reaction against
'enthusiasm'. If religious madness lost its truth, how could poetic
madness maintain its own? In this revaluation, the case of James
Carkesse is highly revealing of dilemmas as to the poet's identity.
Carkesse had been a navy clerk under Samuel Pepys. A casualty
of office politics, he felt himself the target of plots and ended

up locked up in a private madhouse in Finsbury and later in Bethlem under the physician Dr Allen.

Under confinement, he wrote verse, issued on his release in 1679 under the title *Lucida Intervalla*. The fascination of Carkesse's outpourings is that they draw upon the clichés of mad poetry (continuing the great tradition of praisers of folly from Erasmus to Burton, he used the prerogative of lunacy to flay folly), while paradoxically, and rather self-defeatingly, also denying his vocation as a mad poet. The sheer ambivalence of this project appears in contradictory poem titles (one is headed: 'Poets are Mad', another 'Poet no Lunatick'); in the name of the collection (lucid interval: does that not imply that the author is still basically insane?); and in his Burtonian epigraph: *semel insanivimus omnes*: we're all mad.

It's a crazy world, proclaims Carkesse. Physicians are off their heads, but Bedlamites are sane, or at least they would be but for the physician's torments:

> Says He, who more wit than the Doctor had,
> Oppression will make a wise man Mad;...
> Therefore, *Religio Medici* (do you mind?)
> This is not Lunacy in any kind:
> But naturally flow hence (as I do think)
> Poetick Rage, sharp Pen, and Gall in Ink.
> A sober Man, pray, what can more oppress,
> Then force by Mad-mens usage to confess
> Himself for Mad?[93]

Carkesse insists on his own sanity. What is mistaken for lunacy is not lunacy at all, but inspiration:

> Doctor, this pusling Riddle pray explain:
> Others your *physick* cures, but I complain
> It works with me the clean contrary way,
> And makes me *poet*, who are *Mad* they say.
> The truth on't is, my *Brains* well fixt *condition*
> *Apollo* better knows, than his *physitian*:

'Tis *Quacks* disease, not mine, my poetry
By the blind *Moon-Calf*, took for *Lunacy*.[94]

It is thus crucial, Carkesse insists, to distinguish poets from
madmen and so scotch the stigmatising doctrine of *Nullum
magnum ingenium (absit verbo invidia) sine mixtura dementiae*:

It goes for *current truth*, that ever some *madness*
Attends much wit, *'tis strange in sober sadness*:
Hence they are call'd, by *Plot* or *poor* and *rich*,
Madmen, whose *wit's* above the standard pitch;
But sure, when *Friends* and you me *Mad concluded*,
'Twas you your *senses* lost, by th' Moon *deluded*.[95]

Carkesse alleged that Dr Allen (whom he dubbed 'Mad-Quack')
warned him 'that till he left off making Verses, he was not fit
to be discharg'd'. Yet this only proved Mad-Quack's folly. For
poetry was neither the source nor the symptom of madness,
but was therapeutic – why else was Apollo god of both poetry
and healing?

It is hard to evaluate Carkesse, not least because, beyond his
verse, little about him survives. Why was he locked up? He
claimed to have been merely feigning madness, and that the
foolish physician mistook his 'madness in the masquerade' for
a 'senseless condition'; but why he was playing mad in the first
place is not explained. And other details in his story – his boasts
to have been visited in Bedlam by royalty and nobility – alert
our suspicions. Above all, he seems Janus-faced. Steeped in the
learned wit epitomised half a century earlier by Robert Burton,
who had joyously melancholised as a misanthrope ('I am as foolish, as mad as anyone'), he also repudiates the tradition, no doubt
in part because, unlike Burton, he was shut up not in Christ
Church but in Bedlam College. In any case, by the Restoration
madness and incarceration were carrying greater stigma.

Carkesse's abdication from the lineage of mad poet, however ambiguous, was amplified through the succeeding century.

Metaphor and bombast apart, very few Georgian poets seriously offered themselves as inspired from Beyond. There are, of course, exceptions, and they are important. Kit Smart embraced the part, and indeed wrote his greatest poem, *Jubilate agno*, while confined in an asylum. The urge ceaselessly to praise God inspired Smart's vatic vocation. Many features of *Jubilate agno* have long been seen as symptomatic of eccentricity – its fascination with alphabetic sequence, puns, word play, sheer sound and its relentless re-iteration. What has been understood only more recently is the masterly poetic craft Smart exercised over his work, and how its incantatory form – the antiphonal structure of the answering *Let* and *For* verses – sought to recapture what Robert Lowth had shown to be the poetics of the Old Testament. After Smart, Blake of course assumed the mantle of the mad poet, asserting that 'Imagination is the Divine Vision' and claiming to be 'under the direction of messengers from heaven, Daily and Nightly'.

Yet for every mad poet in transports there was another for whom madness lurked as a curse. William Cowper, for example, did not luxuriate in his bouts of insanity. For him it was over-whelming terror; its recurrences, anticipated and actual, were omens of eternal perdition, a doom not a dawn. He took to versifying not, as with Smart, as an outpouring of divine mad-ness, but as a kind of occupational therapy to distract himself from morbid introspection (in G.K. Chesterton's apt phrase, for Cowper poetry was medicine not disease; damned by John Calvin, he was almost saved by *John Gilpin*). It is savagely ironic that Blake was to cast Cowper in the role of the mad poet, recording a vision in which

> Cowper came to me and said: 'O that I were insane always. I will never rest. Can you not make me truly insane?...You retain health and yet are as mad as any of us all – over us all – mad as a refuge from unbelief – from Bacon, Newton and Locke.'[96]

It is the last destiny the anguished Cowper would have wished.

Smart and Blake aside, few disturbed poets saw madness as a
condition of poetic fire. The poems John Clare later wrote while
in High Beech Asylum expressed the deepest loss, both personal
and poetic. Or take the little-known volume of verse by the
Bedlamite the Revd Arthur Pearce, published by John Perceval
in 1851. Pearce's poems, unlike Carkesse's, touch only obliquely
upon the dilemma of his own mental alienation, and certainly
do not claim that madness fired his muse. Quite the reverse.
He apologised that he could offer only 'humble jangling-verse',
because Bedlam's 'hubbub and ding-dong' served to 'scare away
all the Muses of Parnassus'.

Indeed, if the old alliance between Bedlam and Parnassus was
lapsing, it was because a newer poetics was emerging, appropriate
to an age fascinated by inner processes of reasoning. It registered
two chief currents of ideas. For one thing, the true poet was now
increasingly seen as normal rather than possessed or transported.
But also, he was now viewed as intrinsically endowed with powers
– in particular, imagination and judgement – which nurtured
organic genius. And as the terrifying notion of direction from
without was being discredited, Georgian aesthetics were free to
take a more relaxed, though still a measured, attitude towards
imagination itself. Thanks to the vogue for Locke's analysis of
understanding, which showed how order and meaning arose
from processing the atoms of experience, the organic activities
of the mind themselves acquired a mysterious aura, becoming
an alchemical laboratory of infinite ferment.

Vital to these transformations was an evolving conception of
imagination understood within philosophies of mind, taste and
poetics – a faculty regarded as immensely fecund with meaning.
Schools of literary history have often assured us that the Age of
Reason manacled the imagination and hence proved a poetic
waste land until rescued by the Romantic credo (Keats: 'I am
certain of nothing but the holiness of the Heart's affections and
the truth of Imagination'). But that is hardly so. Certainly, from
Hobbes to Johnson, the 'dangerous prevalence of imagination'
generated high anxiety. Mainstream epistemology and aesthetics

– as articulated by Locke, popularised by Addison and poetised by Akenside – championed imagination with increasing confidence as indispensable to generating ideas and thus as a healthy and integral operation of the mind, so permitting profound fears about the morbidity of the imagination to be gradually abandoned. Indeed it was increasingly regarded as a dignifying faculty – as Dr John Gregory put it, 'the pleasures of the imagination [are] peculiar to the human species', or in the words of the American physician, Benjamin Rush:

> The Imagination is a Source of immense delight... Creation is the business of this faculty.[97]

Regarded another way, it was deficiency of the imagination that was diagnosed as a form of disease: that was idiotism.

Thus it would be misleading to imply that the Georgians devalued the creative imagination and as a result distrusted madness as a source of art. It would be truer to say that by constituting imagination as a faculty universal to image-making, they created a model of the poet which made him seem fundamentally sane. Or, put in other words, they denied that rhapsodic transports alone defined the poet. As the psychiatric physician John Conolly summed up these developments early in the nineteenth century:

> No error can be more unjust towards the whole race of poets, than to suppose them to be persons merely distinguished by imagination. It was either Steele or Addison, who, in reply to a correspondent who desired to know what was necessary to a man in order to become a great poet, replied, 'that he should be a very accomplished gentleman;' and the answer, if properly understood, is no less true than it is witty and brief. With the active imagination indispensable to the poet, is conjoined a most vigilant attention, great readiness of comparison, chiefly of resemblances, – a memory most retentive; and a judgement highly correct, and even fastidious.[98]

If, however, in the eyes of Lockian psychology the true poet
was normal, the madman clearly was not. Above all, unlike the
poet, the madman lacked 'judgement', that faculty vital both to
Locke's theory of cognition and to Augustan poetics; indeed Dr
John Monro, physician to Bethlem, deemed 'vitiated judgement'
the defining feature of insanity. Or, alternatively, the lunatic was
abnormal because he suffered from that 'deluded imagination',
which Monro's rival, William Battie, reckoned 'not only an
indisputable but essential character of madness'. The deluded
imagination – grounded, of course, in Locke's doctrine of the
(mis)association of ideas – suffered from harum-scarum hyperactivity. As Dr Thomas Arnold, the Lockian madhouse-keeper,
put it:

> The imagination is too active when it is for ever busily employed
> and led by the slightest associations to pass with facility from
> one object to another; is disposed to arrange and connect, by
> such slight associations, the most dissimilar, and incongruous;
> and to ramble with rapidity through an endless variety: or dwells
> incessantly upon the lively, and indelible impression, of some one
> object of passion.[99]

Galloping imagination, viewed in another light, marked the
failure of the powers of attention or control. As Dr Alexander
Crichton argued at the close of the eighteenth century, imagination must be either voluntary or involuntary. Voluntary
imagination (i.e. that governed by will) begets ideas and art;
involuntary imagination, by contrast, spews nonsense. As John
Conolly later reiterated:

> so long as the association of ideas is not beyond our power of
> suspension and revision, we are not mad:...When the association
> of ideas is so involuntary, so imperative and uncontrollable, that
> we cannot command it, cannot revise and correct it,... then we
> have lost our reason.[100]

Such attempts to explain the divides between art and madness in terms of the use and abuse of imagination were not, of course, confined to psychiatric writers. They were commonplaces of thought. Revealingly, for example, Swift himself suggested that the gulf between voluntary and involuntary imaginative activity formed the acid test both of poetry and sanity:

> the difference betwixt a mad-man and one in his wits, in what related to speech, consisted in this: That the former spoke out whatever came into his mind, and just in the confused manner as his imagination presented the ideas. [The poet on the other hand] only expressed such thoughts as his Judgement directed him to chuse, leaving the rest to die away in his memory... if the wisest man would at any time utter his thoughts, in the crude indigested manner as they came into his head, he would be looked upon as raving mad. [101]

This notion that madness lies in abandoning mental censorship then served as Swift's touchstone for distinguishing true poetry from crazed scribbling. 'I waked at two this morning', he wrote playfully,

> with the two above lines in my head, which I had made in my sleep, and I wrote them down in the dark lest I should forget them. But as the original words being writ in the dark, may possibly be mistaken by a careless or unskilful transcriber, I shall give a fairer copy, that two such precious lines may not be lost to posterity. [102]

What are these lines?

> I walk before no man, a hawk in his fist,
> Nor am I brilliant, whenever I list.

Swift's triumphant irony, of course, lay in the meaninglessness of his inspired 'free association' dream couplet.

Thus opinion among many Georgians converged to rescue true poetry – even sublimity – from what was now seen as the taint of madness. Their characterisations of 'genius' bear this out. . Renaissance Humanism had endorsed the Aristotelian notion of melancholy genius: and, in a later century, the *fin de siècle* movement was to diagnose the genius as 'a great abnormal', degenerate, and even insane. But the Enlightenment argued otherwise, contending for his healthiness. Admittedly, Cheyne and others saw top minds suffering exquisitely from the diseases of civilisation; but Cheyne was not talking about insanity, or even Saturnine melancholy. He championed the healthy sanity of heroes such as Isaac Newton.

What is crucial in eighteenth-century designations of genius is their refusal to identify it with mere imagination *tout court*. As Arnold insisted: 'too great imagination is entirely distinct from genius', for 'genius cannot exist in any eminent degree without judgement; and judgement is the power of regulating the activity of imagination'. Hence, he concluded, it would be folly to equate genius and madness; for it was precisely 'men of little genius and weak judgement' who were 'peculiarly liable to every species of notional insanity', a view later endorsed by Conolly in contending that 'there is much popular error entertained concerning the connexion of talent with madness'.

The Georgian poetics and aesthetics prized genius, but believed that its core lay in balance and organic wholeness. William Sharpe's *A Dissertation upon Genius* (1755), Edward Young's *Conjectures on Original Composition* (1759) and Alexander Gerard's *An Essay Upon Genius* (1774) all esteemed originality, but viewed original literary creation essentially as a product of the healthy psyche, by analogy with the natural growth and flowering of plants. The title of the mind to create through a plastic power of becoming, to kindle fire, could be maintained without dallying with the demonic or morbid. Gerard, for example, specifically defended the organic genius capable of true 'soul' and sublimity from allegations of mere frenzy:

A perfect judgement is seldom bestowed by Nature, even on her most favored sons; but a very considerable degree of it always belongs to real genius... Pindar is judicious even in his irregularities. The boldness of his fancy, if it had been under no control from reason, would have produced, not wild sublimity, but madness and frenzy.[103]

Moreover, this Georgian formulation of genius as healthy was largely endorsed by the Romantics. Romanticism doubtless had its morbid tendencies – Byron's spleen, Keats' love of 'easeful death', Shelley's 'venomed melody'. But its main claim for the artist was not as 'a great abnormal' but as hero – as creator, seer, legislator, god. For Blake, 'art is the tree of life', a far cry from the decadent vision of art as death's double. When Charles Lamb proclaimed 'the sanity of true genius', he was swimming with the Romantic tide.

THE DOMESTICATION OF MADNESS?

Thus the Georgian poet or artist comprises a complex type. If he still has a smack of mystery to him, it is a madness deriving not from Higher Powers but from the secret springs of the psyche itself, from the potentialities of the association of ideas, and from sensibility's faith in the superior capacities of sympathetic genius. The melancholy poet is a man apart. Yet his 'spleen' is precious, delicate; his role as outsider is tolerated, and, like a tame hermit, cosseted; he is easily rendered a figure of fun, as later in Mr Asterias' ruminations on 'the inexhaustible varieties of *ennui*' in Peacock's *Nightmare Abbey*. Politeness and Enlightenment had expunged the true demoniac, the political prophet and the religious Pentecostalist from the players acceptable to the civil stage. The inspired poet, however, was less menacing. Introspectively soliloquising and nervously a-quiver with self, he was an ornament or freak, not a threat. Compared to the wrangling, jangling Carkesse, who would blast the world with his wit, men like Collins, Warton and the stricken deer Cowper represented the mad poet miniaturised down to parlour size.

Andrew Scull has argued that such 'domestication' was thematic in transforming the typing of Georgian madness. In particular, Enlightenment circles relinquished the stereotype of the lunatic as wild beast; bowing to Lockian pedagogics, it yielded to the image of the madman as like a child, maladroit yet capable of education and training. Scull's is a valuable insight, of wider applicability, and I shall explore further features of this remapping in Chapter 4. But one instance of this growing need to relate aspects of 'irrationality' within society – indeed within the home – intimately associated with those cults of sensibility and subjectivity I have just been considering should be mentioned here. It is the changing evaluation of madness among women.

Starkly put, traditional male opinion regarded the female sex as constitutionally prone to irrationality, not least because women were dominated by cold and moist humours, or, later theorists thought, by weak nerves. Such a view of the essence of the feminine was, of course, essentially derogatory as when, for example, the moralist John ('Estimate') Brown condemned English luxury and decadence as 'madness' and 'effeminacy'. But the men who made the characteristic elision between the lady of exquisite sensibility and a kind of mental instability believed they were paying women a compliment, or at least demonstrating solicitude and sympathy.

Following Cheyne, commentators argued that fine feelings and nervous conditions were 'beauty spots' among the more refined ladies of the nation – the 'English milady' readily fell victim to the 'English malady'. Ladies suffered disturbance because their feelings were so readily touched. The fair sex, it was alleged, would even aspire to the vapours or hysteria, to prove their superiority and so capture attention. As Richard Blackmore ungallantly put it, women of quality were commonly 'hypocrites in the spleen', pretending

to this reputable Distemper of the Spirits, with the same Vanity that others affect the Beauty of an unsanguine and sickly Countenance.[104]

This may just be silly chauvinism. But can we simply dismiss all the vast Georgian attention devoted to female nervous disorders as nothing but a load of male twaddle? Many treatises sympathetically depicted how high-pressure social expectations inflamed or frustrated the fair sex: puberty and adolescence (whose symptoms were the green sickness), romantic love, often unrequited or forbidden, the trials of matrimony, the crises of parenthood, or, worst by far, the torments of the old maid. Moreover, anatomy rendered women's destiny doubly trying. Menstruation and childbirth enervated the system and traumatised the nerves with disastrous effects, particularly in view of what was supposed to be the sex's inherently weaker constitution. 'One hour's intense thinking wastes the spirits more in a Woman, than six in a Man', remarks one of Mandeville's characters. Remember that Mandeville's depressive woman, Polytheca, had had ten children by the time she was thirty.

Male opinion, from the *Spectator* onwards, undoubtedly exploited the supposedly supersensitive nature of 'the fair' to create caricatures of them as inconsistent, weak, over-excitable, readily exhausted by activity, and altogether lacking self-control. The fate of Henry Fielding's heroine, Amelia, with its playful mix of condescension and gallantry, is a good example of this typing:

'These Fatigues, added to the Uneasiness of her Mind, over-powered her weak Spirits, and threw her into one of the worst Disorders that can possibly attend a Woman: A Disorder very common among the Ladies, and our Physicians have not agreed upon its Name. Some call it Fever on the Spirits, some a nervous Fever, some the Vapours, and some the hysterics.'

'O say no more', cries Miss Matthews: 'I pity you, I pity you from my Soul. A Man had better be plagued with all the Curses of Egypt than with a vapourish Wife.' [105]

Women, of course were well aware – and often resentful – of this 'invaliding' process. Pondering Richardson's novel *Sir*

Charles Grandison, Lady Mary Wortley Montagu pinpointed how patronising were male attitudes towards female complaints. Richardson, she wrote, should

> be better skilled in physic than to think fits and madness any ornament to the characters of his heroines.[106]

Therapies such as water-shock treatments were sometimes used to break the wills of difficult women in the hope that they would see sense and become 'loving and dutiful'. Yet being vapourish or hysterical were roles (sick roles) which women themselves sometimes adopted – as, of course, did men – to give vent to their feelings and to cope with life's demands. Anne Finch's poignant verses on 'Melancholy' explore the tribulations and frustrations consequent upon Georgian womanhood. She writes how her own talent, poetry, has 'decayed', partly because her verse is ill-received:

> My lines decried, and my employment thought
> An useless folly, or presumptuous thought[107]

(presumably because she is a poetess). As a result, she declares, writing about the spleen does not even prove therapeutic; the condition merely returns with redoubled force. Anne Finch suffered depression as a product of her unrewarding and unrecognised social role; and, in light of the above discussion of a shifting topography of the disorder, it may be significant that she chose to doubt its organic nature. Its seat has not been found in 'the well-dissected body', nor have its 'secret mysterious ways' yielded up their truth. She clearly treasured its enigma.

Some women – like some men – seem to have cultivated melancholy and hysteria more energetically. As her letters show, Mary Wollstonecraft was, even from her early years, all extremes, often exhilarated, sometimes plunged in the depths of despair. Faced with life's sea of troubles, she would take flight in a kind of derangement. At one point she wrote to Henry Gabell: 'My reason has been too far stretched, and tottered on the brink of madness.' Shortly after, she confessed to her sister, Everina:

'That vivacity which increases with age is not far from madness' says Rochefoucault: I then am mad... I give way to whim – and yet when the most sprightly sallies burst from me, the tear frequently trembles in my eye and the long drawn sigh eases my full heart – so my eyes roll in the wild way you have seen them... I sit up very late... 'Tis the only time I live, in the morning I am a poor melancholy wretch – and at night half-mad.[108]

This depiction of the 'strange, inconsistent heart' is not specifically female: men of feeling would also portray themselves on the knife-edge, nerves a-jangle, close to madness. What is distinctive about Mary Wollstonecraft is the identification she makes in her novels between the plight of the mad and the condition of women. Thus in *Maria* she places her eponymous heroine in the madhouse as a 'slave' of her villainous husband, conceiving of her as a superior being by virtue of that persecution which drives her out of her senses: suffering indeed, she writes, is the lot of women.

Certain feminist scholars have interpreted the type of ultra-sensitive woman thus emerging in the eighteenth century as a cry of rebellion: hysteria as the great denial to men. But it is surely wiser, as Elaine Showalter has counter-argued, to treat it more as the mark of impotence, or even of collusion. For in the dominant polite culture developing from the Restoration, women largely lost their independent power base. The great lady ceased to be the direct manager of the house; employment opportunities among middle-class women were squeezed; and not least, the witch was effectively silenced. Whereas until the mid-seventeenth century witches were widely believed to possess lethal power as confederates with the Devil, increasingly they were seen merely as silly old women, cracked in the head. Witches went the way of demoniacs. They were no longer burned, but persecution stopped only as they ceased to be powerful.

Through such processes, women were tight-laced into positions of social subordination. Medical opinion gave strong
reasons, physical and moral, why the weaker vessel was designed
for such roles (they were guardians of the home and private
virtues); and the frustrations and maladies consequential upon
playing second-fiddle doubtless commonly turned such ideology into self-fulfilling prophecies. Thus women, the mad and,
frequently, artists too could all be seen as kindred spirits; blessed
with exquisite sensibilities, acute passions, raw nerves, a vivid
fancy – all had to be protected as privileged inferiors, delicate
ornaments or objects of pity, excluded from, because spared, the
more rational, robust and responsible realm of the men.

Surveying different cultural fields, I have been picking out
important shifts in perceptions of abnormality between the
Restoration and the Regency. Fundamental to these developments in being different was a massive naturalisation of the
understanding of insanity. Disturbance ceased to be thought of
largely in terms of sin or possession by Superior or Infernal
Powers. This paved the way for emergent secular and social
mappings of madness.

These were formulated in the context of the rise to domi-
nance of a brilliant, fashionable, elite culture, elevated above and
in opposition to popular values which it increasingly viewed
as *démodé*, irrational, vulgar, silly and occasionally dangerous.
The elite no longer had cultural room for traditional types of
strangeness: thus the fool or jester figure was discarded by the
enlightened, and even Burton's *Anatomy of Melancholy* began to
seem a very quaint book. Henceforth, high society and low life
would be differentiated as much by distinct sorts of rationality
and madness as by different dress, diet and speech – thanks, in
part, to John Locke's insistence that the great divide in consciousness lay between acute thought (sometimes misguided)
and the vacuities of idiots. Dullness was the *bête noire* of the
Georgian glitterati.

Freed from contamination by the demoniacal and the vulgar,
the elite could luxuriate in the self and toy with mental and

emotional singularities, in so far as these squared with other cultural desiderata such as aspirations to artistic genius, refined sensibility, sublimity, or being an 'original'. Nervous disorders were gentrified and received into good society. As Dr James McKittrick Adair put it, 'Fashion has long influenced the great and opulent in the choice of their physicians'; now, through the nerves, it had 'influenced them also in the choice of their diseases'. So madness was brought down to earth, humanised and domesticated. In this new atmosphere, secular and sympathetic, speculations arose as to how people might indeed be not just organically, but morally mad. Or in other words, as I shall try to show in the next three chapters, thanks to the culture of the Enlightenment a psychiatric space and scenario was opening out.

3

Confinement and its Rationales

PUBLIC POLICY

Madness, I have argued, was traditionally understood in early modern England as a mark of man's fallen state, vitiated by sin, folly, and pride. Morality saw Reason subverted by brutish appetite and the wild man within. Insanity's infection touched all: *semel insanivimus omnes... et semel, et simul, et semper*. Certain embodiments of madness, however – the idiot, the homicidal maniac, the Bedlam beggar, the pretender king, the Mad Maudlin – bore special stigmata for all to see, Providence's warnings to the fortunate to shun the sirens of pride and lust.

A society espousing such beliefs had no special reason to enforce strict segregation of abnormals from the community at large, except where they constituted direct danger to life and limb. Nor, indeed, was there in the sixteenth or seventeenth centuries any wholesale confining of the disturbed, dumb, depressed, and distressed. This was not for want of administrative or technical capacity. In fact, as Slack has shown, strict quarantine measures were mobilised against bubonic plague in Stuart England as well as on the Continent. Rather, the reason why the mad were not automatically locked up was that there were no strong rationales for routine confinement.

In his *Folie et Déraison*, Michel Foucault argued that from the 1660s a 'great confinement' was activated across Europe, stemming from an unholy alliance between the bureaucratic and judicial powers of absolutism and the logic of Enlightenment. Rationality, Foucault averred, came to stigmatise all deviancy willy-nilly as 'unreason'. The crazy, the destitute, feckless, work-shy, vicious, criminal, and the rest of society's flotsam and jetsam – all were anathema to the bourgeois ethos (a morality of labour) and to the Cartesian *cogito* (a rationality of order). Such abominations were shut away together – a critical moment since, for the first time, madness had been reduced to utter negativity, silenced, and made a target of police.

I argued in Chapter 1 that Foucault's term, 'the great confinement', ill describes what happened to mad people in England from roughly the Restoration to the Regency. An unknown but small number of the disturbed had already been under lock and key during the Tudor and Stuart centuries. By the 1810s, official figures indicate that around 2,590 lunatics were confined in licensed houses for the mad, and almost as many again in other places of custody such as houses of correction, workhouses and gaols. The real totals were higher. Even so, it seems gratuitous to invoke the word 'great' to depict this process, particularly when we remember the staggering subsequent acceleration of incarceration.

Foucault thus trips up on scale. But his interpretation fails in a more important respect. His vision of the 'classical age', like that of Klaus Doerner, stresses how central authority acted to sequestrate unreason in all its modes. The course of English developments, however, is almost the reverse. In social discipline, the Restoration of 1660 halted or reversed centralisation, ushering in an era notable for localism and community action rather than programmes emanating from Crown or Parliament. Initiatives in social regulation, welfare and order devolved upon the shires and squires, upon JPs and parish overseers. In contrast to Foucault's ogres of standardisation, rationalisation and intrusion, the key features in England were parochialism and diversity, private expedients but state inertia: the Walpolean *quieta non movere*. This applies to many fields – education, industrial regulation, public health, and not least to insanity. The 'long eighteenth century' produced little legislation for, or central policing of, madness in England. It was, for example, not until 1800 that Parliament first acted to secure criminal lunatics. Managing madness was allowed to remain *ad hoc*, indeed largely private. As in other spheres, this proved both a swamp of scandal and a seedbed of innovation.

In 1660, and still largely in 1800, the English state involved itself in madness in three basic ways. One was a residual expression of feudal paternalism. From medieval times, the judiciary had provided a facility of trusteeship for idiots or lunatics in legal matters – property, contracts, estates, heirships, and inheritance. Until the Civil War, this was handled by the Court of Wards. This service was not restricted to the nobility but was available for a wide range of families where property was at stake. Moreover, the Court did not 'milk' its simpletons, nor – unlike the procedure with wards proper – farm out their estates for exploitation by parasitical courtiers. Rather, it took care to appoint as trustees not adventurers and toadies but local worthies, who might sympathise with the sufferer and have a stake in good family order.

Tests were devised to judge mental capacity to manage life and estate. These were practical, not medical; their aim was not diagnostic or therapeutic but judicial. Criteria of rational competence were kept elementary (did the subject know his name? could he count up to twenty? did he recognise his father and mother? and so forth). As a consequence, the Crown never created a large pool of 'handicapped' or 'subnormal' people legally designated *non compos mentis*.

The Court of Wards was not restored at the Restoration, and its functions for the mentally incompetent fell to Chancery. Petitioned by relatives, the Lord Chancellor would issue a writ *De Lunatico Inquirendo*, and the case would be heard before a jury, stout bulwark against malpractice. If the party were found *non compos* (or popularly, a 'nincompoop'), his estates would pass under Crown protection, to be administered by committee. As the great jurist Sir William Blackstone explained the safeguards,

> to prevent sinister practices, the next heir is never permitted to be this committee of the person; because it is in his interest that the party should die. But it hath been said, there lies not the same objection against his next of kin, provided he is not his heir; for it is his interest to preserve the lunatic's life, in order to increase the personal estate by savings, which he or his family may hereafter be entitled to enjoy.[1]

Doubtless certain families hoped to manipulate Chancery to exploit imbeciles. Yet, given how many legitimate expectations were staked upon property, fears that oddball or half-wit scions would fall under sinister influence and squander estates are understandable. In the various *causes célèbres*, it is rarely easy to adjudicate the rival claims. Take, for instance, the case of Henry Roberts.

Roberts was born in 1717. His father died early. In 1733, the Lord Chancellor judged him feeble-minded, entrusting his estate to his brother-in-law. On coming of age, Roberts sought to obtain from the trustees the profits of his West Indian interests, at which point (so a pro-Roberts pamphlet alleged) they threatened him with a commission of idiocy. This was held in 1743, and after what the pamphleteer called a bullying hearing, the jury found Roberts of unsound mind. A rehearing was secured, and witnesses called. As the pro-Roberts author put it:

> Witnesses of low degree were call'd and examined, who swore they had seen him toss up his Hat, and catch it with his Hands,

and that he used to kick about Pebble-stones. Others, that when he was on Horseback, he could not open a Gate. One Fellow swore that Mr Roberts could not write his Name.[2]

Medical experts do not seem to have been summoned. The jury confirmed the original verdict. At this point, having lost his case, Roberts took his plight to eminent doctors such as Dr James Monro, physician to Bethlem, Dr Frank Nicholls, and Dr Richard Mead. The jurymen, he explained, had fuddled him with their questions:

> They came around me and asked their Questions together, without giving me Time to answer. They asked me what a Lamb, and what a Calf was called at one, two and three Years old. They gave me a Sum of Money to tell, which I miscounted; and then I heard them say, he is not capable of managing his Affairs, we will return him Incapable... [3]

The impression is of pragmatism by the Court in deciding whether Roberts could mind his business. There was no attempt to pin medical diagnoses on him, nor any sign that the family sought to have Roberts committed to an asylum.

However we judge such a case, two conclusions seem clear. First, Chancery proceedings hardly show the state in an aggressively interventionist mood, attempting to police or exploit the subnormal. Rather, the Court offered a means of arbitrating the legal tangles inevitably created by the feeble-minded. Contrast certain other European nations, where absolutism and cameralism dictated more interventionist rationalities. In Russia, for example, Tsarist policy was to commit wrongheaded members of the service nobility to monasteries. Since provincial government depended upon capable, solvent nobles, nitwits posed genuine threats to government. Safe in a monastery, they could neither squander estates nor breed dynasties of simpletons, though they could be esteemed as holy fools.

Second, in Chancery proceedings, the presence of the jury meant that both parties might get a fair crack of the whip. Roberts lost his case, but others won theirs. Most famously, in the nineteenth century, the attempt of William Windham's family to have him declared *non compos mentis* was thrown out by the jury. Windham was a wealthy eccentric of good Norfolk family, who kept company with stable-lads and wenches and dissipated the family fortunes. Yet the jury decided that his profligacy and prodigality were not moral madness but a gentleman's prerogative. Such proceedings probably treated alleged fools and lunatics more sympathetically than the equivalent arrangements in France, where relatives appealed to royal officials for *lettres de cachet* to grant powers over the administration of estates, or to have a family idiot confined. Critics protested that *lettres* were automatically granted on family pressure – there was, of course, no jury – permitting dire abuses. In France, unlike England, the legal status of mad people and fools as the 'children of the King' had the ring of truth.

The second field in which the state encountered the mad was in criminal trials. Inevitably felonies came before assizes in which the understanding of the accused was at issue, and insanity formed the defence. A long history of common law precedents and practice established broad guidelines in such cases. For guilt to be established, *mens rea*, or criminal intent, had to be proven. Unlawful acts committed without *mens rea* should not result in convictions. Summing up such instances in the mid-eighteenth century, Blackstone noted three legal categories. There could first be no *mens rea* where there was 'defect of understanding', the *locus classicus* being actions of children. Nor, second, where there was deficiency of will, i.e. in the case of an idiot or a lunatic, these being

> not chargeable for their own acts, if committed when under these incapabilities; no, not even for treason itself.[4]

This exoneration applied both to those deranged at the time of the crime and to those who had subsequently gone insane, thus preventing their pleading their case. Third, there was no *mens rea* in the case of 'voluntarily contracted madness', which for Blackstone chiefly meant drunkenness. Here, however, intoxication was an aggravation, not an excuse.

In spelling out English practice, Blackstone's general drift is clear: madmen and idiots were not to suffer the rigours of the courts. Yet society also needed protection from such lunatics who

> should not be permitted the liberty of acting unless under proper control...by the vagrancy acts, a method is chalked out for imprisoning, chaining, and sending them to their proper homes.[5]

No exhaustive study has been conducted as to how the law actually handled such pre-nineteenth-century cases, and much of our knowledge comes from possibly unrepresentative instances involving famous people. In 1786 Margaret Nicholson lunged at George III with a dessert knife. Overpowered, she was taken before the Privy Council, examined, agreed to be crazy, and conveyed to Bethlem. There was no trial, no suggestion that she should hang. There was some humanity in the discretion such proceedings permitted. How commonly it was actually exercised is unknown, but criminal lunatics were certainly lodged in several private asylums, such as William Perfect's in Kent, in the eighteenth century.

What happened, however, when crimes came to trial? The most notorious case was that of Lord Ferrers. In 1760 Ferrers murdered his steward, and was arraigned before the House of Lords. He had an unsavoury reputation as haughty and irascible and there was insanity in the family, though before his crime no one suggested that he himself was insane. Horace Walpole described Ferrers' defence before his peers:

> His figure is bad and villainous, his crime shocking. He would not plead guilty, and yet had nothing to plead; and at last, to humour his family, pleaded madness against his inclination: it was

moving to see two of his brothers brought to depose the lunacy in their blood. After he was condemned, he excused himself for having used that plea.[6]

Ferrers was in the impossible position of having to conduct his own expert defence to prove that he was insane. He clearly cut no ice. An eighteenth-century jury would have needed independent evidence of enduring insanity: the monstrous character of his deed in itself would have appeared proof not of madness but of depravity. His demeanour did not help; he seemed captious not crazy, and, as Walpole hinted, his peers probably felt that to show mercy on grounds of insanity would have meant punishing his whole family with its taint.

Indeed, John Bull as juryman had no great difficulty in distinguishing between anger and lunacy, malice and madness. This clarity was to be muddied in Victorian times, when members of the emergent profession of alienists, such as Forbes Winslow, increasingly thrust themselves forward in trials as 'expert witnesses'. From their medical viewpoint, they commonly pleaded that defendants had suffered from perversions of the will exceptionally erupting in fits of 'irresistible impulse' (thus negating *mens rea*). As Roger Smith has emphasised, however, such early psychiatrists, with their implicitly deterministic behavioural model and their dubious expertise aroused suspicion among judges and juries. No such clashes of rival legal and medical readings of insanity arose during the eighteenth century, since it was most unusual for doctors to testify in court. In establishing insanity, the testimony of friends, neighbours, and relatives counted most.

In fact, the star role in the most critical eighteenth-century insanity trial was played not by a doctor but by an advocate, Thomas Erskine. In 1800 James Hadfield, an ex-soldier, fired at and wounded George III. Erskine demonstrated how the defendant had committed the offence in the grip of a comprehensive delusional system. Hadfield had been in contact with 'one Truelock a lunatic', who preached 'that our Saviour's second advent, and the dissolution of all human things, were at hand', precipitating in Hadfield 'the insane delusion... of his own propitiation and sacrifice for mankind... He imagined... that the world was coming to a conclusion... he was to sacrifice himself for its salvation'. Unwilling, for religious scruples, to be guilty of suicide, Hadfield 'wished that by the appearance of crime his life might be taken away from him by others'. Two days earlier, he had attempted to destroy his baby son 'for the benefit of mankind', although he 'knew perfectly well that he was the father of the child; the tears of affection ran down his face at the moment that he was about to accomplish its destruction'.

Thus Erskine pleaded, articulating a psychology broadly derivative from Locke, that delusions cancelled *mens rea*:

> Delusion, therefore, where there is no frenzy or raving madness, is the true character of insanity;... I must convince you, not only that the unhappy prisoner was a lunatic, within my own definition of lunacy, but that the act in question was the immediate, unqualified offspring of the disease.[7]

The defence case – that Hadfield was a religious maniac – was clinched, however, by the fact that Hadfield had suffered a serious head wound while fighting for the king. Two eminent doctors, Henry Cline and Alexander Crichton, testified to its severity, and the likely subsequent brain damage. The organic dimension confirmed, the Lord Chief Justice stopped the trial.

Hadfield's acquittal is of great significance. For one thing it shows how much authority insanity pleas could carry. Despite the enormity of Hadfield's deed, committed at the height of revolutionary war and radical insurgence, the court heeded the insanity plea, accepting that Hadfield's lunacy did not compound but exonerated the deed. The 'psychiatric case' was won long before there were psychiatric experts.

Hadfield's acquittal disclosed a yawning gap in the statute book. For no Act provided for Hadfield's future safekeeping. Parliament – until then so snail-like on insanity – now acted with great despatch, passing an Act for the Safe Keeping of Insane Persons charged with Offences (1800), which provided that if 'any Person, charged with Treason, Murder, Felony' was found 'insane at the Time of the Commission of such Offence' and hence acquitted, 'the Court shall order such Persons to be kept in strict Custody', at Crown pleasure. Hadfield was accordingly committed to Bethlem – as was his fellow religious maniac, Truelock – surviving till 1841, alongside other would-be regicides such as Margaret Nicholson.

The third way public authority regulated the lives of the disturbed was in the domain of public order. Foucault's 'great confinement' notwithstanding, no comprehensive policy for madness emerged in Georgian England. For one thing, Parliament neither built nor even authorised any lunatic asylums. Not till 1808 did an Act even empower local authorities to establish asylums, nor until 1845 did Parliament require counties to found them. In fact Westminster did not direct magistrates to set up any omnibus receptacles for social nuisances. A succession of Acts admittedly facilitated the piecemeal establishment of workhouses, which did indeed hold certain of the mentally disordered; yet, up to the end of the century, little more than a quarter of parishes had acted.

Moreover, hardly any legislation was passed to enhance the general policing of the mad. Only one significant Act found its way on to the statute book. The Act for... the More Effectual Punishing such Rogues, Vagabonds, Sturdy Beggars, and Vagrants, and Sending them Whither They Ought to be Sent (1714) – a consolidating Act – authorised two or more Justices of the Peace to secure the arrest of any person 'furiously mad and dangerous', and his incarceration 'safely locked up, in such secure place' so long as 'such lunacy or madness shall continue'. For lunatics, but for lunatics alone, whipping was specifically forbidden – a point worth noting, since historians have commonly claimed that the Georgians advocated whipping the mad. With paupers, the parish would foot the costs of confinement; otherwise, they would be met out of the lunatic's own estate, or by his family.

This Act was amended in 1744 to include 'those who by
Lunacy or otherwise are so far disordered in their Senses that
they may be dangerous to be permitted to go Abroad'. It also
permitted the detention (with chains if necessary) of such 'dangerous lunatics', by the warrant of two JPs 'during such time...
as such lunacy or madness shall continue'. And it departed in
one small but possibly significant particular from the earlier
Act in providing for the 'keeping, maintaining and curing' of
such people in custody. No mention of 'curing' had been made
thirty years earlier. The Act remained operative throughout the
century.

What were its implications? It made clear that madness was
to fall under the magistrates' gaze as part of the control of the
vagrant poor. Yet the lunatic was to be a problem only if 'dangerous', and dangerous lunacy was expected to be sufficiently visible
to be decided by JPs not physicians. Such nuisances could be
confined in whatever secure place was available, be it workhouse,
lock-up, private madhouse, bridewell or gaol.

No figures are available for how many lunatics ended up in such
receptacles, either before these Acts or as a result of them, until
a Commons Committee of 1807 reported that there were 1,765
pauper lunatics in Poor Houses and Houses of Industry besides
others in Houses of Correction. The pioneering workhouse of
St Peter's in Bristol had taken pauper lunatics since its inception
in 1696, and they had usually – despite Foucault's interpretation
– been separated from sound-minded paupers. Lunatics housed
there may have received conscientious treatment, for a regulation
of 1768 required medical practitioners to visit the 'frenzy objects'
once a week, inspecting new inmates when brought in. On his
pioneering peregrinations of prisons in the 1770s, John Howard
came across a sprinkling of the mad. At Kingston upon Hull bridewell, for instance, he found the same 'poor, raving lunatic' on three
separate occasions between 1774 and 1779, while at the Lancaster
county jail, he saw 'only one poor lunatic, who had been there
many years'. Howard advocated the separation of the insane in
such lock-ups, in the interests of the criminals. Bridewells limited

themselves to securing – rather than curing – the mad, and were, Howard believed, appalling:

> Idiots and lunatics... serve for sport to idle visitants... where they are not kept separate [they] disturb and terrify other prisoners. No care is taken of them, though it is probable that by medicines and proper regimen, some of them might be restored to their senses, and to usefulness in life.[8]

Yet there is no sign of any mass ghettoing of pauper lunatics into workhouses and bridewells. Howard found comparatively few such detainees (why should parishes waste money on lunatics?). In some cases magistrates actually ordered the release of the mad from houses of correction, specifically because they distracted the institution from disciplining real law-breakers. Though Foucault argued that it was *policy* to herd the mad and the bad together, there is no sign that this was so. After all, in London, Bethlem and Bridewell, though managed by the same board of governors, were kept strictly separate, and care was taken to funnel people into the right institution.

When, around the turn of the nineteenth century, the philanthropist Sir George Onesiphorus Paul took upon himself the task of systematising the treatment of pauper lunatics, he found the village sufferer still by and large neglected. Many parishes contained 'some unfortunate human creature who, if his ill-treatment had made him phrenetic, is chained in the cellar or garret of a workhouse'; indeed, most crazy people were not institutionalised at all, being instead 'fastened to the leg of a table, tied to a post in an outhouse, or perhaps shut up in an uninhabited ruin; or if his lunacy be inoffensive, left to ramble half-naked and half-starved through the streets and highways, teased by the scoff and jest of all that is vulgar, ignorant and unfeeling'. For such people Paul wanted public asylums, which would unite 'the police intention' with 'humanity' and 'economy'.

Most disordered people were thus kept at home, boarded out, or left to roam (though John Aubrey stated that wandering Toms o' Bedlam had disappeared with the Restoration). Precisely how badly neglected they were awaits close scrutiny. Piecemeal evidence suggests, however, that parishes commonly made positive arrangements for outdoor relief. Troublesome lunatics would be brought before magistrates, who would bind their families to control them; sometimes they would be boarded on capable parishioners. A few were sent to Bethlem, or delivered as pauper lunatics to private madhouses or to the new public asylums in great towns.

Yet most queer folks remained in their parish, under the watch of family, community and overseers, as Fessler's study of Poor Law administration in seventeenth-century Lancashire, and Rushton's account of the north-east show. In 1654 one melancholy man prowled on the green night after night, and would not enter a house, or eat properly; his head became foully festered, and it was feared that lice had gnawed into his brain. His neighbours managed him firmly but without chains. A woman troubled by a 'virulent lunacy', tearing at herself and her clothes, often had to be bound for her own and other people's safety. In another case, a man's wife, dangerous and suicidal, prevented him from working, but was not apparently bound or confined. Another man under parish care had fallen into a lunatic frenzy with incessant shrieking fits; he was 'bound in Cheanes and Feathers' [sic]. In 1651 a violent woman was fastened to a post, though another, who had plucked out one of her own eyes and was often violent to her family, was allowed to roam. These frantic and sometimes dangerous lunatics generally received no medical supervision, though one man maintained he had done his best to help his wife both by summoning doctors and by chaining her.

Sometimes parish paternalism was active and generous, as in the case of Herman Tayler of Cheriton Fitzpaine in Devon. In 1723 he went wild and decamped to the hills. Brought back at parish expense ('pd for bringing home Herman Tayler from Sparked Downs and cutting his haire and shaving his beard and cleansing the rest of his body... 2s 6d'), for the next two years he was in parish care. £12 1s was spent on maintenance, and Lewis Southcomb, a clergyman-doctor famed for his interest in the mad, received £10 for his 'physeck' and £1 14s 6d for 'warding him', while £2 7s 9d was paid for maintaining Tayler's wife and £5 9s 9d for his children. When Southcomb's treatment proved ineffective, the parish sent Tayler to Dr Spreag at Silverton and maintained him there, paying Spreag £14 for 'cureing Harmon Tayler for a Mallancholy disorder'. By the time Tayler disappeared from the records in 1725, the affair had cost the parish £49 11s 9d – about half a year's Poor Rate expenses for the whole village. His son Andrew was then given a parish apprenticeship and the allowance continued to his widow. Before the advent of large pauper institutions, outdoor relief to the sick was often substantial. Many other lunatics presumably benefited from such policies, which give a glimpse of an important but little-known halfway house between mere neglect or family care and the asylum – *ad hoc* boarding with a cleric or a doctor.

In Georgian times public authorities had no brief systematically to police the mad. Few tailor-made institutions as yet existed for them. When the century dawned there was not a single public asylum for lunatics in the whole kingdom besides London's Bethlem. This dearth was not because more active policies were publicly 'inconceivable'. A 'great confinement' might have been launched, for that is precisely what certain campaigners were actually urging. For example, an anonymous pamphlet of 1700 boldly advocated a comprehensive network of refuges for defectives and unfortunates:

> There should be one General Hospital erected in each County... for the Reception and Maintenance of all poor Lunaticks, Ideots, Blind Persons, Maim'd Soldiers and Seamen, Cripples uncapable of relieving themselves by any Manufacture or Labour, and Bedridden Persons beyond a prospect of Cure, that are or shall be Inhabitants of that County.[9]

Such hospitals should be charged to the rates and overseen by
parliamentary visitors. Along parallel lines, Daniel Defoe urged
Parliament to found a national hospital for natural fools, to be
financed by a special tax upon the learned, for:

> Of all Persons who are Objects of our Charity, none move my
> Compassion like those whom it has pleas'd God to leave in a
> full state of Health and Strength, but depriv'd of Reason to act
> for themselves.[10]

Nothing came of these schemes. We should not be surprised.
Reformers dreamed up endless projects for institutional regen-
eration during the Georgian period, but change was generally
accomplished only in case of gross evil and national emergency.
Centralising schemes such as a national census were overruled.
The mad loomed small in contemporary geographies of fear, and
Newton had demonstrated the force of inertia.

BETHLEM

Thanks largely to the Reformation, early modern England was,
by the standards of comparable nations, singularly ill endowed
with civic and pious institutions for unfortunates. The dissolution of the monasteries and chantries had left little of the
medieval fabric of hospices, almshouses and refuges. Monarchs,
Parliaments, the Church and public alike proved slow to replace
them, though parishes were active in devising *ad hoc* ways of
caring for deserving and controlling difficult people. In 1700,
in a kingdom possessing only two endowed medical hospitals,
London's St Bartholomew's and St Thomas', it is hardly surprising that there was only one public madhouse: Bethlem, at
Moorfields.

The priory of the Order of St Mary of Bethlehem had been
founded in 1247. From 1377 it was used for lunatics. Controlled by
the Crown until 1546, it was then granted to the City. Surviving
the dissolution of the chantries, from 1557 it was jointly managed

with Bridewell, a house of correction at Blackfriars, by a court of governors. The old premises (on the site of today's Liverpool Street Station) were destroyed by fire, and it was reopened at Moorfields in 1676 in a palatial building resembling the Tuileries, thereby increasing its capacity from towards fifty to just over a hundred.

Bethlem the institution was small; 'Bedlam' the image loomed large in the public imagination. 'Bedlam is a pleasant place... and abounds with amusements', commented the deadpan wit, Tom Brown, in 1700. It was traditionally a favourite resort for sightseers. Until around 1770 they simply turned up, Sundays excepted, being expected to drop some coppers into the poor box, and occasionally wreaked havoc. Londoners such as Pepys and Evelyn had all gone along; and provincials up in town would tour Bethlem, together with other shows of London such as the lions in the Tower or Bartholomew Fair. Thus in 1703 the Lancastrian Nicholas Blundell 'walked to Bedlom', and several years later he came back for more:

> I went to Bedlom in Morefields with my Wife and then we went to see the show of the Waterworks but were disappointed they not being to be shewed this night.[11]

Bedlam also had its side attractions, being a haunt of prostitutes. As Ned Ward put it:

> Mistresses, we found, were to be had of all ranks, qualities, colours, prices and sizes... Every fresh comer was soon engaged in an amour; tho' they came in single they went out by pairs... a sportsman, at any hour of the day, may meet with game for his purpose.[12]

But the true lure of Bedlam was the *frisson* of the freakshow. Juxtaposing reason and folly, its meeting of opposites made it a national joke. Thus Ward had a character remark to his friend, on seeing the exterior, 'I conceiv'd it to be my Lord Mayor's Palace,

for I could not imagine so stately a structure could be design'd
for any Quality inferior; he smil'd at my innocent Conjecture,
and inform'd me this was Bedlam, an Hospital for Mad-Folk: In
truth, said I, I think they were Society'.

Spectators thronged to see unaccommodated man. And largely
because Bethlem housed the only collection of mad people
in the nation, it achieved a sort of concentrated notoriety; it
became an epitome of all that people fantasised about madness itself. All this conspired to give Bethlem its lasting dubious
reputation. At best, conveying gloomy horror, it symbolised the
revenge of natural man – Chaos come again – as evoked by an
anonymous poem of 1776:

> Within the Chambers which this Dome contains
> In all her 'frantic' forms, Distraction reigns...
> Rattling his chains, the wretch all raving lies
> And roars and foams, and Earth and Heaven defies. [13]

At worst, Bedlam became a byword for man's inhumanity to man,
for callousness and cruelty – a reputation too often deserved,
and surely retarding improvements by cementing in the public
mind fatalistic associations of madness with despair. Bedlam
had become the focus of public scandal in the 1620s, when
an inquiry revealed gross mismanagement by the eponymous
keeper, Helkiah Crooke. Peculation continued under the steward, Richard Langley, and despite the conscientious labours of its
board of governors, this unsavoury reputation lasted through the
eighteenth century, when four members of the Monro family
were successively physicians in a nepotistic reign which mirrored
that of the four Georges.

Occasional attempts were made to salvage its public reputation, partly through a fund-raising official 'history' penned by the
Revd Thomas Bowen. This work, however, reads as unblushing
panegyric – almost, one might say, as delusion, containing, for
example, the following lines:

To our Governors, due praise be giv'n
Who, by just care, have changed our Hell to Heav'n...
Our Meat is good, the Bread and Cheese the same, Our Butter,
Beer and Spoon Meat none can blame.
The Physic's mild, the Vomits are not such,
But, thanks be prais'd, of these we have not much.
Bleeding is wholesome, and as for the Cold Bath,
All are agreed it many Virtues hath.
The Beds and Bedding are both warm and clean,
Which to each comer may be plainly seen.[14]

Such verses perhaps merely convinced readers that everything touched by Bedlam was crazy, and few can have been surprised when the lid was finally taken off the institution early in the nineteenth century. The precise form the exposures took, however, was somewhat surprising. For one thing, a pamphlet was published by a former Bedlamite, Urbane Metcalf, the first authentic patient's-eye view. *The Interior of Bethlehem Hospital Displayed* (1818) is of great interest. Unlike other revelations by ex-inmates, Metcalf did not clamour against unlawful confinement: he admitted that he had been mad, believing himself heir to the Danish throne. Hence, untypically, he did not allege personal persecution by the physician and staff – and for that reason his charges carry more weight. Rather, he offered a sweeping indictment of a venal and demoralised institution, run for the convenience and profit of the staff, not the patients. Supineness at the top sanctioned callous cruelty below. Metcalf thus presented a cameo of Old Corruption, a fabric rotten with fiddling, oppression, and bullying. He and his fellow Bedlamites suffered not from the evils of psychiatry but from gross neglect by its medical staff.

In this, Metcalf was essentially confirming revelations devastatingly levelled three years earlier before a House of Commons inquiry. The Committee's Report, piloted by reformers, gives the impression that Bethlem had been singled out for blame, in the anticipation that the public disgracing of the kingdom's premier madhouse would carry the more general reform cause. Activists were particularly fortunate in being able to find an epitome of Bedlam's evils in James Norris, a recently demised American sailor confined for eighteen years in a grotesque custom-built harness made of chains and rods, preventing virtually all movement. Despite assurances from John Haslam, the Bethlem apothecary, that such contraptions were necessary and 'merciful', the Committee found it easy to portray Norris' treatment as proof of the institution's barbarity. Norris was engraved by George Cruickshank, and became news.

Moreover, the reformers had a further unexpected windfall. Fiercely cross-questioned, the medical staff broke ranks and began to incriminate each other. In particular, Haslam volunteered that the recently deceased surgeon to Bethlem, Bryan Crowther, had himself long been mad, indeed, 'so insane as to have a strait-waistcoat'. Nor did the staff disguise the physician Thomas Monro's absences. For his part, Monro made it clear that Haslam should carry the can for therapeutic failures.

Even so, Monro had difficulty in parrying the critics. Under questioning, he admitted that he deployed physical restraints such as irons and chains not to cure but to secure; their use was dictated not by medical indications but by rank and money. At Bedlam lunatics were manacled, often to their beds, to reduce staff costs; in his private asylum no such chains were used, being 'fit only for pauper lunatics: if a gentleman were put in irons, he would not like it'. Monro was also forced to admit to therapeutic bankruptcy, treatment amounting to little more than an automatic, indiscriminate spring bloodletting and purge. Though an advocate of physic, he confessed that his medicines were merely those inherited from his father. Though conceding 'the disease is not cured by medicine', he stuck with the antiquated drug treatments, knowing no better.

The 1815 Commons Committee thus heard from the horse's mouth that Bethlem was at best wedded to tradition. Even so, no great reforms followed, though Monro and Haslam found it expedient to resign (Monro made way for his son, leaving

Haslam as the chief scapegoat). Rehoused in new premises in Lambeth, Bethlem gradually faded from the public imagination.

In the light of such disclosures it is all too easy, following nineteenth-century reformers and later historians, glibly to dismiss Bethlem as Hell on Earth, a stage set for a Gothic penny-dreadful. Seriously evaluating Georgian Bethlem is, however, more taxing. For one thing, for all its failings, it may still have been better than its continental equivalents. The anonymous French author of *De Londres et de ses environs* (1788) thought so:

> I stayed for some time in Bedlam. The poor creatures there are not chained up in dark cellars, stretched on damp ground, nor reclining on cold paving stones... no bolts, no bars. The doors are open, their rooms wainscoted, and long airy corridors give them a chance of exercise. A cleanliness, hardly conceivable unless seen, reigns in their hospital.[15]

Certainly, the 'scholars' of Bedlam College escaped some of the worst horrors of confinement abroad, where the use of dungeons and turrets was common. Georgian Bethlem was not overcrowded; each inmate had a cell. And the new hospital built in 1676 was open and airy in ways that impressed visitors. Commenting on 'this fine hospital', César de Saussure noted that

> you find yourself in a long and wide gallery, on either side of which are a large number of little cells where lunatics of every description are shut up, and you can get a sight of these poor creatures, little windows being let into the doors. Many inoffensive madmen walk in the big gallery. On the second floor is a corridor and cells like those on the first floor, and this is the part reserved for dangerous maniacs, most of them being chained and terrible to behold.[16]

Moreover, its broad policies, statutes, and regulations were unimpeachable. Bethlem was a charitable foundation, open to lunatics from the whole kingdom. Applicants would be examined by a court of the governors to ensure their suitability. The suitable patient was the curable lunatic; incurables were not admitted. A lunatic was standardly admitted for a year. If not recovered by that time, he or she would be liable to discharge as incurable though, from the 1730s, provision was made for some who had proved incurable to remain in a special incurables ward. This brisk turnover policy was for the most part maintained, since it accorded with the medical view that cures were obtained either speedily or not all. The aim was that the institution should not silt up with hopeless cases, but rather give as many distressed unfortunates as possible the benefit of its charity. Though historians cavalierly allege that Bethlem cured no one – indeed that nobody expected that patients would be cured – this is clearly erroneous. Indeed, the Committee Book gives plenty of examples of patients discharged, restored to sanity. Thus in May 1710

> Sarah Carter… being this day Called before the Committee she appearing in the Judgment of the Committee and Doctor to be restored to her Senses. It is Ordered That she be forthwith discharged from this Hospital.[17]

She was treated with some generosity:

> And she desiring to goe into Essex where she sayes she has formerly lived Itt is Ordered that forty shillings be given unto her out of Doctor Tyson's Gift thirty shillings whereof is to be laid out by the Steward of this house for Necessary Apparell & Clothing for her and that the remaining ten shillings be given her to bear her Charges into the Country.[18]

Official tabulations of 'cures' must, of course, be taken with a pinch of salt; statistics were probably 'cosmetic', insanity often spontaneously remits, and, in any case, the notion of cure is utterly problematic. Even so it was claimed 'that from the Year

1648 to 1703... there had been in this Hospital 1,294 Patients; of which Number had been cured and discharged 890, which is above two Patients in three'.

Bethlem's governors and their rules were concerned more with house management – maintaining staff discipline and balancing the books – than with therapeutics. Early in the eighteenth century, however, the antiquarian John Strype spelt out a therapeutic ideal ('care and cure'), based on roominess, quiet and decency. Each patient was to have a cell, a bed, and clean straw:

> Those that are fit for it, at convenient Hours, have liberty to walk in the long Galleries, which are large and noble. In the Summer time, to air themselves, there is two large Grass Plats, one for the Men, and another for the Women. And in the Winter a Stove for each apart, where a good Fire is kept to warm them. In the Heat of the Weather, a very convenient Bathing Place to cool and wash them, and is of great Service in airing their Lunacy; and it is easily made a hot Bath for restoring their Limbs when numbed, or cleaning and preserving them from Scurvey, or other cutaneous Distempers. Their Diet is extraordinary good and proper for them, which every Week is viewed by a Committee of the Governors... there is nothing of Violence suffered to be offered to any of the Patients, but they are treated with all the Care and Tenderness imaginable. If raving and furious, they are confined from doing themselves or others Mischief. And it is to the Credit and Reputation of the Hospital, that in so great a Number of Lunaticks that are constantly kept there, it is very rare, and in many Years, that any one Patient makes away with himself.[19]

Thus the gross failings of Bethlem stemmed not from defective aims or regulations, nor from any conceptual fatalism, but from a failure to attend carefully to patients' needs. The standards of treatment adumbrated by Strype were not fulfilled. Thus, despite his talk of stoves, Thomas Monro confessed that Bethlem was excessively cold in winter, causing mortification of extremities;

and Urbane Metcalf indicted the inadequacy of the diet (and this after the house governor had been fired in 1772 for misappropriating provisions). Responsibilities for managing Bethlem were chaotically divided between its governors, its lay officers and its medical staff, and nobody ultimately took responsibility.

But what most discredits Bethlem is its lasting practical therapeutic apathy. None of the physicians in this period investigated insanity or advanced its treatment. This was not through lack of calibre, for they included the pioneer comparative anatomist Dr Edward Tyson; in any case, the Monro succession was able, medically well qualified and, above all, experienced. Yet up to the mid-eighteenth century, no Bethlem physician published a word about insanity – not even to rebut the constant calumnies. This may to some degree have been due to the discretion, not to say secrecy, traditionally surrounding custody of the mad. Yet it is probably because the Bethlem physicians saw their post – which paid only £125 p.a. – if not exactly as a sinecure, at least as somewhat ceremonial. The Monros presumably devoted their time to their own private madhouse, and Thomas in particular absorbed himself in watercolours and art connoisseurship (significantly, he never painted Bethlem).

Considering that the Monros ran Bethlem for 128 years, we know peculiarly little of their philosophy of insanity. Their sole significant publication appeared when John Monro answered William Battie's *Treatise on Madness* (1758). Battie's tract launched a scarcely veiled attack on the management of Bethlem under his father, the late James Monro. Why, Battie asked, was study of insanity so stagnant? Because its treatment was 'entrusted to empiricks, or at best to a few select physicians, most of whom think it advisable to keep the cases as well as the patients to themselves'. James Monro, Battie implied, had engrossed insanity as his private, secret empire. No students were admitted to Bethlem; Monro had not instructed, published or imparted his expertise, or contributed one iota to science. The innuendo, of course, was that the Monros actually had no grasp of madness. Deploring the fatalistic view that insanity was indelible, Battie

condemned hidebound physicians who blindly followed tradition in using 'shocking' but ineffective therapies such as vomits
and venesection.

John Monro was stung into reply, ostensibly in an act of
filial piety to his late father, in his *Remarks on Dr. Battie's Treatise*
(1758). His rebuttal – brusquely condemned by Leigh – painted
a moving picture of the intractability of the disorder ('forever
dark, intricate, uncertain'), contrasted to what he saw as pie-in-
the-sky schemes for its cure. Indeed, Monro's sentiments were
in tune with Samuel Johnson's remarks on the precariousness of
reason shortly to be published in *Rasselas* (1759). But his vision
of the well-nigh ineradicable flaws of human nature ill matched
the optimism of Bethlem's statutes and the rising expectations
of patrons and the public alike in the sunshine years of the
Enlightenment.

Battie's broadside – and the presence of his new model institution, St Luke's, only a stone's throw away – might have been
expected to act as shock therapy on the Monros and Bethlem's
governors, stimulating them into reform. Not so. 1800 came
with Bethlem essentially unchanged from what it had been in
1700. True, from the 1770s casual visiting was ended, a ticket
system being substituted; but the gain produced by ending the
tormenting of patients may have been outweighed by the loss
caused by reduced contact between inmates and the public, and
by diminished public accessibility. Would the evils of Norris'
confinement have taken so long to come to light with the open
access of Old Bethlem? Or in an earlier age, though seen, would
they simply not have been regarded as evils at all?

PUBLIC ASYLUMS

It is remarkable that Bethlem so long remained England's sole
public madhouse, because demand for places greatly exceeded
supply. Yet this lack of mental hospitals merely mirrored the
dearth of general hospitals, in contrast to the wealth of religious and civic refuges dotted across Italy, France and the Low

Countries. Not surprisingly, when public asylums began to be founded in England they chiefly followed in the wake of the voluntary hospital movement, resembling them in their aspirations and management. Indeed, they were sometimes their offspring.

As with voluntary general hospitals, subscription lunatic asylums depended upon personal charity. A substantial gift bought a 'governorship', and governors donated their time and services *gratis*. Voluntary general hospitals proved a signal success. By contrast, public asylums had a much more chequered history.

Individual initiative was the keynote, and early institutions generally owed their origins to a particular activist. In 1713, England's second public asylum was founded in Norwich by Mrs Mary Chapman, in pious gratitude for the preservation of her own reason and in compassion for 'distrest Lunaticks' ('having seen some of my nearest relations and kindred [afflicted] with lunacy'). During the eighteenth century this asylum (known as 'Bethal', or 'sanctuary') generally housed some twenty to thirty lunatics. It never, however, assumed any national importance.

Twelve years later Thomas Guy, the millionaire London bookseller, not only made provision in his will for a general hospital to perpetuate his name but designated that a wing be provided exclusively for incurables, including lunatics:

> Out of such Patients and Persons who shall be discharged out of the Hospital of Saint Thomas, or Bethlehem, or other Hospitals, on account of the small Hopes of their Cure, or the great length of Time for that purpose required or thought necessary.[20]

This was England's first facility for incurable lunatics. A few years later, however, an incurable ward was set up at Bethlem, and another at the French Protestant Hospital.

Subsequent foundations did not rely upon such spectacular individual contributions. Yet founding and financing public asylums remained almost wholly dependent on personal generosity, for donations by corporations or by the churches were paltry, and no block funds came from the Exchequer or the rates. Nor did religious denominations set up their own exclusive asylums, at least before the Quaker York Retreat at the end of the century, and that remained exclusively for Quakers for less than a generation.

Unsurprisingly, the first of the wave of English public asylums – St Luke's, founded by public subscription in 1751 – came in London, where five major general hospitals (Guy's, the Westminster, the London, the Middlesex, and St George's) had all been set up between 1720 and 1750. St Luke's claimed its place in the sun partly on the grounds that Bethlem had a long waiting list (delay wrecked cure prospects). But its true importance lies in the fact that it created a bright new image free of Bedlam's tarnish. For one thing, it called itself not a madhouse or hospital but an 'asylum', with its overtones of sanctuary. For another, it banned casual sightseeing from the outset (Battie condemning the 'impertinent curiosity of those who think it pastime to converse with madmen and play on their passions'), but signalled its commitment to science by admitting medical students – Sir George Baker was one of Battie's pupils.

William Battie, the driving force behind St Luke's, made a bold bid for the public ear by proclaiming in his *Treatise on Madness* (1758) a new therapeutic dawn unknown at benighted Bethlem, illuminated not by medicine but by management. Battie touted the curability of insanity, and the St Luke's annual reports seemed to support him. Even such a sceptic about secular ways with madness as John Wesley was impressed:

> Tues. 21. I had an opportunity of looking over the register of St Luke's Hospital; and I was surprised to observe, that three in four, at least, of those who are admitted receive a cure. I doubt this is not the case of any other lunatic hospital, either in Great Britain or Ireland.[21]

Yet in one respect at least, Battie continued the more dubious practices of the Monros. He doubled serving as physician to St Luke's with proprietorship of his own private madhouse. As

the Monros kept Brooke House, so Battie owned premises first
on the Islington Road, and later in Wood's Close, Clerkenwell,
formerly Newton's Madhouse. Well-heeled patients denied
admission to or discharged from St Luke's were doubtless
funnelled into Battie's own establishment, the public asylum
providing a 'feeder' to the private. Surviving evidence from one
of Battie's invoices, claiming a staggering £749 18s in fees for a
single patient at his private asylum, confirms the contemporary
perception that private asylums were extremely lucrative; Battie's
estate was to be valued at between £100,000 and £200,000.
But if the prestige and publicity of being physician at St Luke's
proved a good venture for Battie, the energetic and popular
Battie also proved a good catch for St Luke's. It flourished. In
1787 it moved to larger, purpose-built premises in Old Street,
costing over £40,000.

The success of St Luke's roused the provinces. First came
Manchester, where the asylum was the offspring of the general Infirmary established in 1752 and largely administered by
its trustees. The Manchester Lunatic Hospital, borrowing rules
from St Luke's including the ban on casual visiting, opened in
1766 with 'cells' for twenty-two inmates. Patients were expected
to pay wherever possible for their keep, though they were to
receive treatment *gratis*. Paupers would be accepted only if their
parish paid. In other words, the Hospital was intended for a
broad clientele, as indicated in 1767 by a trustees' report stating
that one of its aims was to protect respectable local citizens from
the 'impositions of private madhouses'. The standard charge was
to be not less than 10s a week.

Fired perhaps by Battie's optimism, the Manchester trustees
emphasised that their desire was not simply to care but to cure
(a long-term economy, they argued). Coercion would not be
used, except to protect patients from themselves. Mechanical
restraint was authorised, however, in conjunction with a therapeutic menu including bloodletting, blistering, purging and
drugs. Opium was to be given 'in large doses' for maniacs. The
Manchester Lunatic Hospital flourished: already by 1769 some

341 patients were admitted. Yet there is no sign that it pioneered any innovation in treating mental disorder.

Almost contemporaneously, a mental institution was founded in Newcastle. The first plans were laid in 1763 and, two years later, the 'Hospital for Lunaticks for the Counties of Northumberland, Newcastle upon Tyne and Durham' was opened, financed by public subscription including an annual donation from the Common Council. Within a few years, however, it was taken over by its physician, Dr John Hall, becoming a private licensed house known as the Newcastle upon Tyne Lunatic Asylum. Hall, a prominent local physician, had probably always had 'privatisation' in mind, having quarrelled with the governors over the provision for private patients even before the hospital's inauguration, and opening in 1766 his own madhouse – significantly called St Luke's House. After privatisation, the Newcastle Corporation continued to make an annual subscription of ten guineas towards the running costs of the Asylum.

The strained relations between Dr Hall and the Newcastle Council were not unique but a common hazard of public foundations. Such asylums needed paying clients to subsidise charitable ones, but this clearly tempted the physician personally to pocket large fees from the opulent patients. Such tensions stymied attempts to set up an asylum in Gloucester; in Hereford the public asylum was quickly privatised; in York (as we shall see below) they created scandal.

Such problems were less likely to arise when the asylum was tied from the first to a flourishing general infirmary, as at Manchester. A similar link also applied in Liverpool, largely through the energetic advocacy of Dr James Currie. The impetus for the Liverpool Lunatic Asylum (eventually opened in 1797 at a cost of nearly £6,000) came initially from John Howard, who campaigned for it after a visit in the 1780s. But its real begetter was the tireless Currie, who wrote to the newspapers in 1789, arguing from the catastrophe of George III ('A late national distress has... forced the subject upon general attention') to the need for a local asylum. A Liverpool foundation would speedily be followed by several of the principal cities in the Kingdom, and among the happy consequences of the issue of that calamity, future times will probably enumerate a more general provision for and human treatment of this hapless class of our fellow creatures.[22]

Currie advocated linking the lunatic asylum with the Liverpool Infirmary, partly on the grounds of economy and good house-keeping, but also because, in a totally traditional way, he saw madness as quintessentially organic, a medical problem:

> The same offices, apothecary and board of economy will serve both... the institutions themselves are closely allied in their nature; the first affords relief to diseases of the body, the second to diseases of the mind. That these are more nearly connected than is commonly imagined it would be easy to show... The disorder, it is reasonable to suppose on every theory, is seated not in the agent but in the instrument of thought [the brain].[23]

A diametrically opposite point of view about institutional connections prevailed at York, however, where the cultured physician Dr Alexander Hunter argued for the absolute separation of general infirmary and lunatic asylum, believing that

> an Asylum for Lunatics should always be a separate and independent charity; and union with an Infirmary is unnatural.[24]

Empire-building may have prompted Hunter's desire for a separate foundation, but two quite respectable reasons for distinguishing hospital from asylum also stand out. On the one hand, he may have been acknowledging that a public asylum would aspire to a clientele superior in rank to that of a general hospital. The middle classes would receive treatment for general illnesses at home: if deranged, however, their families might be prepared to have them enter an asylum. On the other, he may have been signalling his attachment to more 'progressive' therapeutics than mere medicine, in particular the novel strategy of 'moral management'.

Certainly a whiff of moral idealism attended the formation of the York Asylum, right from the first launch of the project by a series of newspaper insertions in 1772, stating that 'humane persons' desired that 'something should be done for the relief of those unhappy sufferers who are the objects of terror and compassion to all around them'. Opened at last in 1777, the York Asylum seemed for several years the cynosure of enlightened humanity. Its projectors had planned an institution 'where the patients might expect to meet with the most humane and disinterested treatment; and where they might have a chance of being restored to their health'. Early governors' reports paraded its success, and the York Asylum won a good press. For instance, Sir George Onesiphorus Paul was to be lavish in its praise:

> It is about thirty years since a charitable institution was first set on foot at York, having in view the relief and comfort of such Insane Persons as are in low and narrow circumstances. The liberal support given to this institution, not only by gentlemen of the particular county, but of all the northern part of England, has marked the public sentiment on the subject... The relief which the indigent receive is through the increased payments of those in better circumstances for whose accommodation suitable apartments are provided in the same house.[25]

Yet, out of sight, disturbing developments were afoot. For one thing, echoing Newcastle, the public asylum was subject to creeping, clandestine privatisation. Without the governors' knowledge, Dr Hunter and his successor, Dr Charles Best, smuggled personal private patients into the asylum. This was an evident malpractice, since they were leeching upon the donated resources and good name of the asylum to increase their profits. One consequence, of course, was that the accommodation and funds available for the poor were reduced.

Meanwhile the York Asylum, though 'public', also became a place of great secrecy. It is not clear when malpractices crept in. But when in 1790 Hannah Mills, a melancholic Quaker from Leeds, died, a stir was raised because her co-religionists had been refused permission to visit her. The consternation among the local Quaker community led directly to the founding of the York Retreat. A much graver scandal came to light in 1813. Perhaps fired by the publication of Samuel Tuke's *Description of the Retreat*, a zealous magistrate, Godfrey Higgins, began a searching inquiry into the Asylum's management. He and other public-spirited citizens paid subscriptions to buy themselves into governor-ships, securing the right to inspect the asylum and question the physician. Despite sullen obstruction from Dr Best and his underlings (the 'Bestials'), Higgins brought to light evidence of atrocious ill-treatment, profiteering, embezzlement (of at least £20,000) through doctoring the accounts, and concealment (Higgins claimed that 144 deaths had been covered up). Shortly afterwards, the asylum was ravaged by fire, causing the deaths of several patients; arson was suspected, as part of an attempt to destroy vital evidence. The evils of the York Asylum became one of the *causes célèbres* of the House of Commons Committee of 1815. Best's resignation was forced.

It is an instructive episode. It demonstrates how easy it was – as with so many Georgian institutions – for corrupt physicians to feather their nests. Paradoxically, it may have been easier for evils to escape detection in a public asylum than in a private. For after 1774 magistrates at least had the right to inspect private asylums, though not public ones, whereas the panegyric annual reports of supine or trusting governors of public asylums readily created a veneer of perfection which would deflect scrutiny.

What seems clear is that none of the public asylums just dis-cussed pioneered innovations – medical, mechanical, moral, or organisational. The perhaps ornamental presence for a couple of hours a week of an honorary physician, preoccupied with his own private practice, hardly stimulated inquiry or experiment. Altogether, it is one of the oddities of the institutionalisation of insanity in England that public subscription asylums played so small a role, in contrast, say, to Scotland, where they were to become dominant. South of the Border they remained few in number, being overtaken, of course, in the nineteenth century by rate-financed county asylums, and ceasing to be of independent importance.

Why was this? It was not for lack of advocates. Many voices – religious, philanthropic and medical – urged a supportive network of public asylums, typically denouncing the evils of private madhouses. Warning in 1771 of the horrors of the lunacy trade, John Aikin noted how little public provision existed:

> Besides the two in London, there is not throughout the kingdom one that deserves the name of a Lunatic hospital, except a lately erected one at Manchester.[26]

Manchester was a success, and Aikin urged action elsewhere along the same lines:

> I should hope that one hospital in a district of several adjacent counties, would be sufficient to receive all the patients who might offer; and instead of being a burthen, they would be a saving to the community, not only from the relief of private families, but that of parishes which might have paupers afflicted with lunacy.[27]

Currie similarly stressed that public asylums would benefit the whole community:

> The objects of a Lunatic Asylum are twofold – to provide accommodation for the poor suitable to their circumstances, and to make provision for those of superior stations, who are able to remunerate the expense.[28]

Public asylums, he explained, were low-cost compared with general hospitals, because most asylum patients would be fee-paying.

Economical, humane, serviceable, and much touted – why then did public asylums not multiply like general hospitals? Why the gap between promise and achievement? It is hard to be sure. Possibly philanthropic ventures were too public – sited in city centres – to be congenial to respectable families ashamed of the ignominy of the disease. Perhaps few city worthies wanted to draw attention to lunacy by setting up a public asylum: a general infirmary, by contrast, was an unambiguous focus of civic pride. Possibly individual subscribers were less willing to be identified with a disease which wore a badge of shame, rather as lock hospitals for VD sufferers often had financial problems. Overall, institutions for the mad mostly grew up in a more decent, or indecent, obscurity.

PRIVATE MADHOUSES

Herein lies the indispensable, if often shady, service provided by private asylums in the English economy of insanity. It would be an exaggeration to say that private asylums – or, more broadly, the disposal of lunatics through cash transactions – were uniquely English. Fugitive references to keepers of the mad crop up from Renaissance Italy onwards, and private facilities for the rich studded the lunatic landscape of *ancien regime* France. Yet nowhere did they appear in such profusion as in England, or play such a dominant role. They were to prove running sores of scandal: but they also became sites of therapeutic innovation.

The early history of the private 'trade in lunacy' is obscure. Mad-keeping is casually referred to in Elizabethan and Jacobean writings; in Middleton and Rowley's *The Changeling* it is called 'a fine trade'. Shreds of evidence survive from the seventeenth century of a business which – though informal, local and in small units – was probably much larger than commonly recognised. Dr Helkiah Crooke, keeper to Bedlam (1613–34), kept private patients in his own home. When George Trosse went out of his mind in mid-century, he was boarded in Glastonbury with a family experienced in handling the mad. At about the same time the Revd John Ashbourne, a high Anglican, was keeping lunatics in Suffolk; in 1661 he was slain by one of his charges, thus becoming an early psychiatric martyr. Contemporaneously, Thomas Willis was casually referring to a lunatic being placed 'in a house convenient for the business', presumably a reference to a private madhouse. About then, John Newton of Clerkenwell Green was keeping a house for lunatics 'in an excellent air, nere the City', so surviving advertisements assure us. Slightly later, David Irish and Thomas Fallowes were both publicising asylums, and James Carkesse's poems show that before his spell in Bethlem, he had been kept at a private madhouse in Finsbury owned by the physician to Bethlem, Dr Allen.

Such snippets of information indicate that boarding lunatics was well established and that private madhouses existed from before the Restoration. Our information about such houses increases steadily in the last years of the century and through into the eighteenth, a sign both of growing publicity (particularly with the advent of newspaper advertising) and presumably of an absolute rise in their number. We know little about such proto-establishments. This is partly due to poor record-keeping and survival. Like other contemporary institutions such as commercial schools, private madhouses were small, informal, and sometimes ephemeral. Above all, they were pre-bureaucratic. Commonly family businesses, they passed down their therapeutic know-how as a craft skill and their nostrums were prized as family secrets. As in many another family firm, records were kept in the head rather than on paper.

Private madhouses were also in the business of preserving discreet silences. Those contemplating lodging a crazy relative feared publicity, with its implication of madness running in the family. The desire for obscurity was all the greater if placement were occurring under murky circumstances (e.g. attempting to silence a senile parent or bend the will of an heiress). For their part, keepers knew that their livelihood depended upon tactfully pleasing their customers. Thus prudence dictated to them not to keep detailed case records, or to print details of cures involving patients' names – empirics in general medicine by contrast published sheaves of testimonials allegedly signed by 'satisfied customers'. Late in the eighteenth century, even the respectable Revd Dr Francis Willis – restorer of George III – admitted that he did not keep casebooks, and perfectly reputable nineteenth-century asylums such as Ticehurst House resisted what by then were their statutory obligations of maintaining full records, clearly to meet the wishes of patients' families for anonymity.

In short, the early history of private madhouses is shrouded in an obscurity integral to their nature, one which explains both their rise and their enormities. Because there were no legal requirements whatever regulating them before 1774, it is not known how many existed before that date, or when most came into being. For example, in London James Newton's house at Clerkenwell, Thomas Fallowes' at Lambeth Marsh, Mrs Wright's at Bethnal Green (where Alexander Cruden was confined in the 1730s), Brooke House at Hackney – owned by the Monro family – are well-known and long-lasting establishments all in existence by the first half of the eighteenth century. In his *Tour of the Whole Island of Great Britain* (1724), Daniel Defoe stated that there were already fifteen private metropolitan madhouses.

In the provinces it appears that as well as those already mentioned, a madhouse had been set up sometime during the seventeenth century at Box in Wiltshire; another existed at Fonthill Gifford in Wiltshire in 1718; Hook Norton in Oxfordshire dates from about 1725; Fishponds, Bristol, from 1766. Dr Nathaniel Cotton set up his Collegium Insanorum at St Albans, sometime after 1740.

It would be a mistake, anyway, to expect to find clear foundation dates, for many establishments did not spring up suddenly *ex nihilo*, but rather emerged gradually. It is likely that a householder gradually got into the practice of boarding one or more lunatics in an *ad hoc* fashion, and in time formalised the arrangement by advertising his establishment as a madhouse. That, for example, is the origin of Ticehurst House. Its proprietor, the apothecary

Samuel Newington, had been accepting individual lunatics for perhaps thirty years before the House proper opened in 1792.

Particulars of how the earliest institutions were managed are similarly few, and we are mainly dependent on publicity and polemics. On the one hand, we have the angry *exposés* of reformers and patients who savaged them as dens of iniquity. Thus Alexander Cruden's fulminations depict Mrs Wright's madhouse at Bethnal Green as a hive of Dickensian soul-snatchers. On the other, we have their owners' glowing puffs in pamphlets and newspaper advertisements. In time-honoured fashion Thomas Fallowes slated his rivals before depicting his own house as a haven of care:

> The rough and cruel Treatment, which is said to be the Method of most of the Pretenders to this Cure, is not only to be abhorr'd, but on the contrary, all the Gentleness and Kindness in the World, is absolutely necessary, even in all the Cases I have seen;... I have never us'd any Violence to any Patient.[29]

Indeed, Fallowes promised a veritable pudding-time to his clients:

> Such Entertainment as is fit for Persons of any Degree or Quality, in my House, in Lambeth-Marsh. The Conveniences may be easily observ'd upon view; the Situation is in an Air neither too subtle and thin, nor too gross; the Gardens to the House are Commodious, Large and Pleasant, into which the Patients are admitted, in their Intervals, and with a Person to attend them. There is as much Privacy as can be desired, and very good Rooms, and 'tis within such a Distance from the City as any Patient may be visited by their own Physician or Chirurgion, if they think fit; for I shall be ready to admit them.[30]

Not least, he claimed, cold-bathing facilities were available, as well as the famed Lambeth Waters nearby.

This may, of course, tell us nothing about how Fallowes actually treated his patients. Indeed, he has the unsavoury honour

of having been the first mad-doctor convicted for illegal confinement. It does, however, say much about the face a private
proprietor felt he should wear. Even by 1700 the trade in lunacy
was evidently making 'large promise' of curative therapy, gentleness and comforts – good accommodation, air, exercise and diet.
There was little left of mere 'humanity' for later moral therapy
enthusiasts to add: all that was needed was the implementation
of such ideals. Whatever the popular stereotypes of madmen as
brutes, every proprietor knew he could not cash in by harping
on the severity of his treatments, or on his talents as a whip-
master.

In a nation where custody of lunatics increasingly fell to private enterprise, entrepreneurs of madness clearly had to adjust
to market forces, meeting explicit demands and creating fresh
ones. One consequence of this was the extreme diversity of the
private sector. The public foundations in Manchester, Newcastle,
Liverpool etc. discussed above largely cloned each other, and
were derivative from St Luke's in London (the first keeper and
matron at Liverpool were both recruited from St Luke's). But
what characterised private madhouses were their variations – in
size, opulence, the social rank of their charges, the qualifications
and skills of their proprietors, and their notions of treatment.

Many began, and remained, extremely small. Parry-Jones'
exemplary studies of two Oxfordshire madhouses, Witney and
Hook Norton, showed that they catered for no more than
about a dozen patients. The Revd John Lord's house at Drayton
Parslow in Buckinghamshire – which seemed to have specialised
in Oxford University breakdowns – was smaller still. Anthony
Addington's madhouse in Reading had 'from 8 to 10 Patients...
at a time'. As late as 1800 there were only seven asylums outside
London exceeding thirty patients, and between ten and twenty
with fewer. Indeed, at the smaller end of the market it is hard
to say – at least before the advent of formal licensing – whether
there was a minimum size of establishment properly called a
'house', as distinct from informal 'boarding'. It was in any case a
common practice to lodge a single lunatic with a keeper under

the general charge of a physician. This, for example, was the fate at the end of the eighteenth century of the watercolourist J.R. Cozens, supervised by Dr Thomas Monro. Because the law chose not to meddle with 'single lunatics', the practice throve in the nineteenth century.

Given such smallness, it is significant that the standard eighteenth-century term for such institutions was mad*house*, or just *house*, or after 1774 'licensed *house*', for most indeed were integral or adjacent to the owner's residence. One of the main claims to fame of the York Retreat was that it capitalised on the therapeutic virtues of domesticity, retraining patients for family life. But most eighteenth-century madhouses spilled over in any case into the households of the proprietors. Before the opening of Brislington House and the York Retreat, themselves designed to resemble country houses, purpose-built private madhouses were hardly known. Distinctively institutional asylum architecture, with its elaborate therapeutic, sanitary, and panoptic rationalities, was a nineteenth-century science pioneered by the Scots William Stark and Andrew Duncan, with Jeremy Bentham as its patron saint.

Even prominent institutions mostly remained very modest in scale. In the twelve-year period from 1801 to 1812, Fishponds Asylum in Bristol had just 183 admissions, or an average of about one new patient every three weeks. Most had far fewer. Thomas Arnold's house at Shrewsbury had ninety-six. Over the same span, Hook Norton took just fifty-six new patients, and the Willises' establishment at Greatford in Lincolnshire a mere forty-six. Even lower are the figures for William Terry's house at Sutton Coldfield, which appears to have taken only eleven new clients between 1793 and 1812. This level of new admissions is explained not by protracted stays but by overall smallness.

Thus the large private asylum was highly exceptional. Up to the end of the century there were perhaps no more than three in the whole country, all huddled just beyond the City of London: Whitmore House (which became known as Warburton's), Hoxton House, run by Sir Jonathan Miles, and Holly House.

By 1815, Hoxton House had 486 patients. Among them were a few genteel recruits (for instance, Warburton housed the son of the Duke of Atholl, who reputedly paid £1,500 a year); but they predominantly took two types of patient. On the one hand there were parish lunatics, contract boarded at a fixed charge per person (around 10s a week). The sum was rather higher than for the workhouse; but, as Warburton explained to the Commons Committee in 1815, it was not sufficient to cover treatment and medicines as well as keep. On the other hand there were members of the armed forces, placed through contracts with the War Office. The Revolutionary and Napoleonic Wars caused their numbers to rocket, and by 1815 the Hoxton madhouses were warehousing some 500 patients in conditions of overcrowding, squalor and profiteering.

Nevertheless, the worst evils of the eighteenth-century madhouses were not that mix of gigantism and long-stay demor-alisation − 'institutionalisation' − which rendered Victorian aspirations for the asylum nugatory. Indeed, some of the most horrifying − for example, that at Box in Wiltshire visited by Edward Wakefield and shamed before the Commons Committee of 1815 − were the tiniest: 'I never recollect to have seen four living persons in so wretched a place', reported Wakefield. Protesters such as Alexander Cruden and Samuel Bruckshaw had no end of complaints; yet they had a cell to themselves, were not regimented, and were quickly released.

Thus madhouses came large and small. They also came cheap and dear. As indicated above, parish lunatics were commonly boarded in private asylums for sums between 7s 6d a week and half a guinea. They would be housed separately from individual private patients, in a detached wing or even in stables, receiving a scanty diet and little attention. Often they slept on straw more than one to a bed. In themselves, such conditions were not exceptional hardships to Georgians (servants, apprentices and labourers often fared worse). But reformers deemed them utterly undesirable for lunatics, who were often dirty and incontinent and easily communicated disease and delinquency one to another.

Doerner has argued that eighteenth-century confinement was essentially of the poor. But the trade in lunacy – like other trades – depended upon its middle-class clientele. Certain proprietors, for example, Dr Charles Best at his private asylum at Acomb in Yorkshire, stressed that their houses were 'for persons of condition only'; this explains how William Belcher was able to brand such proprietors as 'smiling Hyenas' who 'ravish the rich'. Private asylums profited from paying patients whose families would foot the bill, the typical fee for middling folk rising to about a guinea a week by 1800. Proprietors would also angle for exceptional patients who would receive special treatment (plusher rooms, greater attendance, richer diet, or, perhaps, greater secrecy) and would be charged correspondingly higher. A few asylums in any case standardly operated with stiff tariffs. For example, the Revd John Lord charged male patients £200 p.a., and Dr Nathaniel Cotton at St Albans billed three or five guineas a week per patient (five guineas was approximately the annual wage of a maid servant). Charges, however, were not fixed but flexible, depending on individual needs. Thus, in more opulent houses, patients would bring their own personal servants, paid for separately by their families, but whose accommodation would go on the bill. Medicines and treatment were commonly itemised as extras.

One form of differentiation of madhouses – one which later became highly controversial – was the question of medical proprietorship. Before 1828 there were no statutory requirements stipulating that madhouses had to be attended by medical personnel.

Some had almost no medical presence, others a high medical profile. Prominent physicians, such as Anthony Addington, the Monros, William Battie, Nathaniel Cotton, Thomas Arnold and Edward Long Fox, all kept private houses. Samuel Newington, the founder of Ticehurst House in Sussex, was a surgeon-apothecary, and his son and successor, Charles, a physician. Indeed, most asylums whose names remain famous nowadays were headed by medical practitioners, reflecting the fact that it was chiefly they who published in the field – witness works such as Thomas Arnold's *Observations on the Nature, Kinds, Causes and Prevention of Insanity* (1782–6) and William Perfect's *Select Cases in the Different Species of Insanity* (1787). Yet there were exceptions, as is shown by the York Retreat, founded by a philanthropic tea merchant, William Tuke, whose grandson Samuel published the most influential 'asylum' book of all, *The Description of the Retreat* (1813), a work sceptical of medication.

In fact, before the nineteenth century there was no real quarrel between medically and non-medically managed madhouses. Some practitioner proprietors, such as the surgeon William Finch, actually made more play of 'humanity' or even 'providence' than of physick. Witness his advertisement:

CURE LUNATICS

WILLIAM FINCH of MILFORD, near Salisbury, [has] for many years had great success in curing people disordered in their senses... the many cures he has performed on Lunatics... can be attested by the greatest satisfaction he can say, that every person he has had charge of, has, with the blessing of God, been cured and discharged from his house perfectly well. The friends of such unfortunate persons who are committed to his care, may depend on their being treated with the greatest tenderness and humanity, by their faithful humble servant,

WILLIAM FINCH, Milford [31]

By contrast, Thomas Bakewell, the highly respected 'empiric' proprietor of Spring Vale in Staffordshire, stressed the propriety of medication and boasted a secret family recipe, whose contents he could not, in fairness to his descendants, divulge.

Interestingly, many family asylums began by being lay-run, but were eventually to take on a medical character. For instance, Fishponds near Bristol was founded in the mid-eighteenth century by George Mason, a man without medical qualifications who, drawing possibly on his Baptist background, claimed to run a humane and homely establishment; his family took tea and held prayers with the patients. Later members of the family, above all Joseph Mason Cox, received a medical education, however, and their publicity stressed medical treatment, including a rotating chair. The major scandal in Fishponds' history occurred in 1848 when it was under the control of Dr Joseph Bompas, who had studied medicine at University College, London.

Did the public want asylums to be run by doctors? The 'empiric' Thomas Bakewell told the House of Commons Committee that clients primarily valued humanity and experience. And the Committee itself clearly underwrote the moral managers' and moral therapists' claims that medicine possessed no master-key to madness. The contrast between the shifty Dr Best at the York Asylum and the honest Quaker Tukes at the York Retreat was not lost on the Committee.

If the public truly harboured fears about the ways machinating medical men manipulated the mad for private profit, these would certainly have been inflamed by Benjamin Faulkner's *Observations on the General and Improper Treatment of Insanity* (1790). Faulkner – a layman – who from 1785 owned a private madhouse in Little Chelsea, appealed to the public against the evils of physician-owned premises. These, he claimed, lay in an improper amalgamation of function, rendering the physician simultaneously both medical adviser and hotelier. This created irreconcilably divided loyalties. The duty of the physician was to cure speedily; but, as 'hotel keeper', his interest lay in prolonging the stay. The outcome, Faulkner suggested, was that the physician would consult his pocket, pervert his physic, and the patient's confinement would be unnecessarily protracted:

> It requires no uncommon faith to believe, that the desire of profit and the accumulation of advantages resulting from expensive board and lodging, will, with too many, have more weight than the reputation of an early cure.[32]

Deeming that the liberty of a subject required the separation of powers, Faulkner advocated splitting the 'hotel' function from the clinical. The madhouse-keeper should solely provide accommodation. The patient and his family should have free choice of practitioner:

> Let them consult a Fordyce, a Baker, a Warren, or a Reynolds; men whose knowledge cannot be surpassed, whose integrity is unimpeachable, and who can derive no advantage from the local situation of the afflicted.[33]

Such doctors, unencumbered by madhouse ownership, would have no pecuniary motive for unnecessary confinement. Faulkner's proposed system – a 'free house' – aimed to put paid to two damaging evils. On the one hand, detention beyond necessity. On the other, families' presumed reluctance to despatch crazed relatives into madhouses, lest they never got out. This meant they often delayed treatment until it was too late. By contrast, claimed Faulkner, his scheme would encourage early confinement and prompt treatment, since release would always remain easy. It was vital for sufferers that asylums be easy of access and egress.

Thus a broad spectrum of asylums became available on the market, some good, some bad, some indifferent. All proprietors protested, of course, their humanity, care, and power to cure. An early 'quacks bill' mouthed promises which were to become the platitudes of the trade:

> In Clerkenwell-Close, where the Figures of Mad People are over the Gate; Liveth one, who by the Blessing of God, Cures all Lunatick distracted or Mad People, he seldom exceeds 3 Months in the Cure of the Maddest person that comes in his House, several have been Cur'd in a Fortnight, and some in less time; he has cur'd several from Bedlam and other Madhouses in and about this City, and has Conveniency for People of what Quality soever. No Cure no Money.[34]

Caveat emptor. But utterly reputable proprietors too made roughly comparable claims. Good cheer, invigorating surroundings, and care – all were paraded as the essence of the asylum, as by David Irish, at the dawn of the eighteenth century, who was offering

> good fires, Meat and Drink, with good attendance, and all neces-
> saries far beyond what is allow'd at Bedlam, or any other place he
> has yet heard of and cheaper, for he allows the Melancholy, Mad,
> and such whose Consciences are Opprest with the sense of Sin,
> good Meat every day for Dinner, and also wholesome Diet for
> Breakfast and Supper, and good Table-Beer enough at any time:
> They have also good Beds and Decent Chambers.[35]

Indeed, the hallmark of the madhouse as generally presented to the public consisted in such classical 'non-natural' virtues as 'air' and 'hospitality', rather than any specific clinical regimen. Highly characteristic was Faulkner's appeal to 'comforts':

> Proper objects and amusements to engage and invigorate the
> mental faculties, proper exercise and proper diet are the grand
> restoratives in this malady. For the accomplishment of all these
> my house is peculiarly calculated.[36]

Moreover, despite a contemporary bad press which historians have hardened into gospel truth, the signs are that certain Georgian asylums were indeed humane. For instance, Dr Nathaniel Cotton was respected for the care provided at his private Collegium Insanorum at St Albans. When William Cowper became suicidal in 1763, he was sent there. Although he records few specific details of his treatment, he was neither immobilised nor subjected to violence, and was allowed to read. Cotton cared:

> I was not only treated with kindness by him when I was ill, and
> attended with the utmost diligence; but when my reason was
> restored to me, and I had so much need of a religious friend to

converse with, to whom I could open my mind upon the subject without reserve, I could hardly have found a fitter person for the purpose. The doctor was as ready to administer relief to me in this article likewise, and as well qualified to do it, as in that which was more immediately in his province.

The treatment Kit Smart received at Potter's madhouse in Bethnal Green was also considerate. As his biographer puts it,

Provided with pen and ink and paper, allowed visitors, digging in the garden playing with and talking to his cat, reading books and periodicals, possibly even allowed a few hours' accompanied freedom... Smart spent almost exactly four years in the private madhouse at Bethnal Green. Part of each day... was ritually devoted to the composition of one, two, or three pairs of lines that were then written down neatly in the document he entitled Jubilate Agno.[37]

John Wesley was impressed by conditions in the 1780s at Hanham madhouse near Bristol, run by Richard Henderson, and Edward Long Fox was managing an obviously humane madhouse at Cleeve in the 1790s, before going on to found Brislington House in 1804. One of his co-helpers was Katherine Allen, who became wife to George Jepson, an early superintendent at the York Retreat. Of the Hoxton asylum where Mary Lamb was confined, her brother wrote, 'the good lady of the Madhouse, and her daughter,... love and are taken with her amazingly'.

In respect of 'humanity', the House of Commons Report of 1815 is highly revealing. As is well known, it painted a glowing portrait of the York Retreat, lauding its humane 'moral therapy', and broadcasting its impressive cure statistics. But several other asylums were also singled out for praise, including some of the old school such as William Finch's near Salisbury, which primarily provided a hospitable environment. Publications by such late eighteenth-century madhouse-keepers as Thomas Arnold, William Perfect and Thomas Bakewell, with their rich case histories and claims to high cure rates, seem to bear witness to attentive care; while right at the close of the century a clutch of select asylums such as Ticehurst were building reputations as superior receptacles for the mad.

Of these, the York Retreat clearly won the palm, and I shall explore its 'moral therapy' regime in the next chapter. But here it is relevant to note that from its inception the Retreat encouraged serious observers, and that practically every visitor brought away glowing reports. As one American visitor, Louis Simond, put it:

> There is near York a retreat for lunatics, which appears admirably managed, and almost entirely by reason and kindness; it was instituted by the Quakers.[38]

It is not hard to see why the Retreat made such a good impression. Unlike practically all other contemporary asylums, it was purpose-built (at a cost of £3,869), being designed to combine security with the façade of a genteel country residence. Clever devices helped to unite these two functions; there were no window bars, but the panes of glass were retained not by wooden but by metal slats. It basked in eleven acres of well-laid-out estate, without forbidding retaining walls. Its staff-patient ratio was enviable at about one to ten. Visitors to Ticehurst and Brislington House (also specially built, at an ultimate cost of some £35,000) were similarly impressed. The trade in lunacy produced palaces as well as pigsties.

CONFINEMENT AND ITS ABUSES

Throughout the century, private asylums remained tainted with accusations of neglect and corruption. Early on, the prime grievance was wrongful confinement. It became almost proverbial that keepers were sharks, and the sane were improperly sequestered in private asylums. The evil had got to such a pitch, Defoe claimed in *The True Born Englishman*, that private madhouses, mushrooming around London, had become far worse than 'a clandestine inquisition'. 'Is it not enough,' he demanded, 'to make anyone mad, to be suddenly clapped up, stripped, whipped, ill fed, and worse used?'. 'If this tyrannical inquisition... be not sufficient to drive any soul stark-staring mad... I have no more to say.'

Defoe's recommendation was simple:

> In my humble Opinion all private Madhouses should be suppress'd at once, and it should be no less than Felony to confine any Person under pretence of Madness without due Authority. For the cure of those who are really Lunatick, licens'd Madhouses should be constituted in convenient Parts of the Town, which Houses should be subject to proper Visitation and Inspection, nor should any Person be sent to a Madhouse without due Reason, Inquiry and Authority.[39]

His attack found support. An anonymous pamphlet of 1740, *Proposals for Redressing Some Grievances Which Greatly Affect the Whole Nation*, echoed his calls:

> Several are put into Madhouses, as they are called, without being mad. Wives put their Husbands in them that they may enjoy their Gallants, and live without the Observation and Interruption of their Husbands; and Husbands put their Wives in them, that they may enjoy their Whores, without Desturbance from their Wives; Children put their Parents in them, that they may enjoy their Estates before their time; Relations put their Kindred into them for wicked Purposes.[40]

Particular cases were adduced to clinch the point:

> I know of a Gentlewoman of substance who lived at Windsor, who was flattered by her roguish Apothecary into the Management of her Fortune, and when he had fixed himself in her Opinion and did all her Business for her, he decoyed her into a Madhouse not far from London on the Bank of the River Thames, where

he took care that she was so ill used, that she, after a while, was
made really mad in good earnest, and the Apothecary enjoy'd
her Fortune, and took care that no Relation or Acquaintance of
hers should have access to her, or visit her.[41]

These allegations, increasingly embroidered in fiction, as in
Tobias Smollett's novel *Sir Launcelot Greaves*, were clinched by
cases which came to the courts. In 1714, as mentioned above,
a 'Dr Fellows' (presumably Dr Fallowes) was convicted for the
wrongful confinement of a sane person as a lunatic. Just four
years later the notorious Mrs Clark's case showed how easy it was
for a family to sequester one of its members in her own house,
as if mentally incompetent, purely on its own say-so. Fortunately
for her, Mrs Clark was rescued by her friends; her case was
heard before the Lord Chief Justice and she was 'set at liberty'.
Longer-running and more spectacular altogether, however, was
the saga of Alexander Cruden.

A Presbyterian proofreader, Cruden was confined in private
madhouses on three separate occasions between the 1720s and
1750s. Once he contrived to escape, still wearing his ball and
chain, scaling a wall and running off to present himself before the
Lord Mayor of London. Over this period, he produced a stream
of publications vindicating his sanity, alleging persecution by
enemies, who had confined him out of mere malice, and offering
himself as a classic example of a free-born Briton deprived of
his citizen's rights by the tyranny of private asylums. Cruden's
outpourings, notably *The London-Citizen Exceedingly Injured: or
A British Inquisition Display'd, In an Account of the Unparallel'd
Case of a Citizen of London, Bookseller to the late Queen, who was
in a most unjust and arbitrary Manner sent on the 23rd of March last,
1738, by one Robert Wightman, a mere Stranger, to a Private Madhouse,
containing, I. An Account of the said Citizen's barbarous Treatment in
Wright's Private Madhouse on Bethnal-Green for nine Weeks and six
Days, and of his rational and patient Behaviour, while Chained, Hand-
cuffed, Strait Wastecoated and Imprisoned in the said Madhouse: Where
he probably would have been continued, or died under his Confinement,*

if he had not most Providentially made his escape (1739), did not, perhaps, convince anyone of his normality, so obsessed was he with his own Job-like misfortunes. Yet he made his 'persecution' the basis of an eloquent plea 'to the legislature… plainly showing the absolute necessity of regulating Private Madhouses in a more effectual manner than at present'.

Indeed, no 'effectual manner' whatever of regulating private madhouses then existed, and no legislation governed the trade in lunacy. Families might lawfully commit relatives to private asylums; if that procedure were challenged, recourse to *habeas corpus* was – in theory at least – available, and the party might be released, as happened with Clark. Many cases showed, however, that people in their right minds were easily dumped in such madhouses with little prospect of redress. This made news in 1761 in the case of Rex *v.* Turlington. Mrs Deborah D'Vebre had been confined to Turlington's Asylum in Chelsea by her husband. Her relatives sued *habeas corpus*, and the court granted that a physician and her nearest relative should be permitted to see her. The physician judged her perfectly rational; when she was brought before the court, his finding was confirmed and she was released.

Mrs D'Vebre obtained justice. But her case brought to light fresh instances of injustices unrestored. As Parry-Jones notes, discussing the mid-century Chelsea asylum:

Perhaps the most striking revelations were those made by King, Turlington's 'agent' at the Chelsea house, where the rule was to admit everyone who was taken there. King stated that he had 'admitted several for drunkenness, and for other reasons of the same sort, alleged by their friends or relatives bringing them in, which he had always thought a sufficient authority'… he frankly confessed that out of the whole number of persons whom he had confined he had never admitted one as a lunatic during the six years he had been entrusted with the superintendency of the house.[42]

A tide of opinion now urged action to prevent further abuses. In 1754 the College of Physicians was asked by Sir Cordell Firebrace, MP for Suffolk, to consider a bill recommending that the College should regulate private madhouses. Hostile as always to outside interference in medical affairs, it demurred. The agitation did not subside, however, and the case for regulation was forcefully restated in 1763 in an anonymous article in the *Gentleman's Magazine*, that crucial organ of Georgian opinion:

> When a person is forcibly taken or artfully decoyed, into a private madhouse he is, without any authority or any farther charge than that of a mercenary relation, or a pretended friend, instantly seized upon by a set of inhuman ruffians, trained up to this barbarous profession, stripped naked, and conveyed to a darkroom. If he complains... the attending servant brutishly orders him not to rave, calls for assistance, and ties him down to a bed, from which he is not released until he submits to their pleasure... next morning, a doctor is gravely introduced who, taking the report of the keeper, pronounces the unfortunate person a lunatic, and declares that he must be reduced by physic.[43]

Cornered thus, it became progressively difficult for such a patient, once confined, to prove his sanity:

> If the patient, or rather the prisoner, persists in vindicating his reason, or refuses to take the dose, he is then deemed raving mad;[44]

In particular, patients would be subjected to depletive medicines. Refusal to comply would be seen as a mark of perversion. But taking them would have a depressive effect, 'until the patient is so debilitated in body that in time it impairs his mind'. The indictment closed with an appeal to humanity:

> What must a rational mind suffer that is treated in this irrational manner? Weakened by physic, emaciated by torture, diseased by

confinement, and terrified by the sight of every instrument of
cruelty and the dreadful menaces of an attending ruffian, hardened against all the tenderness of human nature... [45]

The upshot of this public consternation was a parliamentary
committee, which took evidence from leading mad-doctors,
including Monro of Bethlem and Battie of St Luke's, who admitted that wrongful confinement occurred. Indeed Battie stated,

> it frequently happened, and related the Case of a Woman perfectly
> in her Senses brought as a Lunatic by her husband to a House
> under the Doctor's Direction, whose Husband upon Doctor
> Battie insisting he should take home his Wife, and expressing
> his Surprise at his Conduct, justified himself by frankly saying,
> he understood the House to be a Sort of Bridewell, or Place of
> Correction.[46]

At this point, the College of Physicians again used its muscle
to block regulation (fellows had a large financial stake in metropolitan madhouses), and it was not until more bills had been
lost, and a further eleven years elapsed, that legislation was finally
passed policing the lunacy trade for the first time.

The Act for Regulating Private Madhouses (1774) was a legislative landmark. Its fundamental stipulation was that private
madhouses should be licensed. Outside London, the licensing
body was to be the justices at assizes. Licences would be valid for
only a year, and would specify the maximum number of patients
to be admitted. Proprietors were required to keep patient registers. Moreover, legal confinement of all but paupers would
require certification from a medical practitioner (paupers could
still be confined by magistrates according to the Act of 1744).
Finally, private madhouses were to be liable to inspection. In the
provinces, this was to be by magistrates; in London, a five-man
commission of the College of Physicians was to serve.

The Act was important in many ways, not least because by
requiring the keeping of registers and providing for inspection,

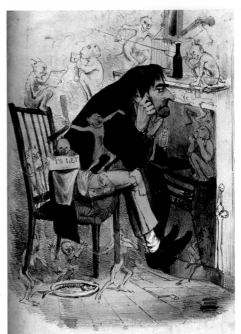

1 A wretched man with an approaching depression, here represented by the encroachment of little devils. Indeed, Burton labelled melancholy as the 'Devil's instigation', supporting the popular view that madness, temporary or otherwise, was due to diabolic possession.

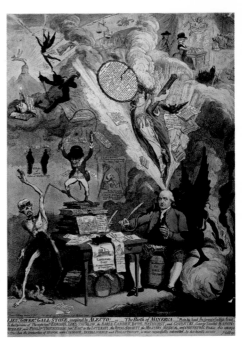

2 The author and eccentric Philip Thicknesse writing at a table, surrounded by demonic apparitions representing aspects of his life. Many seventeenth- and eighteenth-century patients, including the much-chronicled George Trosse, claimed to experience the turmoil of inner 'demons'.

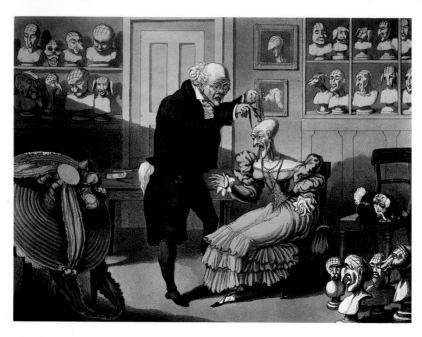

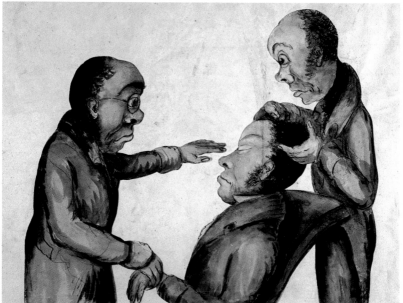

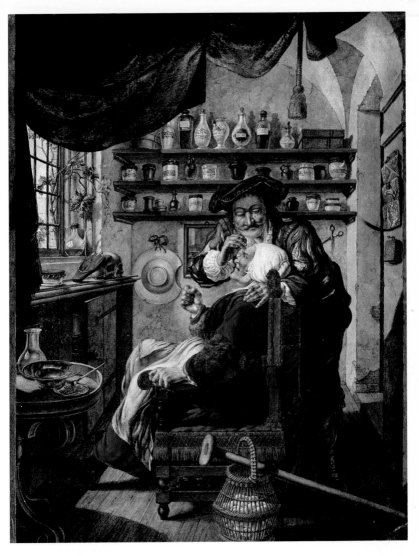

Opposite above: 3 Franz Joseph Gall (1758–1828) measuring the head of a patient. Gall was a chief proponent of the would-be science of 'phrenology', which maintained that the seat of the mind was the brain, whose configuration both determined and displayed the personality.

Opposite below: 4 Franz Joseph Gall and his partner in 'phrenology', Johann Caspar Spurzheim, examining a patient.

This page: 5 A surgeon extracting stones from a grimacing patient's head; symbolising the extraction of 'folly' (insanity).

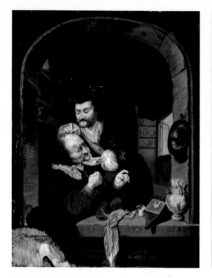
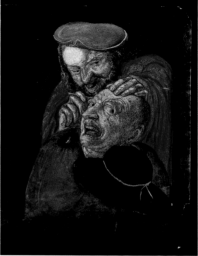
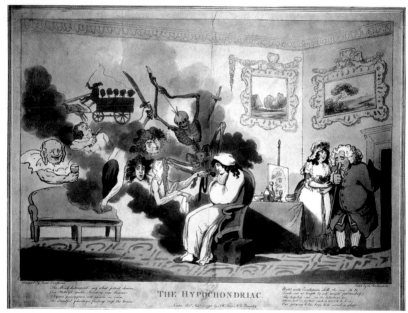

Top: 6, 7 More grimacing patients having stones extracted from their heads.

Above: 8 A hypochondriac surrounded by doleful spectres. In late Stuart and early Georgian times, there was a blossoming of eminent melancholic and hypochondriacal intellectuals, including Robert Hooke, Isaac Newton, John Locke and William Whiston.

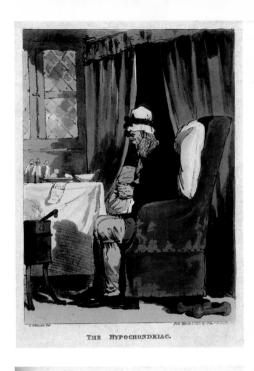

THE HYPOCHONDRIAC.

OH! THERE'S SOMETHING IN MY EYE!

I wish you'd take it out.
There's always something the matter with me!

9, 10 Eighteenth-century mad-
doctors discouraged the 'mad talk'
of hysterics and hypochondriacs.
It was believed that attending
to the imagined illnesses of
hypochondriacs would lead to
them 'talking themselves into
further ills'.

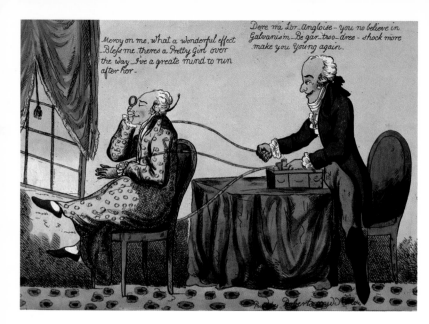

Above: 11 An affluent man receiving electrical therapy. Electrical therapy for the mad became one of the 'great hopes' of the Georgian era, and was advocated by enthusiasts such as John Wesley.

Below: 12 The Hospital of Bethlem (Bedlam) at Moorfields, London. This is the second building of the hospital designed by Robert Hooke and built in 1675–76. Its showy exterior was the subject of much satirical comment.

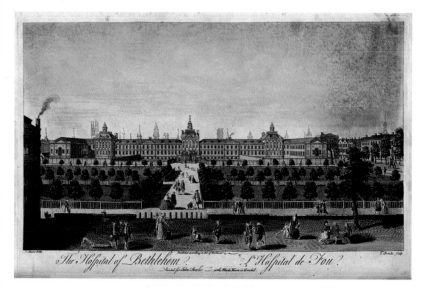

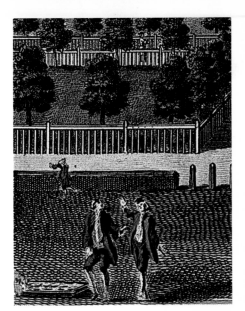

13 Lunatics capering about in front of Bethlem, c.1771.

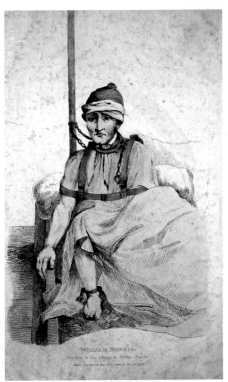

WILLIAM NORRIS

14 James Norris restrained by chains at the neck and ankles in Bethlem hospital. An anonymous critic described the London madhouse as a 'school of misery'.

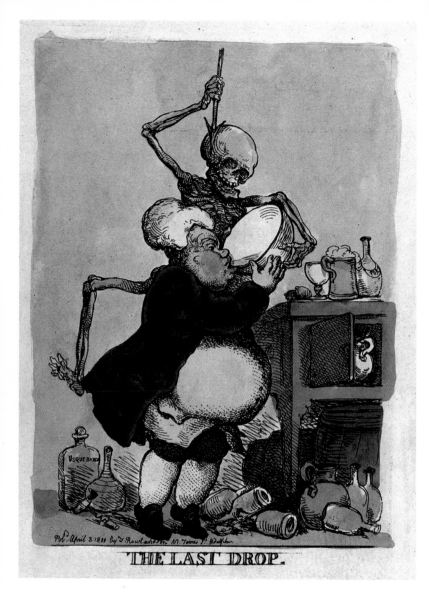

THE LAST DROP.

15 Satire of a man drinking himself to death. Alcoholism was bound together with mental illness in the eighteenth century, and the term 'alcoholism' was coined around this time. Samuel Johnson himself kicked the habit, stating, 'I can't touch a little, child, therefore I never touch it. Abstinence is as easy to me as temperance would be difficult.'

it tore the veil of secrecy traditionally shrouding private mad-houses. In principle, it would thereafter be possible to know precisely who and how many people were being confined, and for asylum interiors to become public knowledge. Moreover it offered due safeguard – clinical judgement – against unlawful confinement, at least of non-paupers. Whereas previously there had been no machinery to prevent the sane being confined (redress had come, if at all, after the event, by *habeas corpus*), henceforth the public should be protected by physicians' integrity, mediating between family and sufferer.

How far the 1774 Act provided real safeguards is hard to say. Its scope was limited. It did not police public asylums, 'single lunatics' privately boarded, or Chancery cases. Moreover, it was toothless. No penalties were appended. There was no provision for punishing abuses or infringements. Nor were criteria established for granting licences. It is not clear that magistrates even had the power to reject a licence, and there is no evidence that one ever was refused. It might thus be argued that the Act's tendency was perhaps to *license* the abuses of the status quo, rather than eradicate them, just as (arguably) the patient himself, confined post-1774 under the sovereign authority of a medical certificate, would find pleading for release even more arduous than before. Not least, we have few signs that magistrates were zealous in fulfilling their responsibility of inspecting madhouses. Equally, as the 1815 Commons Committee brought to light, College of Physicians' visitations of metropolitan asylums were extremely peremptory, and conducted upon the narrowest of briefs. Several madhouses were visited in a day, and the commissioners contented themselves with checking patient registers. So long as the asylum population tallied with the register, the house was reckoned proper. No case is known where the conduct of any private asylum was changed through agitation from magistrates or College. Indeed, many thought the Act nugatory, and the visitations a farce.

Notwithstanding the recent regulations [argued William Pargeter] there are many private madhouses in the neighbourhood of the metropolis, which demand a very serious enquiry. The masters of these receptacles of misery, on the days that they expect their visitors, get their sane patients out of the way; or if that cannot be done, give them large doses of stupefying liquor, or narcotic draughts, that drown their faculties, and render them incapable of giving a coherent answer. A very strict eye should be kept on these gaolers of the mind; for if they do not find a patient mad, their oppressive tyranny soon makes him so.[47]

These limitations are not very surprising, for the 1774 Act was framed solely to forestall the unlawful confinement of the sane. It was not a general measure of regulation or reform. It gave no brief to evaluate therapy, judge cure rates, criticise standards of hygiene, health, restraint, care or whatever. It was not until the setting up of the Metropolitan Commissioners in Lunacy in 1828, a body not made national till 1842, that a panel of experts had incentive and authority for protecting the public against defective asylums. In the eighteenth century Parliament's concern ran at best to safeguarding constitutional liberties, not to enhancing the quality of care. It might license market arrangements but did not set up an optimal system of refuges for the mad.

What, then, was the impact of the 1774 Act? As the evidence laid before the 1815 Parliamentary Committee amply showed, it did not end the evils of private madhouses. But it did put them on the agenda of public concern. Later reformers such as Edward Wakefield, who bombarded the 1815 Committee with so much devastating information, were able to make their investigations because, at last, the requirements of keeping admissions registers and allowing inspection had been established. Thanks to the 1774 Madhouse Act, whatever other horrors the 1815 Report revealed, the discovery of hordes of illegally confined people was not among them.

Indeed, the criticism levelled against private asylums gradually shifted. Originally illegal confinement had been the cardinal evil. This source of outrage still, of course, continued into the Victorian age, as campaigners such as Louisa Lowe revealed.

Indeed, once certification by a physician was mandatory, professional authority grew and release perhaps became more difficult, because the more enlarged ideas about insanity held by physicians carried greater weight. Take, for instance, a case discussed by James Parkinson. In 1807 Parkinson, medical attendant to Hoxton House, had certified one Mary Daintree. Supported by relatives, she protested her sanity and secured her release. Parkinson justified his conduct by contending that though to lay eyes she had appeared rational when he certified her, the veneer of normality often concealed latent or recurrent madness. The physician had to protect the public – and his own reputation – against the possibility of a former inmate, prematurely or over-optimistically released as cured, committing some heinous outrage. Safety first was the watchword; thus the 1774 Act could easily generate rationales for extending confinement.

Hence questions of certification remained contentious. Yet the primary issues changed. Public concern shifted from the wronged individual to the institution at large. Agitation grew over the rising tide of confinement, and a vocal minority began to express its fears. Thus the surgeon Andrew Harper argued in 1789 that far from solving the insanity problem, the new asylums were intensifying it, by confirming the mad in their madness. The asylum was utterly counter-productive:

> big with ignorance and absurdity. [Confinement] 'tis true, may answer the purpose of private interest, and domestic conveniency, but at the same time it destroys all the obligations of humanity... confinement never fails to aggravate the disease. A state of coercion is a state of torture from which the mind, under any circumstances, revolts.[48]

Similar anxieties were voiced by Dr Erasmus Darwin. For him the traditional yardsticks for confinement remained right and proper. Was a man a threat to others, a danger to himself, or helpless? If so, confine him. If not, not. For, all too often, 'confinement retards rather than promotes their cure'. Darwin argued that the old criterion – judging insanity by behaviour not secret thoughts – remained sound:

> If every one, who possesses mistaken ideas, or who puts false estimates on things, was liable to confinement, I know not who of my readers might not tremble at the sight of a madhouse.[49]

Darwin foresaw with trepidation the developments soon to occur, by which the criterion of insanity became a medical diagnosis and families and physicians would concur in a tendency to put the disturbed away not because they were dangerous, but because they were mad, in the hope that they might be cured. Whereas in 1660 it had been exceptional for a lunatic to be put in a madhouse, by the beginning of the nineteenth century confinement was becoming increasingly normal, indeed the resort progressive opinion was recommending.

AN APPROVED RECEIPT TO MAKE A LUNATIC?

One major development during the 'long eighteenth century' was clearly the increase in the number of madhouses, a slow growth through most of the century, accelerating quite rapidly after about 1780, partly in line with aggregate national population growth. Official figures record that there were sixteen metropolitan licensed madhouses in 1774, but forty by 1819; between 1802 and 1819 the total of provincial licensed houses rose from twenty-two to forty-nine. Many were also growing in size. One social implication of this, increasingly marked over time, was a widening segregation of the mad from the sane in the belief that such a policy represented lunatics' best interests. If people became crazed in society, then they must be sequestered 'far from the madding crowd' (Gray knew all about disturbance). By the nineteenth century, this was psychiatric orthodoxy. 'There is no general maxim', opined George Man Burrows in 1828, in the treatment of insanity wherein medical practitioners, ancient or modern, foreign or domestic, are so unanimous as that of separating the patient from all customary associations, his family, and his home.[50]

For Burrows, the battle for confinement had already been won:

Few of the medical profession require arguments or proof to convince them of the great utility of separation. When the friends of any insane person have a doubt, and have not confidence in the advice or probity of their physician, they should consult the works of authors who have treated of insanity, and who can have no interest in the question.[51]

Indeed, by the beginning of Victoria's reign psychiatric doctors were even representing the asylum as, potentially at least, more rational, harmonious, and civilised than society itself. 'Conceive a spacious building', invited W.A.F. Browne,

resembling the palace of a peer, airy, and elevated, and elegant, surrounded by extensive and swelling grounds and gardens. The interior is fitted up with galleries, and workshops, and music rooms. The sun and the air are allowed to enter at every window, the view of the shrubberies and fields and groups of labourers is unobstructed by shutters or bars; all is clean, quiet, and attractive. The inmates all seem to be actuated by the common impulse of enjoyment, all are busy, and delighted by being so. The house and all around appears a hive of industry... There is in this community no compulsion, no chains, no whips, no corporal chastisement, simply because these are proved to be less effectual means of carrying any point than persuasion, emulation, and the desire of obtaining gratification.[52]

The asylum eventually became the preferred medicine for the sickness of civilisation. Yet until the close of the eighteenth

century, its rise was slow, limited and piecemeal, and it is argu-
able that the term 'system' which has occasionally been applied
to this development may be misleading. After all, as late as early
Victorian times, the nation had only a patchy coverage of madhouses, even in heavily populated areas, and despite the passing
of the 1808 Act permitting counties to establish rate-supported
asylums, a mere twelve had acted up to 1845. The eighteenth-
century madhouse map reveals less a coordinated system than
a highly uneven spattering of heterogeneous establishments
– big and small, private enterprise and charity, subscription and
proprietary. The term 'system' hints at a misleading uniformity.
Diversity remained of the essence. Some establishments were
genuinely appalling, as the House of Commons Committee of
1815 heard. But were all so bad? Take Edward Wakefield's reaction to Norman House, a female madhouse in Fulham: '[I] was
delighted with the manner in which they were treated'. Or what
of St Patrick's in Dublin, founded by Jonathan Swift? 'It contains
nearly 200 persons', reported Henry Gray Bennet in 1815,

> 51 of whom are boarders and pay for their treatment...The whole
> clean and in good order; the galleries long, having cross windows;
> cells in the side, and a large window in the end, commanding a
> cheerful view...The cells were 10 feet 8 inches long, 8 feet broad,
> and 12 feet high; the bedsteads wooden; the bedding found by
> the boarders...All the others were paupers, and were maintained
> at the expense of the charity, and to these were found mattress,
> sheets, etc., which were clean and good.[53]

Moreover, if the asylums as a whole did not form a connected
system, individually it would be wrong to think of Georgian
madhouses as manifesting the evils of 'total institutions' in
Goffman's sense. The units were simply too small. Under the
1774 Act, many private asylums were licensed for at most a dozen
people. Also, in contrast to High Victorian times, most private
patients were short-stay. Parry Jones' analysis of late eighteenth-
and early nineteenth-century patients at Hook Norton asylum

in Oxfordshire found that no fewer than sixty-eight per cent of them stayed for less than six months. Similarly, in the early years of Ticehurst, the average patient stay was just a month: the asylum was used for crisis care not routine care.

Not least, the institutions themselves remained low-profile. The Georgian mind looked to the hospital, general or mental, not as a panacea, but as an expedient. Characteristically, in appealing for funds, St Luke's argued pragmatically, 'the principal end of establishing hospitals is that the expense is lessened by providing for a number together'. And distaste for putting people away remained strong. Dr Johnson famously deplored the shutting up of his fellow-poet Kit Smart. 'His infirmities were not noxious to society', Johnson argued, 'He insisted on people praying with him, and I'd as lief pray with Kit Smart as any one else. Another charge was that he did not love clean linen, and I have no passion for it'. Nevertheless, the fact that Smart's family had him confined is surely a significant straw in the wind.

Of course asylums multiplied, and their proprietors took pains to make them attractive to paying clients. But few people before 1800 saw institutions as sovereign remedies. The therapeutic action-centre remained much more personal, emanating from the *virtù* of the proprietor, his family and attendants. Take the Revd Dr Francis Willis, called in to treat George III. Debates will continue as to whether his therapy for the king was brutal or a form of enlightened encounter psychiatry. The real point, however, about his strategy – imperious yet trusting, fixing his royal patient with the eye, using strait-waistcoats and blisters, yet allowing the monarch a razor for shaving and *King Lear* to read – was that it was man-to-man, totally personal. Willis belonged to no medical corporation or 'ism', and wrote no books. He presented himself as a man of mystique, a charismatic healer.

In short, before the nineteenth century it was not the institution that was expected to cure. Madhouses grew up largely as places of safekeeping or as living space. Their rules were principally about diet and duties, not applications of institutional psychiatry. They were as yet underdetermined resources, empty vessels waiting to be filled by new rationalisations, establishments still lacking positive roles. It was not until Bentham had planned his Panopticon penitentiary, Bell and Lancaster the monitor school (the steam engine of the moral world) and Robert Owen his ideal factory environment that the lunatic asylum discovered its destiny within an ideology of salvation through system.

By the time of the Victorians, John Perceval's *Narrative* (1838) was to give the patient's view on how the asylum had become a total psychiatric institution. What of its eighteenth-century precursor? We have a few first-hand accounts – unrepresentative, of course, and almost all written by highly literate males – but better than nothing. Unlike Perceval's, these earlier narratives are not preoccupied with combating psychiatric systems of surveillance; they record no encounter with panoptic control or the surrogate moral family. The autobiographical lucubrations of Alexander Cruden, Samuel Bruckshaw, William Cowper, William Belcher and others are the accounts of men for whom confinement meant not intrusion but exclusion, being left alone in their own cells, and hardly subject to constant spying. When their letters were intercepted, they were enraged; but the narratives of eighteenth-century inmates reveal that, though confined, they actually enjoyed extensive contact with the outside world. They had little to do, however, with fellow patients. With the exception of Metcalf, they depict no Goffmanesque underlife or subculture. So much was Cruden left on his own that he was able to hack his way through the bedstead leg to which he was chained.

Perceval's abiding recollection of Brislington in the 1830s was that Dr Fox's psychiatric regime required that for eventual emancipation he had to accept his role as madman and then play the part to the letter. When, by contrast, earlier ex-patients denounced their confinement, their complaints had little to do with insidious psychiatric oppression. Their anguish and anger were about detention, infringed rights and injustice. Cruden and Bruckshaw saw themselves not as psychiatric guinea pigs but as John Bull in chains; not as patients but as prisoners. Eighteenth-century fiction agreed. In Smollett's *Sir Launcelot Greaves*, the hero, confined by trickery, reflected on the British Bastille:

> People may inveigh against the Bastile in France, and the Inquisition in Portugal; but I would ask if either of these be in reality so dangerous or dreadful as a private madhouse in England under the direction of a ruffian... In England, the most innocent person upon earth is liable to be immured for life under the pretext of lunacy... and subjected to the most brutal treatment from a low-bred barbarian, who raises an ample fortune on the misery of his fellow-creatures, and may, during his whole life, practise this horrid oppression, without question or controul.[54]

Thus the madhouse was criticised principally in terms not of psychiatric regime but of individual rights. Asylum life shared the common coin of other Hanoverian institutions – prisons, public schools, bridewells, the army – epitomising Old Corruption rather than being a panoptic, rational, centralised system of discipline.

Nevertheless, the last third of the century did bring one key shift, the emergence of a 'leading sector' of more presentable, prestigious asylums. This was partly because by then some, such as Fishponds in Bristol, had already existed long enough, passed down in the family from proprietor to proprietor, to have built sound reputations. Moreover, madhouse-keeping was growing entrepreneurial, more confident and conspicuous. Some madhouses were emerging from the shadows. They were being advertised intensively in the newspapers; a few solicited visits and were the subject of active publicity – classically the York Retreat, the first asylum actually to have a full length book devoted to it, doubling as advertisement and scientific report. In his *Description of the Retreat* (1813) Samuel Tuke incorporated comments on the Retreat by visitors, staked its claims, and wrote its history. The glowing reports in the *Edinburgh Review* and elsewhere echoed the optimism of Tuke's book itself. Here, for the first time, was a lunatic asylum of which Britons could be proud.

In other words, an important change finally came over the public face of certain private madhouses. Some became notorious as Augean stables, needing their parliamentary Hercules (he proved extremely tardy). Others, however, began to 'come out', achieving prominence and respectability, establishing the asylum's place in the sun. The result was that by the early nineteenth century what was on the agenda was not (*pace* Rothman) the discovery of the asylum, nor indeed its abolition, but rather its reform.

WAS MADNESS INCREASING?

From Georgian mad-doctors to Victorian psychiatrists, the consensus was that insanity was on the increase, in fact mushrooming quite disproportionately beyond the net surge in population. Numerous early nineteenth-century authors, such as Dr William Blacks, attempted to prove this by figures, capitalising on the data yielded by Bethlem's records, the new Town and Country Register of Madhouses, and by House of Commons Reports. Moreover, their conclusions carried conviction, because their notion of an epidemic of insanity coincided with common experience (were there not more madhouses appearing to meet the need?), with certain sensational events (above all the extremely public 'madness' of George III), and with Jeremiads about social disintegration. In a hybrid lamentation drawing both on Classical Humanism and on the Cheynian sociology of the English malady, affluence and luxury were blamed for fermenting epidemic madness. Commenting on the 'truly astonishing... progress of insanity', Benjamin Faulkner judged:

> The rapidity with which the disorder has spread over this country, within the last fifty years, may be attributed, in a great measure, to the encrease of luxury,... inordinate desires, and the indulgence of inordinate passions, not unfrequently subjugate reason, and produce insanity.[55]

In blaming rampant individualism, he was echoed by William Rowley:

> The agitations of passions, [and] this liberty of thinking and acting with less restraint than in other nations, force a great quantity of blood to the head, and produce greater varieties of madness in this country, than is observed in others. Religious and civil toleration are productive of political and religious madness.[56]

These late eighteenth-century strictures were often repeated. Thus in 1824, Alexander Morison argued that 'insanity increases with civilisation'. It is

> stated to be very small in South America, and among the Indian tribes, &c. and to be very considerable in China. It is therefore probable, that the increasing civilisation and luxury of this country, co-operating with hereditary disposition, tends rather to increase the numbers in proportion to the population.[57]

And so ultimately, such views primed the pump for *fin-de-siècle* degenerationism. Yet although the medical response to this tide of insanity could itself be quite hysterical ('Madness, strides like a Colossus over this island', boomed the London physician John Reid in 1808), the data fuelling this alarm look quite modest to us. Official data found only a couple of thousand confined mad people. George Man Burrows was to stress how readily a rise in madness' visibility might be mistaken for its real increase; perhaps what was mainly rising was alarm. But voices like his were a minority.

So *was* madness striding Colossus-like? Dr Edward Hare has recently attempted statistically to show that there was an authentic epidemic of madness at this time, hinting at a secular rise of organic schizophrenia. Scull's sceptical rejoinder, however, rightly casts such doubt upon the reliability of the figures and of our capacity to extrapolate from them, as to render the exercise speculative in the extreme. Scull endorses Burrows' insight that the data tell us much more about psychological reactions than about any epidemic 'real presence'.

Nevertheless, various scholars have echoed the mad-doctors, contending either that there was a genuine explosion, or at least that violent social disruption was making insanity increasingly impossible to handle any longer by traditional, largely informal means. Above all, this alleged growth of disturbance has typically been blamed on capitalist economic dislocation. Industrialisation, Doerner hypothesised, caused profound psychic trauma by alienating people from Nature and from traditional communities, destabilising face-to-face relations, and casting people into the cash-nexus rat race. Competitive individualism lived off anxiety – after all, Locke had written that 'the chief spur to human industry and action is uneasiness'. And this created an artificial, false world of the imagination, of 'speculation', South Sea Bubbles and bank crashes. Moreover (Doerner argues) the Protestant ethic enshrined neurotic attitudes towards work, driving some to distraction, while making the work-shy and the workless seem sub-rational. As Foucault would see it, within the bourgeois moral economy, rationality sided with labour while, on the other hand, idleness became unreason. These repudiating the bourgeois duties of labour did so at their own peril.

All such extrapolations seem too schematic and doctrinaire. Ultra-rapid industrialisation and factory labour remained extremely localised, directly disrupting only a tiny fraction of the population. There is no decisive evidence that urbanisation either created traumatic anomie or reduced communities' ability to cope with disturbed people. The regions most conspicuous for asylum-building were not the industrial boom-towns. Georgian private asylums commonly sprang up away from dense population centres, in Kent, Sussex, Wiltshire, Gloucestershire etc.; and their catchment areas were quite restricted. Many heavily urbanised manufacturing regions, such as the West Midlands, were slow to get licensed houses or, after

1808, county lunatic asylums. Lancashire was particularly thinly supplied with private asylums.

It is a plausible hypothesis that industrialising processes which disrupted life and work rhythms would also disturb minds; that new relations of production which alienated man from man, workers from Nature, capital from labour and reduced whole people to 'hands' would also cause alienation of mind. But, when scrutinised in detail, the supportive evidence remains unconvincing. As Michael Anderson has shown, rapid migration into factory towns could renew social and familial solidarity as much as jeopardise it. John Walton's pioneering empirical studies of the problems of handling disordered people in industrialising Lancashire indicate that there was no catastrophic crisis in the abilities – or willingness – of families or communities to look after their disturbed folk.

The hypothesis that the steam-pressures of a market-dominated and putatively more nerve-racking economy were driving more people insane remains unproven. It receives little obvious support from scrutiny of the life circumstances of patients committed to asylums in the eighteenth century. We will never have anything resembling full profiles of them, but casual sampling indicates that an immense scatter of different ranks and occupations ended up confined for a constellation of reasons. It is first worth noting that male admissions notably outstripped female, a pattern reversed in county asylums after the mid-nineteenth century. Georgian asylum admissions lend no support to the view that male chauvinist values were disproportionately penalising women with mental disorders, or indeed that the asylum was significantly patriarchy's device to punish difficult women.

In the eighteenth-century asylum, it must next be stressed, patients from the middling or well-off classes were probably disproportionately represented as compared to the poor. The Victorian public asylum was later, no doubt, a 'technological fix' to process the mad poor; indeed by the 1880s something like ninety per cent of all asylum inmates in England were officially

'paupers'. But although Foucault and Doerner have asserted
that the eighteenth-century madhouse was 'specifically for the
poor insane', Georgian private madhouses were social micro-
cosms which commonly included a ballast of parish paupers
(providing a dependable income base for the owner) but also
tradesmen, widows, clergymen, and farmers. Proprietors angled
to raise the social tone, hence fee level, of their patient intake.
Thus when Ticehurst opened in 1792, the typical patient was
the one-guinea-a-week person. Within a decade, its growing
prestige had put the average patient into the two-guinea-a-
week bracket. The Georgians had better sites than the asylum
for disciplining the mob.

If the asylum was not bulging with the indigent, or with
victimised women, who was inside? The case notes which
mad-doctors such as William Pargeter and William Perfect published show a spread of social strata and occupations: crashed
businessmen, melancholy clergymen, old-maidish spinsters,
rebellious teenagers, *soi-disant* princes and popes, drunken
labourers, senile servants, religious fanatics, and so forth. Some
had been driven to distraction by financial problems (it was
said that the South Sea Bubble's boom unhinged more than its
bursting). Others were haunted by noises in the head, above all
religious despair and suicidal impulses. And many had collapsed
under the miseries of family and personal crises – a bullying
spouse or tyrant parents, an unhappy love affair, acute loneliness
or a bereavement. William Perfect's patients and their ailments
would have been familiar to Richard Napier a century and a
half earlier. Wards full of sufferers from general paralysis of the
insane, the senile and demented and sexual offenders were a
Victorian development.

Above all, there is little to suggest that the 'long eighteenth
century' unleashed 'witch-hunts' against the mad, concerted
drives to put deviants under lock and key. Of course it was
said that society was endangered by 'madness'. Thus Dr Johnson
characterised London:

Here malice, rapine, accident conspire. And now a rabble rages,
now a fire;[58]

Such events as the Gordon Riots would be dubbed mad conta-
gions inflaming the minds of the mob, and Coleridge called the
French Revolution 'the Giant Frenzy'. But – notwithstanding
Pope's *Dunciad* – there was no practical fear that silent armies of
the insane or perverts were sapping the very sinews of society,
comparable to the way in which, from the mid-nineteenth
century, degenerationist scares seized the social imagination.
In so far as the masses were seen as 'mad', it was essentially as
'fools' – bovine bumpkins, disqualified, of course, from society,
but hardly threats to its survival.

If, then, the evidence for any real disproportionate epidemic
of disturbance is doubtful, how should we explain the growth
of madhouses? It was not due to Parliament: public legislation
and money were not to come until the nineteenth century.
Collective philanthropy also remained of scant importance.
Rather, the main growth-sector was the private one: people
were being confined on the initiative of friends and family
rather than by the authorities.

The rise of this Georgian lunacy trade can best be regarded
as one aspect of the emergence of a thriving service sector in
the *laissez-faire* economy at large. In a buoyant market, entrepreneurs sprouted in many fields, from mills and music to
madness, combining business acumen with technical skills, to
provide services for which there were at least potential buyers.
Madhouses and mad-doctors arose from the same soil which
generated demand for general practitioners, dancing masters,
man-midwives, face painters, drawing tutors, estate managers,
landscape gardeners, architects, journalists and that host of other
white-collar, service, and quasi-professional occupations which
a society with increased economic surplus and pretensions to
civilisation first found it could afford, and soon found it could
not do without. In the 'birth of a consumer society', one growing item of consumption was the services of madhouses, not

because affluence drove people crazy, but because its commercial ethos made trading in insanity feasible.

Just as Wedgwood had to use astute salesmanship to create a demand for his ceramics ('vase madness'), so madhouse-keepers likewise had to prime the pump. There was as yet no high Victorian professional etiquette hindering advertising in the press. As the Prussian von Archenholz remarked of English advertisers:

> One person informs you that his MAD-HOUSE is at your service; a second keeps a boarding-house for idiots; a good natured man-midwife pays the utmost attention to ladies in certain situations, and promises to use the most scrupulous secrecy. Physicians offer to cure you of all manner of disorders, for a mere trifle.[59]

When Ticehurst was founded, custom was initially a mere trickle, indicating that demand had to be 'created' or at least nursed, rather than being a dammed-up lake seeking outlet. Nevertheless, once a 'supply' was created, demand soon rose to capacity. Indeed, Benjamin Faulkner lamented how readily the places available were filled:

> The number of unhappy objects seem to have increased in proportion to the increase of houses licensed for their reception.[60]

A poignant example of how cases might become suitable for asylum places where none had existed before is offered by the fate of a wandering female simpleton near Bristol in 1776. Known as Louisa, she lived rough, begged food, and slept in a haystack:

> Some ladies in the vicinity having become acquainted with her condition, she was supplied with food, but neither solicitations nor threats induced her to sleep in a house... and as her mental

derangement increased she was removed to St. Peter's Hospital in Bristol. How long she was detained there is unknown, but she regained her liberty in 1777 or 1778, and immediately returned to the stackyard at Bourton, where, strange to say she remained nearly four years, receiving food from the neighbouring gentry, but obstinately refusing the protection of a roof, even in winter.[61]

Rather like the Wild Boy of Aveyron, however, Louisa proved no match for Bristol's do-gooders, who clearly, by the 1780s, were of a mind to think that such misfits needed the protection of the asylum:

In 1781, the condition of the poor woman excited the interest of Miss Hannah More, who with the assistance of friends had her removed to a private lunatic asylum at Hanham.[62]

Thus public authorities showed little zeal for confining a harmless lunatic (she was, after all, released from St Peter's), but humanitarians proved more determined.

Nursing this new demand, a clutch of madhouses arose largely through the speculative activities of their proprietors. Though often anticipating demand, asylums, once established, finally flourished. The founding of county lunatic asylums in the early nineteenth century merely echoed the process. When they were first legalised in 1808, there was widespread bleating that they would prove white elephants. Indeed some did briefly operate half-empty. They quickly filled up, however. Create an institution and it soon becomes indispensable. Rather as with geriatric homes in the twentieth century, initial moral repugnance was papered over with plausible moral rationalisations.

The prime movers in this process of articulating a market were thus the 'mental entrepreneurs' who founded the madhouses. What led them to do it? Those laypeople, men and women, who set them up were simply carving out a more specialised sector of the vast contemporary board-and-lodging business, both private and underwritten by funds from the Poor Laws. Boarding the mad, though perhaps unpleasant, was surely lucrative. And it could be argued that, among medical proprietors, career prospects weighed particularly heavily. The pool of medical practitioners was spreading during the century. In a congested occupation, specialisation made sense. Some became venereologists or obstetricians; some army, navy, or colonial surgeons; other opportunists went in for anatomical lecturing or medical authorship. Among these new niches was that of the madhouse proprietor.

Prospects were bright too. Studies have shown how rich the pickings were for successful operators such as William Hunter in that often calumniated medical specialism, man-midwifery. The same is true for madhouse proprietorship. William Battie got rich from his private madhouse, as did the Newington family from keeping Ticehurst. Madhouses promised profits denied to general practitioners. The owner was guaranteed a constant income for every patient, and he could charge not just for medical services but for lodgings, laundry, food, attendance, and many extras. As John Gregory commented, no diseases were 'so lucrative as those of the nervous kind'.

Thus the key development, accelerating in the second half of the eighteenth century, was the emergence of a cadre of ambitious, able people – increasingly, medically qualified men – aiming to make a living, and more than that, a career and a name, through asylums. According to Thomas Bakewell, as late as the mid-eighteenth century, the mad-doctor had still been commonly regarded as a 'conjurer', practising the 'black art'. This changed. In time madhouse-keeping became an object of pride not shame; helping, not hindering, a medical career. William Battie rose to become President of the Royal College of Physicians; Anthony Addington, who had kept a madhouse in Reading for five years, became physician to George III and father to a prime minister. Building respectable reputations, doctors such as Thomas Arnold at Leicester and Edward Long Fox at Brislington helped to disarm public suspicion, and put the madhouse on the map. It would be misleadingly premature to talk of the rise of the psychiatric profession, for up to the close of the century, no *esprit de corps* had formed among them. They operated in isolation, highly individualistically, as the Battie-Monro feud or the unseemly rivalries over the treatment of George III reveal. With French disdain, Pinel curled his lip at it all with his phrase 'empiric psychiatry', and John Haslam did not mince his words when he later termed it 'a species of farming'. Not till the 1840s did professional organisations and journals appear. All the same, the emergence in England of institutions for the mad is best regarded not as an act of state, nor as a work of social control or medical police, nor even as bowing to necessity – the sheer pressure of madness! – but rather as the triumph of these captains of confinement.

What was the impact of the increasing presence of the 'respectable asylum' by the early nineteenth century? Did the availability of madhouses constitute sufficient rationale for confinement? Did the institution change attitudes, eroding social tolerance for the disordered, creating a marginalisation of the mad? Was the net of madness being cast more widely than before? The situation is complicated. In some ways little had changed. In 1800 as in 1700 the prime criterion for confinement was danger rather than psychiatric benefit. By 1850 things were different. By then, even erstwhile libertarians such as Dr John Conolly had come round to the view that screwballs were best treated in the asylum.

Yet, already in the eighteenth century, the availability of private madhouses was leading to the confinement of people who were essentially just social nuisances or embarrassments – provoking Dr Johnson's heartfelt defence of Kit Smart's liberty. Johnson feared that his own abnormal mannerisms might one day cascade into the kind of derangement which would lead to confinement; hence his celebrated delivery of a padlock to Hester Thrale. No man such as Johnson, dreading the uncertain continuance of reason, would countenance Bethlem. Yet great oddity was in fact still widely tolerated, and there is scant evidence, during the years of Revolutionary wars, of the use of the madhouse as a weapon against plebeians or radicals. In the eighteenth century, as the contrast between Smart and Joanna Southcott shows, it was family rather than the state which took action over the disturbed. And many families clearly still believed it was more caring – or less ignominious – to keep people at home than in an asylum.

4

The Making of Psychiatry

TRADITIONS

When and whence psychiatry? Hunter and Macalpine thought there had been *Three Hundred Years of Psychiatry*, 1535–1860. By contrast, Sir Aubrey Lewis plumped for an epiphany around the 1790s, with Tuke, Chiarugi and Pinel, thanks to whom the mad could finally be treated 'on medical rather than moral lines. They could at last speak for themselves. Psychiatry was thus born'. Behind the trivial matters of semantics and anachronism which these discrepancies raise, real issues are at stake, posing the problem of how distinctive bodies of knowledge and sets of practices came about.

Of course, 'psychiatry' is as old as the hills if we treat it as a portmanteau term for all attempts to 'minister to minds diseased'. High and low cultures alike have needed remedies, time out of mind, for the sick in head and heart. Hundreds of such traditional cures were collected in Burton's *Anatomy of Melancholy*, ranging from the 'spiritual' such as music ('a tonick to the saddened soul'), to polypharmaceutical therapies. Suffering from 'head melancholy'? Then 'Take a Ram's head', advises Burton,

> that never meddled with an Ewe, cut off at a blow, and, the horns only take away, boil it well skin and wool together, after it is well sod [i.e. boiled], take out the brains, and put these spices to it, Cinnamon, Ginger, Nutmeg, Mace, Cloves, in equal parts of half an ounce, mingle the powder of these spices with it, and heat them in a platter upon a chafing-dish of coals together, stirring them well, that they do not burn; take heed it be not overmuch dried, or dryer than a Calves brains ready to be eaten. Keep it so prepared, and for three days give it the patient fasting, so that he fast two hours after it... For fourteen days let him use this diet, drink no wine, &c.[1]

Best of all, however, in Burton's view are regimen and mirth, and his parting words to the melancholic are: 'Be not solitary, be not idle'.

Over the next centuries, advice poured off the presses telling the sick at heart how to keep their minds healthy within healthy bodies. When George III became delirious loyal subjects sent in remedies by the score, ranging from crab's claw powder to ground ivy, from electricity to asses' blood, not forgetting the application of lambskins. With all his rustic omniscience, William Cobbett also dished out words of wisdom. Paramount in 'the management of babies', he argued, was the matter of preserving '*sanity of mind*':

> [Many] become insane from the misconduct or neglect of parents, and generally from the children being committed to the care of servants. I knew, in Pennsylvania, a child as fine, and as sprightly, and as intelligent a child as ever was born, shut into a dark closet by a maid servant, in order to terrify it into silence. The thoughtless creature first menaced it with sending it to 'the bad place,' as the phrase is there; and, at last, to reduce it to silence, put it into the closet, shut the door, and went out of the room.

> She went back, in a few minutes, and found the child in a fit
> [and it]... was for life an idiot.[2]

However homespun, Cobbett's wisdom chimed with Locke's notion of how madness arose from false associations of ideas. Similarly, through aiming at a higher social class, George Cheyne spelt out simple living as a prophylactic against hypochondriasis.

But what if remedy was needed, not prevention? The range of madness cures available in the common mental medicine chest was quite staggering. In the seventeenth century Thomas Sydenham recommended Venice Treacle and venesection for mania, while at a more popular level, Nicholas Culpeper thought that herbal remedies such as water pimpernel and marsh marigold were best, and folk wisdom was still advocating the use of holy wells and pools. Magical charms retained their supporters. John Wesley detailed many such remedies in his *Primitive Physick* (1747), and put some to the test:

> Give decoction of agrimony four times a day. Or, rub the head
> several time a day with vinegar in which ground-ivy leaves have
> been infused.

> Or, take daily an ounce of distilled vinegar. Or, boil the juice
> of ground-ivy with sweet oil and white wine into an ointment.
> Shave the head, anoint it therewith, and chafe it every other day
> for three weeks. Bruise also the leaves and bind them on the head,
> and give three spoonsful of the juice, warm, every morning. This
> generally cures melancholy. The juice alone taken twice-a day
> will cure. Or, be electrified. (Tried.)[3]

Medication, using kitchen physick, was thus every bit as central to the 'little tradition' as it was to the faculty's armamentarium. But another popular mode of healing consisted of words of comfort to troubled souls, to soothe and lift the spirits. Timothy Bright's *A Treatise on Melancholie* (1586), the first major English tract on the subject, is explicitly addressed to a victim – real

or fictitious – named 'M'. Like many later treatments, such
as Timothy Rogers' *A Discourse Concerning Trouble of Mind
and the Disease of Melancholy* (1691), Bright's book was itself
written by a sufferer. Such manuals characteristically urged
gentleness and sympathy. 'Look upon those that are under this
woful Disease of Melancholy with great pity and compassion',
Rogers stressed:

> Do not use harsh Speeches to your Friends when they are under
> the disease of Melancholy... They may fret and perplex, and
> enrage them more, but they will never do them the least good...
> If you be severe in your speeches, they'll never be persuaded that
> it is in kindness, and so not regard at all what you say.[4]

Above all – contrast Freud! – trust was vital:

> You must be so kind to your Friends under this Disease, as to
> believe what they say. Or however, that their apprehensions are
> such as they tell you they are; do not you think that they are at
> ease when they say they are in pain.[5]

Rogers took the same line as physicians such as Richard
Blackmore – that it was countertherapeutic to dismiss melancholy as mere imagination:

> It is a foolish course which some take with their Melancholy
> Friends, to answer all their Complaints and Moans with this, That
> its nothing but Fancy; nothing but Imagination and Whimsey.
> It is a Real Disease, a Real Misery that they are tormented
> with...[6]

Instead, he contended, melancholy ought to be regarded like any
regular somatic malady:

> Suppose when you have the Toothach, or Headach, and people,
> when you complain, should tell you 'tis nothing but Fancy, would

not you think their carriage to be full of cruelty? and would it
not vex you to find that you cannot be believed?[7]

Yet was it wise to encourage melancholics to pour out about
their troubles? That was hotly in dispute, and many thought
that articulating and dwelling upon morbid fears merely
compounded them. Indeed, doctors and laymen alike typically
preferred diversions. Thus Samuel Johnson strove to convince
the hypochondriacal James Boswell that it was useless to try to
'think down' one's anxieties:

> Make it an invariable and obligatory law to yourself, never to
> mention your own mental diseases; if you are never to speak of
> them you will think on them little, and if you think little of them,
> they will molest you rarely.[8]

Johnson urged instead an almost frantic syllabus of distraction
for the distracted person:

> Let him take a course of chymistry, or a course of rope-dancing,
> or a course of anything to which he is inclined at the time. Let
> him contrive to have as many retreats for his mind as he can, as
> many things to which it can fly from itself.[9]

Forms of 'talking cure' had their advocates, such as Dr Bernard
Mandeville in his *A Treatise of the Hypochondriack and Hysterick
Passions* (1711). In this fascinating fictional dialogue, Mandeville
depicts a nuclear family effectively curing itself of 'nervous disorders' simply through 'now let's talk about me' sessions with their
sagely taciturn physician. All the indications are that sufferers in
practice sought mutual reinforcement and exchanged advice.
For example, early in the eighteenth century the edgy Dudley
Ryder confided to his diary some tips against depression:

> Tuesday, March 20. Met... Mr Whatley and Mr Smith... Mr
> Whatley showed us a paper which he had writ for the cure of the

vapours. Mr. Whatley proposes that a man should fix to himself
one determined end, whether it be riches or wisdom or whatever
it be, that he should keep this habitually in view. [10]

The need to focus one's energies was a common theme of self-
help advice, though this could lead to obsession, which was just
as dangerous. Boswell in particular – despite Johnson's warnings!
– loved to blab about his own anguish, albeit guiltily, suspecting
that it was an indulgence which confirmed rather than lifted
the melancholy fit:

> Breakfasted with Seward, and was a little relieved by talking of
> melancholy and hearing how often he was afflicted with it. I was
> sensible it was wrong to speak of it. But the torment was such
> that I could not conceal it. [11]

Thus popular maxims and treatments for the disturbed formed
part of medical self-help culture of early modern England. Yet in
addition to these vernacular salves for the sad, specialist expertise
was also crystallising. Indeed, by the last third of the century,
perhaps some thirty to fifty practitioners were primarily in the
business of treating the disturbed, many of them owning madhouses. Boswell himself enthused over Dr Thomas Arnold of
Leicester, a physician whose name was familiar to George III
and whose writings were read by Hester Thrale. Without much
anachronism, we might call such people embryonic professional
psychiatrists. Their rise marked a change. For until then, victims
of frenzy or melancholy would typically seek aid from people
who did not deal exclusively in mental disorders. They might,
of course, highly exceptionally, get help from another strange
person – a jesting fool, imparting *Pills to Purge Melancholy*; a
holy fool, to bless; or even a witch, to purge a curse. More
likely, however, if they could afford it, they would have gone
to a regular physician who, regarding the complaint as organic,
would probably have prescribed medicines and regimen, as is
shown by many cases of Thomas Willis, practising in Oxford

as a young physician around the 1650s. General physicians of course went on treating mood and thought disorders. Thus the letters of Dr Erasmus Darwin between the 1760s and 1790s are full of advice, friendly and practical, to his hypochondriacal friends and clients.

Clergymen too had traditionally been consulted by sufferers, especially conscience-racked souls seeking solace and succour. A few might even perform exorcism, though in the Anglican Church this had been forbidden by the Canons of 1604.

Or – a further possibility – sufferers might seek out unortho-dox healers, astrologers, cunning-men, wise-women, or quacks. With their implicit or explicit appeals to 'faith', or at least to the sick person's mind or will, 'irregulars' made a speciality of treating those intractable disorders – increasingly called 'nervous' – which baffled regular physick. Stuart monarchs healed by the 'royal touch'; later 'sex therapists' such as James Graham tack-led impotence; Mesmeric healers made their presence felt; and nostrum vendors such as Wilham Brodum and Samuel Solomon marketed potions (such as the 'Balm of Gilead') for nervous depression. Most such irregulars made great play of special techniques of somatic healing – e.g. the action of Mesmer's animal magnetic fluid. Thus Michael Herwig's *The Art of Curing Sympathetically or Magnetically, Proved to be the Most True Both by its Theory and Practice* (1700) claimed special powers in the 'Cure of Madness'. Investigators and critics divined that in so far as their healing actually worked, it was because they drew upon some ill-understood, even occult, powers of sympathy. Skilfully deploying suggestion, yet doing so through the medium of somatic therapies and material medicaments, such charismatic healers claimed good success rates.

These distinct modes of healing just mentioned were not mutually exclusive. In Jacobean England, the Revd Richard Napier combined the callings of physician and parson; well over a century later, John Wesley viewed insanity as diabolical possession yet was also eager to make use of drugs and medi-cal machines, not least electric shock treatment for the mad.

Wesley's contemporary the Revd Dr Francis Willis, George III's mad-doctor, was a beneficed clergyman who had moved into medicine and become a madhouse proprietor. Before the mid-eighteenth century, hardly anyone specialised exclusively in mental disorders, either as a vocation or as a livelihood. Rather, it was a sideline.

In this chapter, I shall plot the emergence of a cluster of healers – exclusively male – who pioneered speciality practices in treating the disturbed. This development went hand in hand with new ways of thinking, among laity and professionals alike, which increasingly regarded disturbed cognition and conduct as posing distinctive problems beyond the province of both traditional divinity and general physick. In particular, currents in metaphysics and medicine were proposing fresh paradigms of mind and body, behaviour and self, and thereby opening a new field eventually to be denominated the psychiatric. For this, the catalyst proved to be the associated emergence of bricks-and-mortar institutions for lunatics; for the presence for the first time of concentrations of patients, isolated in madhouses, encouraged close 'scientific' surveillance of delusions and delinquencies, stirring the clinical 'psychology' of the disturbed. This hitherto unparalleled scrutiny of lunatics under controlled conditions, particularly while interacting with keepers, formed the matrix for the practical (experimental) discipline of managing madness.

These developments will be dealt with in the chapter. But two pointers may initially be helpful. First, the emergence of specialisation. Around 1700, the top practitioners for the disturbed were all-round physicians: within a century they were specialists. Certain early eighteenth-century practitioners, such as Cheyne, Blackmore, and Mandeville, of course gained fame for their attention to nervous complaints. But they also wrote copiously about gout, fevers, plague, diet, general regimen and myriad other complaints, and cultivated large general practices. This was to change. There still remained many general physicians esteemed for their astute handling of disordered minds, as for example Sir Richard Warren or Sir George Baker, physicians to George III.

But by their time, specialists in insanity had emerged – men such as Thomas Arnold, William Perfect, Samuel Newington and Joseph Mason Cox – whose expertise commonly went hand in hand with owning a madhouse. Mad-doctoring came of age on the day in 1788 – 5 December in fact – when the failure of the king's physicians-in-ordinary to master George III's delirium was acknowledged by the summons to the specialist, if very much despised, mad-doctor Francis Willis.

This is not to imply that these emergent specialist mad-doctors as yet formed a coherent cadre. They were generally self-trained in their expertise, and close teacher–pupil relations were uncommon. In the lunacy trade, blood was thicker than water and craftskills were typically passed down from father to son in family businesses. As yet, mad-doctors had won no professional identity, association or influence. They did not unite to form pressure-groups to lobby Parliament or save the nation. Instead, each was his own man in matters of theory and therapeutics. Early specialist mental medicine was eclectic, pluralist and divided. The unreformed state saw no use for an expert corps.

In general medicine, 'fringe' and quack doctors were typically allowed to practise in peace in the Georgian age, with little interference from the state or medical colleges, and this applies particularly for mad-doctors. Anything went, from Mesmerism to heroic purging, from swing chairs to country walks. Doctors, as well as the laity, publicly touted a great range of remedies for restoring George III – Betsy Sheridan spoke of 'Great Wars and Rumours of War among the medical Tribe' – in the eyes of critics, discrediting the experts' pretensions out of their own mouths. Although this chapter surveys the emergence of 'psychiatry', we should not expect to find a neat and tidy professional cohort emerging.

Second – and a related point – Georgian physicians of the mind were primarily interested in madness at an individual, clinical level, within the framework of general practice or the lunacy trade. Especially in the first half of the century, they were mainly dealing with patients still living within the community like the fictional gentry family depicted in Mandeville's *Treatise*, or the recipient of Timothy Rogers' advice. Later, the asylum patient becomes the focus of attention. Few Georgian mad-doctors centrally addressed themselves to larger questions of state policy, national mental hygiene, legal reform, or the threat of pauper lunatics. They did not set themselves up as bureaucrats of madness. Before 1800 there was almost no jurisprudential discussion of lunacy and the courts. Nor was medicine for the mad yet considered worthy of a university chair – not even at Edinburgh – nor of recognition by the medical colleges. As yet, the art had no collective face.

THE ANATOMY OF THE NERVES

New 'mad-doctors' meant new knowledges. Major developments occurred during the 'long eighteenth century' in medical, scientific, and philosophical explanations of human nature and behaviour both normal and pathological, providing resources enabling the treatment of the mad to become a distinctive body of theory and practice. Among these changes, innovations in gross anatomy and physiology provided an initial impetus, by forefronting a model of the animal economy laying more stress upon the solids than the fluids, upon local organs and lesions rather than general metabolic equilibrium, and specifically upon the brain rather than the abdomen.

At least until the mid-seventeenth century, humoralism was still prominent among physicians and laymen alike. Gradually, its capacity to provide satisfying explanations of disturbed thoughts and actions fell under a cloud. 'Science' denied that the womb could wander, and found no evidence that the spleen's function was to absorb black bile. Instead, new hypotheses of the metabolism more consonant with the chemical or the mechanical philosophy commanded attention. Thus when Thomas Willis explained how low spirits could issue from the guts, he invoked not humours but chemical pathogenesis:

The learned Dr Willis [reflected Richard Blackmore] has formed
a Theory on this Subject... by which he accounts for all these
Effects, by the good or bad Disposition of a Leven or Ferment;...
while it remains in a regular State, is a great Assistant and Refiner
of the animal Spirits, and when it is perverted, and becomes too
sowre and austere, he makes it the chief, if not the sole Cause of
Hypocondriacal Symptoms.[12]

Indeed Blackmore himself, early in the eighteenth century,
largely accepted Willis' interpretation, arguing that intestinal
ferments agitated the nerves and disordered the brain:

If the Juices... contained in any of the Bowels, degenerate, and
become immoderately acid, sharp, pungent and austere, they urge
and vellicate the Nerves so much, and irritate and scatter the
Spirits in such a violent Manner, that the whole intellectual and
animal Administration is violated and disturbed, while the Mind
is deprived of proper Instruments for its Operations.[13]

Above all, humoralism was succumbing to new physiologies
which emphasised the network of fibres forming the nervous
system. Exactly how the nerve mechanisms organised sensation
and motion baffled agreement. Particularly in Boerhaave's ultra-
influential teachings, the prime model was hydraulic: nerves were
seen as hollow pipes, filled under pressure by a fluid composed
of the subtlest of bodily particles. This hydraulic theory readily gained credence, not least because it could incorporate the
old Galenist doctrine of animal spirits, those superfine agents
mediating between body and soul. Graphic and easy to visualise,
it pictured depression and disorientation as corporeal plumbing
failures. If the tubes became clogged – if, for instance, 'heavy'
diet and low habits were indulged – the fluids grew sluggish,
causing 'heaviness' and 'lowness'.

Gradually, however, this hydraulic model was in turn challenged in popularity by theories seeing the nerves not as hollow
pipes, but as wires. Communication along these strings might be

seen as by electrical impulse, or more commonly through the
active medium of ill-defined 'animal spirits'. Good spirits would
be ensured by the uninterrupted rapidity of their passage, itself
a measure of the tone of the fibre in tension.

Yet minute controversies over the precise mechanism of the
nerves mattered less in reorientating interpretations of mental
disturbance than did the alternative geography of anguish and
action all of them implied. Thomas Willis' neuroanatomy, developed from the 1660s, proved seminal, being widely quoted and
debated, if rarely thoroughly accepted, in the next generations.
Pervading the body and gathered along the spine, nerves passed
through the neck to the cortex, where – and this was Willis' particular claim – distinct sectors of the brain performed a division
of labour. The corpora striata served the function of perception,
the corpus callosum was the seat of imagination, the midbrain
the site of the instincts; vital centres were focused in the cerebel-
lum, and memory in the cerebral cortex. Consciousness was an
attribute of the brain. Whereas in the old humoral physiology the
power-house of the animal economy seemed to depend upon
the stomach, the liver, the heart, the blood, following Willis it
was the head that dominated. Of course, the viscera remained
of extraordinary importance within the new neuroanatomy,
through their resonant sympathies with the brain. As the clinician William Heberden was still emphasising at the close of the
century,

> The nerves of the stomach and bowels have so great a domain
> and controul over the whole nervous system, and these parts are
> so generally disordered in hypochondriac and hysteric patients,
> that, in my judgement, the best medicines will be such as correct
> their acidities... [14]

Nevertheless, in the new physiology understanding pain and
response, sensation and reaction, was increasingly a matter of
tracking the pathways of the nerves; and a proper 'neurologie'
(the term was Willis') demanded explanations relating to the

brain. The possibility was opening for the anatomy of melancholy to become a specialist field for nerve and brain experts,
the latter-day neurologists.

This emphasising of the nerves suggested that mental disturbances had a distinct pathology, perhaps quite specifically
in lesions of the brain. The nerves also assumed a further
importance. In the mid-century physiologies of Robert Whytt,
Alexander Munro II and William Cullen in particular, the
nervous system became pivotal to the thinking dominant at
that great 'nerve centre' of Enlightenment medical education,
Edinburgh University. Cullen argued that, strictly speaking, all
diseases without exception are 'nervous', all being mediated
through nervous excitation. Above all, he coined the term 'neurosis' to refer to those particular diseases of the nervous system
causing sensory-motor alterations, that is to say,

> all those preternatural affections of sense and motion, which are
> without pyrexia as a part of the primary disease; and all those
> which do not depend upon a topical affection of the organs,
> but more upon general affection of the nervous system, and of
> those powers of the system upon which sense and motion more
> especially depend.[15]

In Cullen's nosology, one of the key subdivisions of neuroses
were the species of insanity. Viewed thus, insanity took its place
in the classification as a distinct disease entity, rather than merely
as a bundle of abnormal symptoms.

Particularly pregnant for the future was Cullen's notion that
mania and melancholy were functions of the intensity of the flow
of nervous impulse, or of abnormal fluctuations of excitation:

> Delirium may depend... upon some inequality in the excite-
> ment of the brain... for... our reasoning or intellectual operations
> always require the orderly and exact recollection or memory of
> associated ideas; so, if any part of the brain is not excited, or not
> excitable, that recollection cannot properly take place, while at

the same time other parts of the brain, more excited and excitable, may give false perceptions, associations, and judgments... [16]

This doctrine – which may be said to 'physiologise' Locke's associationism – that mental 'up' or 'down' swings registered oscillations of nervous excitement and prostration was eagerly developed by other influential authors, particularly those, such as Erasmus Darwin, who had studied in Edinburgh. Addressing the problem of the interplay of organic life with consciousness, Darwin envisaged a continuum of stimuli leading from elemental physical irritations, up through sensations and volitions, to the association of ideas, all mediated through nervous reflexes. Discrepancies between organic excitations ('irritation') and their enregistration in consciousness ('volition', 'association') commonly found expression in mental disorders. Comparable ideas were also central to the popular system of Cullen's pupil, John Brown, who made excitability the master-key to health. For Brown, mania was a state of overexcitation, melancholy of underexcitement (technically 'sthenic' and 'asthenic' conditions). Brown recommended counterbalancing treatment by opposites. Mania needed sedatives (opium in particular), melancholy required stimulants – opium might work here as well, but Brown largely prescribed alcohol. Brunonian psychiatry was mainly expounded in Britain by Robert Jones and George Nesse Hill.

This emergence of 'neurology' had a dual importance. Scientifically, it encouraged new thinking about the body and consciousness in the animal economy. Exploration of the related but distinct phenomena of irritability and sensation stimulated a new understanding of reflexes, instincts and habits. Classifying such processes as blushing, respiration and the pulse had traditionally posed difficult questions. Were these kinds of responses automatic? Or were they under the control of the conscious will? How much autonomy did the lower nerve centres themselves possess? These, of course, had traditionally been functions ascribed to the 'vegetable' and 'animal souls', but – Enlightenment physiology pondered – were not these formulations just verbal smokescreens?

In this intricate debate relating consciousness to behaviour – one critical for the status of time-honoured faculties such as 'Reason' – the extreme positions were taken up by continental savants. On the one hand, Stahl argued that all body activity was directed by the soul – i.e. an independent governing principle, probably immaterial, autonomous and ultimately transcendental; on the other, Haller contended that localised irritable responses (e.g. blinking) formed self-contained reflex-systems triggered by outside stimuli. A fruitful *via media* between 'animism' and 'mechanism' was elaborated in Edinburgh by Robert Whytt, who argued that a particular repertoire of purposive vital motions, including blushing, flushing, erection, and a variety of other 'nervous tics', neither fell directly under conscious will nor yet were automatic like heartbeat. Such 'involuntary' motions of which 'we are no way conscious' rather formed a behavioural stratum, perhaps originally under the immediate control of consciousness but having in course of experience become, through Lockian processes of association and acculturation, habitual, and so 'unattended with consciousness'.

Whytt's suggestive perception, with its dynamic and ontogenic overtones, enlarged the map of mind-body relations. It inserted levels of activity which constituted neither mere local reflex responses to external stimuli, nor independent acts of conscious will. The mind, it seemed, could perform purposive acts which were nevertheless unconscious. It might thus operate on distinct planes of awareness, being more layered and integrated rather than a simple unity. Whytt's physiology had a rich potential for explaining features of mental abnormality such as amnesia, compulsive behaviour and obsessions. It squared with the association of ideas, which explained philosophically how, through experience and learning, habit would in time direct activity without constant individual deliberative acts. Along similar lines, his contemporary David Hartley would argue that 'mad persons... lose that Consciousness... by which we connect ourselves with ourselves', and Erasmus Darwin explored the mental processes behind such conditions as speech defects. Itself the product of a new climate of sensibility, this neurology of unconscious action was also supportive of the contemporary idea of organic 'vegetative' genius, and suggestive for explaining disturbed behavioural states, such as those involved in dreaming, sleepwalking and trances. Indeed, Whytt's model of action seemed to find instant literary embodiment in Laurence Sterne's hero, Tristram Shandy, who puzzled how his own behaviour was but partially under his own command, being activated by strange impulses which nevertheless clearly arose from his own nature.

Furthermore, this doctrine of nerves, founded thus in new currents of medico-anatomy, provided a language immensely fruitful for discussing the mind/body and thought/action mediations. Supplementing and replacing the increasingly *démodé* humoralism, it met the criteria for public plausibility in an age when doctors still had to make themselves intelligible to the public. It was new and fashionable. Yet it also translated into common-sense images: nerves, like fiddle-strings, needed to be kept in tune. The relaxed nerve, like the slack string, performed flat. By contrast, the overstretched fibre was 'sharp', scratchy, highly strung. Neurology thus gave a scientific dimension to common talk of being 'up' or 'down', just as humoralism had made much of being cold, hot, wet, dry etc. (i.e. sanguine or phlegmatic, choleric or melancholic), or suffering from excess or deficiency. Talk of nerves keyed experiences of disorder into the *soma*, and hence pre-empted imputations of mere malingering, imagination, or a pathological state of the will itself.

Neurology also provided a choicer physical seat for disorders than had humoralism. For in the cultural iconography of sickness, the disturbed guts, so crucial to humoralism, had always been utterly equivocal, ever vulnerable to a misanthropic, Swiftian physio-pornography. Nerves by contrast were like gossamer, fine and filmy. Far from gross, they were the media of the most delicate sensations, channels of those exquisite vibrations de rigueur in the age of sensibility, especially for the man or woman of feeling. Not

least, nerves pointed directly up to the brain. Georgians wished
to be people of feeling rather than arid rationalists; they did not,
however, wish their feelings to be low 'gut reactions' but rather
uplifted and high-minded, bathed in memories, imagination, and
consciousness-soaked associations. Numerous physicians went into
print instructing the public of the mingled delights and dangers
of these nervous disorders, culminating in Dr Thomas Trotter's
View of the Nervous Temperament (1807). Trotter's aim was to bring
Cheyne's *English Malady* up to date. 'The last century had been
remarkable for the increase of a class of diseases but little known
in former times,' he explained:

> They have been designated in common language, by the terms
> Nervous, Spasmodic; Bilious; Indigestion; Stomach Complaints;
> Low Spirits; Vapours, &c... In the present day, this class of diseases
> forms by far the largest proportion of the whole, which come
> under the treatment of the physician.[17]

In short, reflecting the new physiology, 'nervous complaints'
came into vogue. As Dr James McKittrick Adair, one of Whytt's
pupils, reminisced:

> Upwards of thirty years ago, a treatise on nervous disease was
> published by my quondam learned, and ingenious preceptor, Dr
> Whytt, Professor of Physick, at Edinburgh. Before the publication
> of this book, people of fashion had not the least idea that they had
> nerves; but a fashionable apothecary of my acquaintance, having
> cast his eye over the book, and having often been puzzled by
> the enquiries of his patients concerning the nature and causes of
> their complaints, derived from thence a hint, by which he cut the
> gordian knot – 'Madam, you are nervous'; the solution was quite
> satisfactory, the term became fashionable, and spleen, vapours and
> hyp, were forgotten.[18]

Doctors such as Adair affected to despise these wafts of diagnostic fashion. Yet such tastes were manna to ambitious physicians

eager to provide authentic medicalisations of disturbance – here neuroanatomy proved a godsend – yet insistent that the nerves and the brain formed a specialised (indeed, superior) branch of medicine, beyond the grasp of routine physicians. Such medical tactics were deliciously caricatured by Smollett in *Sir Launcelot Greaves*:

> 'Doctor, (said our hero) if it is not an improper question to ask, I should be glad to know your opinion of my disorder –' 'O! sir, as to that – (replied the physician) your disorder is a – kind of a – sir, 'tis very common in this country – a sort of a –' 'Do you think my distemper is madness doctor?' –'O Lord! sir, – not absolute madness – no – not madness – you have heard no doubt, of what is called a weakness of the nerves, sir... '.[19]

Thus major foundations were laid from the mid-eighteenth century for a specialist mental medicine. Many physicians, such as William Pargeter, William Perfect and William Rowley and then – after 1800 – George Nesse Hill and John and Thomas Mayo, emphasised its authentic organic status, sometimes invoking the graphic evidence of skull damage and brain tumours. Above all, classifications of nervous complaints were developed, generally deriving from Cullen's nosology. Such attempts to pigeonhole madness within anatomy or a disease taxonomy remained, however, highly controversial. They formed, many critics argued, an essentially artificial, specious – or, worse still – dangerous schematisation. Thus Thomas Beddoes complained that such classifications descended into crazy hair-splitting verbalisings:

> Modern nosologists have so entirely departed from the original principle of distinction, by which melancholy madness was characterised according to the appearances of what is vulgarly called melancholy in sane people, that they now give us no other criterion than the partial nature of the insanity. 'Insanity' says Dr. Cullen, 'consists in such false conceptions of the relations of things, as lead to irrational emotions or actions. Melancholy is

partial insanity without indigestion – Mania is universal insanity'. According to this account, the partition between the two
is thin indeed.[20]

Though distrusted, such nosologies were nevertheless strategi-
cally important to their proponents for putting mind disorders
on the map as real diseases no less than fevers, while showing that
they also constituted a quite separate disease terrain (Cullen's
'vesaniae'), demanding specialist knowledge and care.

The standing of these 'nervous' mad-doctors remained unsure.
They were confident, on the one hand, that their physiology,
aetiology and nosography were all of great explanatory power.
Patients who suffered head wounds, abused alcohol, endured
post-partum convulsions, or enervated themselves with high
living were all perfect grist to their mill. But the gap between
the new organic physiology and therapeutic efficacy remained
as wide as ever.

PHYSIC FOR THE MAD

Physic for mania and melancholy had, of course, a long pedigree.
Medication had taken many forms and possessed a multitude of
rationales. Certain treatments, particularly those containing iron,
aimed at consolidating shattered spirits and reinforcing the fibres.
Bloodlettings, emetics and purges sought to purify, which was
also one rationale of cold-water immersion. Blistering constituted a counter-irritant or shock. Drugs were meant to stimulate
or pacify. Calomel, saline draughts, antimoniacs, cathartics, vale-
rian, blisters, purges – all had their particular advocates. 'Bleeding
and purging are both requisite', believed John Monro.

Alongside such traditional strategies, surgical and drug therapies for mental disorders multiplied during the eighteenth
century, and many new treatments were touted. The apothecary Cromwell Mortimer – incidentally, Secretary of the Royal
Society – had his own secret powder, an evacuant, for which he
claimed dramatic successes in self-advertising case histories:

*The Case of Mr Martin, at Nurse Wood's, in Tyburn-Road, near Soho–
Square. A Mania or Madness cured by three Doses.* This Gentleman
had lived well; but, thro' Misfortunes, coming to Decay, Grief had
brought on Epileptic Fits for some Years past: At length, being
seized with a Mania, he was carried to this Nurse's, till his Friends
could get him into Bethlem. April, 1742, a Relation of his Wife's
desired me to visit him. I found him chained down in his Bed,
Hands and Feet, quite furious, not knowing any body.[21]

Fortunately, Mortimer was ready with his nostrum:

I gave him four Pills, which vomited and purged him several
times; upon which he was much better. The next Day but one, I
saw him sitting up in his Bed, calm, and with his Hands at Liberty.
I repeated the Pills, which operated as before; In a few Hours he
came quite to his Senses; knew People; and was unfetter'd. Four
Days after, he took a third Dose of the Pills, was quite well... This
is a true Account of the speedy Cure of this Patient, upon his
taking the above-mention'd Medicines, he being all the while
under my Care.[22]

Various other drugs came into vogue. Opiates in particular
became popular for nervous conditions. Like the camphor
oil recommended by Kinneir and George Nesse Hill, opium
chimed with the new nervous physiology, for both prepara-
tions were thought to stimulate the nerves when taken in
small quantities for depressive conditions, while being sedative
if given in large concentrations, and thus indicated for mania.
Physicians such as Erasmus Darwin prescribed opium in quite
heroic doses.

Another novel treatment, also harmonising with theories of
the nerves, was electricity. As experiments increasingly indicated
that electricity charged the nervous system, conveying sensory
information and stimulating the brain, defects in internal electric circuits or supply were plausibly blamed for hyperexcitation
or depression. Particularly for melancholia, medical electricity

became one of the great hopes of Georgian therapy, both among enthusiasts such as John Wesley and with regulars.

All the therapeutic optimism about wonder drugs and machines, however, produced a mouse: applied to the mind they met little lasting, reliable success. Even apparent cures might be equivocal, for practitioners such as Peter Shaw candidly recognised that recovery often owed more to the healing power of Nature (natural remissions) than to the surgeon's or apothecary's bag of tricks. All in all, the anatomical advances which forwarded explanation and perhaps diagnosis did not directly bear fruit in successful therapeutics. As William Heberden could note gloomily at the close of the century, apart from opium, the *materia medica* was futile: 'I have observed nothing which has been of any service in removing this great affliction'.

It is, of course, nothing new in medicine for theory to outrun therapy, and such situations have not generally discredited the art. But here it created a dilemma. In the face of failure, the proponents of somaticism were particularly vulnerable. The unpredictable ravings and remissions of the maniac, the bizarrely wandering pains of the hypochondriac, the ceaseless howls of the lunatic, the seizures of the hysteric, the self-destructive fits of the melancholic – all taunted medicine's authority. Madness remained mysterious, catastrophic, arbitrary. As Young put it,

> I have seen some women seized with an hysteric vomiting, or colic, as often as they ere under any disappointment, anger, or vexation, tho' the minute before in perfect health both of body and mind; yet one slight affront has set them immediately a vomiting, with great difficulty of breathing, and the whole train of hysteric symptoms.[23]

Young recommended opium; but he was forced to throw up his hands and ask, almost biblically, 'What can opium do here? What will our juleps do, and draughts of *sal* and *suc. limon*? What will all our stinking or heating nervous medicines avail?' All physic could do, he argued, was to soldier on:

> To such patients we are often called, and we go through the
> fashionable practice till their passion of mind subsides; and then...
> the disease is cured, and we come off with the applause both of
> ourselves and others... I confess I have, thro' ignorance, given
> hysteric pills, when I might as well have given pills to purge folly
> and make my patient wiser.[24]

All in all, Young was melancholy about prospects. For mental
disorder was indeed a will-o'-the-wisp, so double-dealing that,
paradoxically, it sometimes proved that the only medicines
which actually worked were strictly speaking useless ones, mere
placebos: 'I do not mean', he explained,

> that when the patient complains grievously of a pain in her head,
> she should be told that she has none; for she really feels it, but
> mistakes the cause, when she thinks it independent of her anger.
> She will not be satisfied unless the physician prescribes; and he
> may do it with this comfort, that whatever innocent thing he
> orders, it will generally succeed; for the passions will subside in
> time, either with or without medicine.[25]

Indeed, the bankruptcy of traditional medications grew more
patent both to physicians and to the public. In his *Treatise on
Madness* (1758), William Battie excoriated the Bethlem therapeutics of bloodlettings, blisters and, above all, routine vomiting
(he termed it 'shocking'). John Monro managed quite a spirited
defence of the old ways; yet half a century later, cross-questioned
by the House of Commons Committee, his son, Thomas, had to
confess that the Monro therapeutics were just family heirlooms.
They availed little, but he 'knew no better'.

A crisis was brewing. Mental disturbance was calling forth
a specialist branch of medicine, focused upon the nerves. This
development had left general ('humoral') therapeutics archaic.
Yet the new specialism did not produce new cures. In any case,
scientific research into nerve and brain functions remained very
patchy. Cranial anatomy, for example, was not systematically

pursued in eighteenth-century England. Thomas Willis' hypo-
thetical localisations provoked much scepticism, but it took
nineteenth-century experimental neurology to advance much
further. There were no systematic autopsies on lunatics' brains,
and those post mortems which the surgeon Bryan Crowther
conducted at Bethlem perplexingly failed to highlight differ-
ences between maniacs and the sane. Brain surgery likewise
contributed little to understanding madness.

In the long run, of course, organic approaches were to rule
the roost. During the nineteenth century, physicians persuaded
Parliament that mental disorder was at bottom a medical preserve,
and the asylum was statutorily medicalised. Doctors entertained
the dream that in the fullness of time, experimental neurology
and chemistry would indeed unveil insanity's secrets. By the
late nineteenth century, neurophysiology was in the driving
seat and, as Bynum and Clark have demonstrated, psychiatry
was thrown onto the defensive (what it dealt in was 'delusion').
Yet in the late eighteenth century the most confident of those
specialising in handling the mad were not the somatists but the
proto-psychiatrists, those practising the arts to be dubbed 'moral
medicine', 'moral management', and 'moral therapy'.

THE EMERGENCE OF MENTAL APPROACHES

Who were the pioneers of 'moral' or 'mental' approaches? On
which intellectual traditions did they capitalise? To explain this,
we must return to the metaphysical crisis of the seventeenth
century and trace its traumatic impact upon ideas of the right-
and wrong-thinking mind. Medieval scholasticism, Thomism in
particular, had enshrined Reason as the citadel of knowledge.
A universal attribute, Reason possessed innate truths, partici-
pated in eternal and natural law, and could garner knowledge
about the mundane world. Divine Wisdom guaranteed the
reliability of Reason, its ability to find truth and follow the
moral law. Scholasticism was scarcely all plain sailing (forever
racked by debates about words and things, nominalism and

essentialism), yet it throve till the novelties of the Renaissance and Reformation, the discovery of the New World, the New Learning and the New Science all shook the foundations. The old certainties challenged, the spectre of scepticism loomed, and there were few people who felt as comfortable with Pyrrhonism as did Montaigne.

Aiming to move from doubt to certainty, Descartes advanced his *cogito*, an irrefutable, immediate, divinely guaranteed source from which knowing could proceed. In England, however, relentlessly mechanistic Cartesianism seemed intellectually crass and religiously unacceptable. Instead, an empiricist epistemology won the day whose champion, *par excellence*, was Locke.

For the Locke of the *Essay Concerning Human Understanding* (1690), there was no divinely illuminated, *a priori* Right Reason, no certain logic of truth, no innate verities. Rather, Locke presents mind initially as a *tabula rasa*. Knowledge is composed from unit sensory inputs which mental operations assemble into conceptions, ideas, and finally lengthier thought-chains. Neither are values – both moral and aesthetic – inborn, but they too are built up from responses to the sensations of pleasure and pain resulting from experience. Both thinking and feeling were fruits of the education of the senses. Depending on the success of these processes, a mind might become filled with natural ideas and normal judgements, or it might end up cognitively and emotionally disorientated. Nothing was certain.

Want of certainty, however, was no disaster, for probability in beliefs would do for the business of life. Probable knowledge was generated out of the interplay between mental energies and the world outside, mediated via the senses. Thus the problem of knowledge became a problem about how minds worked, and metaphysics and syllogistic logic were elbowed out by what in time would be called epistemology and psychology, but which was then termed 'experience'.

Locke's philosophy of experience left mind in the balance. Rational certainty was a chimera; yet there might be progressive paths to reliable enough knowledge. Our senses were deceptive, indeed they often lied; yet experience could be consolidated by regular habits of thinking. Nevertheless Locke's empiricism set a chasm between consciousness and the essence of things, one bridged only by those none too trusty servants, 'sensations'. Thought would always be uncertain, because knower was cleft from the known, and the go-betweens, the senses, were irrevocably equivocal. So there was a radical edge of contingency about Locke's model. Man was in effect a self-creation, the product of his education and experience, a progressive being who was always becoming. Optimistically, this meant he was not radically flawed by Original Sin, or by elemental strife between Reason and appetites. Man's grasp on reality was doomed to be precarious.

Locke did not conflate the conscious, thinking faculty with the immortal soul; nor did he reduce mind to brain. By grounding knowing in the senses, his philosophy hinted at a close, if ill-defined, affinity between consciousness and cortex. It would not be inconceivable, he notoriously commented, for God to have created matter which could think – a suggestion variously taken up during the eighteenth century, conspicuously in the radical materialism of the French Enlightenment but also in the theological monism of David Hartley and Joseph Priestley.

Locke's formulations were at once highly challenging, yet also a collection of commonplaces. They proved profoundly suggestive for understanding how knowledge was gained, and what reliance might be vested in it; for showing the origin and status of the passions and of moral belief; for analysing learning, character and development; for delving into the secret springs of consciousness. Being so suggestive, they were adopted by educated and enlightened thinking for the next century, much as Darwin's or Freud's later. When Laurence Sterne conceived *Tristram Shandy* as a train of free associations on Locke, he could assume that everyone would see the joke.

In several cardinal ways Locke transformed common perceptions of *homo rationalis*. Right Reason was dissolved and the business of thinking now became paramount. No longer was

Reason a divinely illuminated faculty as, say, for the Cambridge Platonists, or a certainty-guaranteeing logic engine. What counted, rather, was how the workaday mind dynamically responded to sensory inputs, those fleeting, fragmentary atoms of experience. There was no escaping an irreducibly subjective, provisional element to consciousness. Lacking ultimate innate truths, the order of the day lay in probability, opinion and belief: every mind had to remake the world for itself. As Locke remarked,

> There is scarce any one that does not observe something that seems odd to him, and is in itself really extravagant, in the opinions, reasonings, and actions of other men. The least flaw of this kind, if at all different from his own, every one is quick-sighted enough to espy in another, and will by the authority of reason forwardly condemn; though he be guilty of much greater unreasonableness in his own tenets of conduct, which he never perceives, and will very hardly, if at all, be convinced of.[26]

In thus depicting the understanding, Locke carved out a natural, secular realm of consciousness, a space for thinking beneath the immortal soul (with which he did not meddle). The problem of how mind worked, and why it all too frequently misfired – producing, but also rectifying, error – was to dominate post-Lockian philosophy.

For Locke's theory of knowledge clearly had dramatic implications for the sense of ego. In Descartes' *cogito*, Right Reason and the self, thinking and being, were logically all of a piece; analytically, they stood together. But Locke's *tabula rasa* notion of mind rendered the nature of the ultimate self potentially puzzling. So what price the common sense of personal identity? On what was it based? Locke thus made a problem of the formation and standing of 'personality'. No longer might character be automatically assumed to be innate and fixed, flawed by Original Sin, determined by humours, beset by ruling passions. Instead, it was something generated. The answer to Tristram Shandy's 'Who are you?', was to become a question of development, for, as Sterne hinted, Locke's *Essay Concerning Human Understanding* was indeed a 'history-book', the history of 'what passes in a man's own mind'.

Locke envisaged a consciousness whose operations were intricate, dynamic, and liable to erroneous as well as true beliefs. He also specifically formulated – if perhaps by way of afterthought – a massively influential theory of madness. For traditional moral philosophy, madness meant Reason ambushed by appetite. Locke demurred. For one thing, he did not see the passions as intrinsically blind and tumultuous. They had their own histories: educated by experiences of pain and pleasure, they evolved, grew refined, and were duly accommodated into the larger self and society. Feelings were friends to virtue, not its foes. For Locke, as for later Enlightenment philosophers such as Shaftesbury, Hutcheson, Hume and Bentham, passions should not automatically be blamed for madness.

On the contrary, Locke believed that the key to insanity lay not in the overthrow of Reason but in reasoning itself. Madness was a misconception grounded in false consciousness; it was marked by an incongruency between a person's picture of the world and outside reality, produced by the misconstrual of experience, often exacerbated by the mischief of the words which clothe our thoughts. In other words, madness was essentially delusion and the custom-built chains of activity consequent on such hallucinations. This Locke clarified by spelling out the distinction between idiots and the insane:

> A fool is he that from right principles makes a wrong conclusion; but a madman is one who draws a just inference from false principles... A madman fancies himself a prince; but upon his mistake, he acts suitable to that character; and though he is out in supposing he had principalities, while he drinks his gruel, and lies in straw, yet you shall see him keep the port of a distressed monarch in all his words and actions.[27]

How then did such crazy 'false principles' arise in the first place? Locke's explanation was grounded in association. Ideas were conglomerates of sensations, and sensations were necessarily frail:

> For, methinks, the understanding is not so much unlike a closet wholly shut from light, with only some little opening left, to let in external visible resemblances... would the pictures coming into such a dark room but stay there, and lie so orderly as to be found upon occasion, it would a very much resemble the understanding of a man, in reference to all objects of sight, and the ideas of them.[28]

Sights, sounds, tastes etc. thus filtered into the sensorium, and ideas were assembled from trains of sensations linked by associations (e.g. similarity, contiguity). If such links were ill-forged at the outset, perhaps through the treacheries of words, the final outcome of a chain of reasoning in belief or action would prove delusory. Misconception was thus the marrow of madness.

Locke's formulations proved extraordinarily influential throughout the eighteenth century. For instance, the eminent psychiatric doctor Alexander Crichton was to acknowledge in his *Inquiry into the Nature and Origin of Mental Derangement* (1798) that he had received 'much assistance' from 'our British Psychologists, such as Locke', as also from Locke's own successors, 'Hartley, Reid, Priestley, Stewart and Kames'; Crichton became a great advocate of Locke's method of 'analysis'. Both Battie and Samuel Tuke also acknowledged their debts. Not that Locke's view was accepted wholesale or by all. It was often challenged. Thus when Battie (who, as a student in Cambridge, surely studied Locke) advanced the Locke-derived theory in his *Treatise on Madness* (1758) that insanity lay in deluded imagination, John Monro rebutted him by contending that most madmen showed no signs of false *ideas*; their insanity lay in perversion of moral will – not in hallucination, but in 'vitiated judgment'.

The Humanist doctrine of the madman as passion's slave had likened the mad to brutes. Locke's stress on error, by contrast, viewed them more as infants, incapable as yet of thinking straight. As with the educability of children, the mad could, given instruction, be reconditioned for civilised life. Of course, such an image of insanity as educable became popular because it meshed with Enlightenment pedagogy – indeed with the pedagogics of Locke's own *Some Thoughts Concerning Education* (1693) – and its links with later moral therapy will be explored in detail below. If, however, in these respects Locke's model of madness was emancipatory, its potential for regarding all intellectual irregularity as a mode of insanity was to prove far more equivocal. For if madness is error, error becomes madness. In contrast to Pope's lapsarian pity ('To err is human'), Locke's associationism had a sinister potential for invalidating all wrong thinking ('to err is mad'). As already indicated in cases of 'religious insanity', Georgian ideologues were not slow to dub as mad those thought-systems which did not square with their own.

Locke's philosophy was thus Janus-faced in its implications. Congruent with the new culture of the 'English malady' discussed earlier, Locke removed reasoning about madness from the theological (his philosophy had no place for authentic divine madness or for Reason as the candle of the Lord) and from the man–beast dilemma (no longer the civil war between Reason and passion). Madness was thus humanised. Sympathy was due. With the effective metaphorisation of Original Sin, madness was a blemish which could be rectified, indeed cured. However, the other face of this secular optimism was an insistence upon the mind's fragility, the ease of becoming trapped within webs of misassociation, subjectivity and solipsism, the potency of error, fed by delusions.

Locke's agenda for understanding the operations of the mind, both normal and abnormal, was widely adopted as the most promising path for explaining insanity. For experts such as Battie and Arnold, intellectual delusion became the definitive feature of lunacy. Arnold for instance posited two sorts of insanity: *notional*, in which the sufferer formed misconceived ideas about things really existing; and *ideal* insanity, which involved pure delusion. It must not be supposed, however, that the developments in neuroanatomy discussed earlier, on the one hand, and the appeal of Lockian epistemology, on the other, created two rival schools, one essentially medico-organic, the other 'moral' or 'mental'. Above all, it would be simplistic to imply that it was the latter which became 'psychiatry'.

Of course, polemics flared through the century about the aetiology of madness. Thus Dr Nicholas Robinson, though valuing Locke's associationism, encased it within an aggressive somatism: 'Every Change of Mind, therefore, indicates a Change in the bodily Organs'. Faulkner thought likewise: 'If the intellect appears to be disordered, it is the business of the physician to attend to the habit of the body', and Thomas Bakewell wrote, 'The primary disease is corporeal'. Others, particularly later in the century, contended for mentalist explanations. For example, Andrew Harper – surprisingly, one might think, for a surgeon – claimed that it was

> an unquestionable axiom, that the cause of [insanity] must depend upon some specific alteration in the essential operations and movements of the mind, independent and exclusive of every corporal, sympathetic, direct, or indirect excitement, or irritation whatever.[29]

And, slightly later, William Hallaran was to argue that authentic mental alienation was distinct from somatic frenzies:

> The hallucination of the mind, as primarily the seat of the disorder, [should not be confused] with the delirium, which is the associate of corporeal suffering.[30]

For Hallaran, the two sorts of sickness must be distinguished, and the independent ontology of mental disease recognised:

> I have long entertained in a practical point of view, a distinction between these two species of insanity, [involving] opposite modes of treatment... the malady of the mind which is for the most part

to be treated on moral principles, should [not] be subjected to the operation of agents altogether foreign to the purpose; and that the other of the body, arising from direct injury to one or more of the vital organs, may escape the advantages of approved remedies.[31]

By the early nineteenth century in the polemics of Harper, Hallaran and George Nesse Hill – who regarded mentalistic accounts of madness as little better than delusions themselves – there was, perhaps, an explanatory polarisation. At an earlier stage, however, it was more common for writers to make play of their uncertainty as to how to demarcate between or integrate anatomy and intellect. The whole question of mind/body dialectics seemed overwhelming, for, as Sir George Baker put it, from earliest times physicians and philosophers

knew that it was impossible for the mind to suffer without the body becoming sick also, or the body to be ill without the mind being associated with it in the distemper.[32]

Operating within a sensitive psychosomatic and somatopsychic framework of reference, Baker stressed the indispensability of shrewd clinical judgement in the individual instance:

In how many cases is the mind at fault when a hodge-podge of medicines composed of almost all the elements collected from every source is applied to the stomach; surely here the best medicine is no medicine... In such diseases it is Socrates' medicine, not Galen's which ought to be applied... The saying of the old man of Cos was not rashly made; 'The philosopher is a god-like physician.'[33]

Moreover, what was at stake, of course, in these rival theorisings of insanity were not just matters of neutral observation and abstractions, but a tangled fabric of values concerning human nature, personal responsibility, and the authority to treat. Thus

Harper's idealist aetiology was embedded in a polemic about the condition of George III. Insanity, Harper syllogised, was of the intellect; the king clearly had serious organic symptoms and afflictions; therefore the king was not, properly speaking, mad. All the same, new observations and interpretations played their part, even if they essentially brought to light still further mysteries of the mind/body continuum. Thus Whytt's studies of 'sympathy' between particular organs (how anger, for example, quickened breathing and heartbeat and violent passions often terminated in convulsions, catalepsy, epilepsy, or death) led to many notable explorations of the devious dealings of the stratified consciousness and its somatic manifestations.

THE MYSTERIES OF THE MIND

The deeps of the mind were similarly explored by John Haygarth and William Falconer. Investigating somatic cures apparently wrought by such therapies as Perkins' Tractors or Mesmer's animal magnetism, they insisted that such techniques were scientifically bogus. Certainly they cured, but they worked only by 'the impression... made upon the patient's Imagination', thus confirming the alarming power of the mind to affect the body. To understand this, Falconer called for a new 'anatomy of the mind'. In the secularised climate of the late Enlightenment, such mental mysteries had been demoted from Satanic terrors to medical nuisances, curiosities, or problems for further inquiry. As the London practitioner Sayer Walker argued, in dealing with nervous symptoms such as palpitations it was not enough to explore 'the corporeal functions':

> It will [also] be necessary to pay some regard to the state of
> the mind, which, we have seen, is often very nearly concerned
> with these diseases... to determine whether the state of the body
> is to be attributed to that of the mind, or the latter to the
> former.[34]

For the nervous avenues were two-way:

> It is well known that any unpleasant affection of the mind, long
> continued, will have a very considerable influence on the state of
> the animal frame, and more particularly on the nervous system.
> On the other hand, it is equally true that different diseased states
> of the animal function will be productive of some affections of
> the mind. If, therefore, we can discover to which of these sources
> different symptoms are to be traced, we shall have a more clear
> indication of cure.[35]

Even David Hartley, whose theory of corpuscular vibrations
('vibratiuncles') in some ways physicalised Locke's associationism, had denied that he was a simple monist or materialist,
contending for a more bifocal approach:

> The Causes of Madness are of two Kinds, bodily and mental. That
> which arises from bodily Causes is nearly related to Drunkenness,
> and to the Deliriums attending Distempers. That from mental
> Causes is of the same Kind with temporary Alienations of the
> Mind during violent Passions.[36]

All investigators urged redoubled attention to the subtle dynamics of mind and body. And as the century progressed, medical
opinion seems to have been increasingly inclined to blame the
recesses of the mind for a widening range of recalcitrant maladies. Take for instance hysteria, typically regarded, around 1700,
as organically sited. The keynote of case studies during the eighteenth century lay in an increasing fascination with individual
and personal precipitants. Within a Lockian framework, the hospital physician Robert Bree examined how it could principally
be associations of ideas which generated the physical symptoms
of hysteria:

> Impressions thus linked in the mind by association, will become
> a train of sensations, the individual parts of which successively

introduce each other. When this association is established, the same animal motions may be repeated from apparent dissimilar causes, but these are remote causes of the immediate sensation inducing the disease.[37]

This helped explain how life-history associations could cause the organic symptoms of hysterical paroxysms. For instance:

> A lady had been thrown into a paroxysm of terror by a footpad, and for the first time sustained a series of hysteric fits. Her consti-tution became feeble and acutely sensible. The hysteric affection recurred on smaller occasions of alarm for many years afterwards, but more particularly was excited by the renewal of slight cir-cumstances which referred to the attack, though entirely distinct from the outrage. After the interval of three years, during which she had diversified her impressions in a distant neighbourhood, she passed in a carriage along the road, and by the spot where the assault was made, and affected by the chain of ideas and her attention to them, she relapsed into strong convulsions.[38]

Abundant parallels are offered in John Ferriar's copious and per-ceptive studies of what he called the 'conversion of diseases'.

In all these areas, the key development was the heightened perception of mysterious, treacherous, inner faculties capable of disturbing – and even disorientating – the individual, indepen-dently of rational will. When humoralism ruled, the disposition corresponding to physical distemper had been a public language, visible on the surface ('complexion'). There was nothing very individual about the rage of the traditional choleric man or the joviality of the sanguine. But increasingly doctors found themselves forced to point to a mental faculty responsible for such disorders as asthma, convulsions or hysteria, which were uniquely individual, difficult to pin down, control, or indeed rectify.

This transition – a growing sense of 'self' or 'personality' as a ghost in the machine, a growing use of 'mentalist' explanations

– was vital to the emergence of the 'psychiatric'. What was at stake, in terms of skewing the play between the moral and the physical, is particularly clear in Georgian discussions of vice-ssociated maladies. Drink disorders offer a good example. No doctor doubted the physical damage done by hard drinking. Erasmus Darwin (who, personally finding that Bacchus and Venus did not mix, gave up Bacchus) warned:

> Mark what happens to a man who drinks a quart of wine or
> of ale, if he has not been habituated to it. He loses the use both
> of his limbs and of his understanding! He becomes a temporary
> idiot, and has a temporary stroke of the palsy!… is it not reasonable
> to conclude that a perpetual repetition of so powerful a poison
> must at length permanently affect him?[39]

Few demurred. Medical texts by the score praised alcohol's cordial properties but decried its abuse, listing the great train of dysfunctions hard drinking caused, from flatulence and dyspepsia to dropsy, gout and cirrhosis, newly described by that expert clinician, Matthew Baillie (it 'would seem to depend upon the habit of drinking… most commonly found in hard drinkers'). Indeed, many mad–doctors blamed dram–drinking for lunacy. As Ferriar concluded at the close of the century:

> The most general causes of insanity which I have had occasion
> to notice, are hard drinking accompanied with watching; pride,
> disappointment, the anguish arising from calumny; sudden terror
> [etc.][40]

At first the deleterious effects of drink were slight. As John Bond noted, typical nightmare sufferers were 'the luxurious, the drunken and they who sup late'. Nightmares often led to hypochondriasis, followed by madness proper among indulgers in 'frequent intoxication [and] the constant use of narcotics', as Andrew Harper put it. Benjamin Faulkner similarly judged that 'habitual intoxication' produced insanity; frenzy was the consequence of 'freely Drinking of strong liquors', and this dread downward spiral of the Sot's Progress was sure (thought Thomas Arnold) to bottom out in despair, and even suicide, so dire were the

> distressful feelings both of body and mind – known to hard drinkers by the appellation of the horrors – arising from excessive indulgence either in wine, or opium, as... to render life a burden;[41]

Particularly by the beginning of the nineteenth century, psychiatrists began to flesh out these stereotypes of the destructiveness of drams with personal tragedies, often taken from their records, as for example this warning case of the twenty-eight-year-old 'J.R.', presented by George Nesse Hill:

> An active farmer thin and small, but capable of hard labour, having met with a disappointment... became drunken, which excess had for some time no other consequence than common. At length during sober intervals he began to complain of depressing pain at his breast, accompanied or rather soon followed by pain across the forehead with confusion of thought, to relieve which he drank brandy. The mental derangement seemed to commence with the disappointment and to increase after every act of inebriety which now had but few intervals. After a long drinking bout as he termed it he became furiously maniacal.[42]

These visions of the demon drink fitted traditional images of madness like a glove. They confirmed, on the one hand, the age-old judgement that madness was the wages of sin and the drunkard's just desserts, while also tallying with the fundamental belief that insanity was somatic, seated in the viscera. Physiologically speaking, as William Sandford pointed out, alcohol corroded the stomach, ardent spirits thereby ruining the sufferer's own spirits.

Georgian medicine condemned liquor itself as the cause of all manner of disease, physical and mental. But did it regard the craving for drink and habits of drunkenness as diseases themselves? In particular, when did it first see such desires as diseases of the mind, inducing dependence and enslaving? As standard histories state, the identification of habitual drunkenness as a disease was without a doubt present by 1804, when Thomas Trotter published his *Essay Medical Philosophical and Chemical on Drunkenness*, based on his Edinburgh MD thesis of 1788. Described as 'the first scientific investigator of drunkenness', Trotter stated point-blank that the 'habit of drunkenness was a disease'; indeed, a 'disease of the mind', 'like delirium'. 'Are not habits of drunkenness more often produced by mental affections than corporeal diseases?' Moralists and parsons, he asided condescendingly, had been well-meaning in damning drunkenness as vice or sin, but now at last it had been set within its rightful domain, medicine, to be managed by 'the discerning physician'. Contemporaneously in America, Benjamin Rush was also calling chronic drunkenness a 'disease', a 'derangement of the will'. Drinking, Rush argued, began as an act of 'free will', descended into a 'habit', and finally sank into a 'necessity'.

And from its birth with Trotter and Rush, historians have traced the progressive emergence of the psychiatric idea of alcoholism (a term coined in 1852), noting how *delirium tremens* was described by Thomas Sutton in 1813, how Esquirol saw compulsive drinking as a mode of monomania, how Bruhl-Cramer formulated 'dipsomania', Magnus Huss 'chronic alcoholism', and LeGrain and Morel incorporated alcohol addiction within 'hereditary degeneration'. Clearly, around in 1800 in the work of Trotter and Rush, alcohol addiction could be conceptualised as a mental disease within the domain of emergent 'psychiatry'. These thought-strands actually stretched back into the eighteenth century, despite Trotter's own claim that 'I have not any precursors in my labours'.

For Trotter was not the first to term habitual drunkenness a 'disease'. Thomas Wilson's *Distilled Spiritous Liquors* (1736) was already so calling it; and many Georgian doctors readily fitted drunkenness into their disease grids without any sense of novelty or incongruity. Thus in his *Commentaries on the History and Cure of Diseases* (1802), William Heberden gave a contents list of diseases, sandwiching Drunkenness between Diabetes, Diarrhoea and Dropsy above, and Dysentery, Disorders of the Ear and Epilepsy beneath.

If, then, there was nothing new about labelling habitual drinking as a disease, was there anything about Trotter's particular concept of chronic drunkenness which was radically novel? Certainly Trotter powerfully grasped the ravages of dependence, showing how in severe cases it finally reached a 'gulph, from whose bourne no traveller returns'. But such ideas were being voiced previously. Before him, John Coakley Lettsom had already traced progressive dependence, showing the fatal cycle leading from tippling for stimulus, relief, or exhilaration, to low spirits, which were its inevitable after-effects; which in turn could be obliterated only by further bouts of yet heavier drinking. He cited those who

> have endeavoured to overcome their nervous debility by the aid of spirits; many of these have begun the use of these poisons from persuasion of their utility, rather than from love of them; the relief, however, being temporary, to keep up their effects, frequent access is had to the same delusion till at length what was taken by compulsion, gains attachment, and a little drop of brandy, or gin and water, becomes as necessary as food; the female sex, from natural delicacy, acquire this custom by small degrees, and the poison being admitted in small doses, is slow in its operations, but not less painful in its effects.[43]

Eventually, such dependence would set in that neither threats nor persuasions were powerful enough to overcome it. But there was nothing new in Lettsom's account either. Before him, Thomas Wilson had depicted progressive enslavement, that headlong plunge in which alcohol gave stimulus, stimulus was followed by depression and stomach disorder, and these in turn could be expunged only by still more powerful draughts, until victims were so 'habituated' they 'could be justly reckoned among the dead'.

And before Wilson was George Cheyne, who also revealed how old soaks succumbed to 'cravings':

> They begin with the weaker wines; These, by Use and Habit, will not do; They leave the Stomach sick and mawkish; they fly to stronger Wines, and stronger still, and run the Climax from Brandy to Barbados Waters, and double-distill'd Spirits, 'till at last they find nothing hot enough for them.[44]

Thus the penal servitude of 'Necessity upon Necessity' set in, whereby 'Drams beget more Drams… so that at last the miserable Creature suffers a true Martyrdom'. And even before Cheyne, Mandeville had told the same story, his character 'Misomedon' offering this sorry tale of how drink brought its own punishment. Misomedon began by praising the bottle god:

> It has laid my pains, appeas'd my Soul, made me forget my Sorrows, and fancy over-night, that all my Afflictions had left me; But the next Morning, before the Strength of the Charm has been quite worn off, they have in Crowds return'd upon me with a Vengeance and my self paid dearly for the deceitful Cure. 'Tis unspeakable in what Confusion and Horror, Guilt, Fear, and Repentance I have wak'd, in what depth of Grief, Anguish and Misery my Spirits have been sunk, or how forlorn and destitute of all Hopes and Comforts I have sometimes thought my self after the Use of this fallacious remedy.[45]

Such diagnoses from Georgian physicians mirror lay testimonies as to alcohol dependence. Not least, of course, Samuel Johnson's, who – unlike Boswell – kicked the habit, telling Hannah More,

> I can't touch a little, child, therefore I never touch it. Abstinence is as easy to me as temperance would be difficult.[46]

During the Georgian century the evils of drink were adumbrated by doctors as a disease involving the power of the will as well as the grape. Physicians routinely spoke of men 'addicting' themselves, implying assumptions of irresponsibility and dependence, as when Dr Rollo described the case of someone who had died of drink, having 'addicted himself to the use of rum in large quantities'.

Perceptions of the evils of drink also changed in nature. No longer just a failure of 'temperance' or moderation within the old humoral model, nor even simply a mark of physical malady, hard drinking was gradually reconstituted during the eighteenth century as a disease of the mind, entailing disastrous psychosomatic consequences for the whole person.

The conceptual frontiers between mental and somatic aetiology, agency and responsibility shifted, responding to explanatory pressures in which the findings of experience, the professional ambitions of doctors, and the moralisings of the public all played their part. Parallels to this 'psychiatrisation' of alcohol-related maladies can be found in other spheres of consciousness and conduct, particularly those conceptions of sickness inseparable from notions of vice and responsibility. Changing conceptualisations of the maladies associated with love and sex offer a further revealing instance. Being a noble affection of the elevated mind, love had always been linked, romantically and tragically, with madness (*vide* Shakespeare's 'The lunatic, the lover and the poet/Are of imagination all compact'); and the annals of insanity, not least asylum records, abundantly testify to those driven out of their minds by unrequited passion.

Within traditional humoralism, as espoused by doctors and laity alike, sex was not seen as a particular trigger of insanity, nor excessive eroticism as a mental disease. Sex was a normal desire and discharge, fulfilling the biological purposes of reproduction. Performed, like other functions, in due moderation – neither too much nor too little – it constituted a healthy evacuation, not altogether different from bloodlettings or purges. Indulged to excess (so warned advice manuals such as Nicholas Venette's

The Mysteries of Conjugal Love Reveal'd and *Aristotle's Master-Piece*)
it would, of course, prove debilitating. Sexual intemperance was
traditionally regarded as stemming chiefly from material causes,
being, for instance, triggered by spicy food, aphrodisiacs, excessive wine, or genital irritation; and gross venery was viewed as
primarily physical in its consequences, leading to exhaustion,
infertility, baldness and premature decay. Unnatural sex denial
was also thought to produce essentially physical disorder, as when
Ebenezer Sibly near the end of the eighteenth century described
the effects of green sickness or chlorosis on teenage girls:

> This disease usually attacks virgins a little after the time of puberty,
> and first shews itself by symptoms of dyspepsia or bad digestion.
> But a distinguishing symptom is, that the appetite is entirely viti-
> ated, and the patient will eat lime, chalk, ashes, salt etc... In the
> beginning of the disease, the urine is pale, and afterwards turbid;
> the face becomes pale, and then assumes a greenish colour: some
> times it becomes livid or yellow, the eyes are sunk, and have a livid
> circle round them; the lips lose their fine red colour; the pulse is
> quick, weak, and low, though the heat is a little short of a fever,
> but the veins are scarcely filled [and so forth].[47]

Thus sex was not intimately and dramatically linked with alienation of mind in traditional medico-moral discourse, and sexual
aetiologies loom small in eighteenth-century treatises on insanity, as also in madhouse admissions.

As is well known, all this had changed by the Victorian age.
Nineteenth-century opinion waxed eloquent about the perils
of sex, and this was not least because Victorian psychiatry came
to regard sexual abuses or deviations not as simply physically
induced, but as welling up from subterranean psychopathologies
defined within a whole range of newly formulated perverted
types. As Foucault argued:

> From the end of the eighteenth century to our own, they circu-
> lated through the pores of society; they were always hounded, but

not always by laws; were often locked up, but not always in prisons; were sick perhaps, but scandalous, dangerous, victims, prey
to a strange evil that also bore the name of vice and sometimes
crime. They were children, wise beyond their years, precocious
little girls, ambiguous schoolboys, dubious servants and educa-
tors, cruel or maniacal husbands, solitary collectors, ramblers with
bizarre impulses; they haunted the houses of correction, the penal
colonies, the tribunals, and the asylums; they carried their infamy
to the doctors and their sickness to the judges. This was the
numberless family of perverts who were on friendly terms with
delinquents and akin to madmen. In the course of the century
they successively bore the stamp of 'moral folly', 'genital neurosis',
'aberration of the genetic instinct', 'degenerescence', or 'physical
imbalance'.[48]

Thus sex was well and truly 'psychiatrised' in the nineteenth
century – or, as Foucault put it, 'sexuality' was invented. But was
this purely a nineteenth-century vision, or can this psychiatrisation of sex – like that of 'alcoholism' – be traced back into the
Georgian age? To some degree. For example, it was then that the
panic about masturbation began, signalled by the publication in
1710 of *Onania*, a tract certainly attributing the evils of self-abuse
in part to inflamed imaginations. Yet, although Georgian opinion
undoubtedly thundered against masturbation, it was not directly
linked – unlike later – with insanity.

Few nineteenth-century psychiatrists doubted that masturbation caused madness. In Esquirol's word, 'masturbation is
recognised in all countries as a common cause of insanity'; or
as Henry Maudsley put it, 'the development of puberty may
indirectly lead to insanity by becoming the occasion of a vicious
habit of self-abuse'. Indeed, David Skae specifically claimed that
masturbatory insanity was even a distinct species of mental disease. Not surprisingly then, masturbation became a reason for
confinement. For example, of the 157 males admitted to Colney
Hatch Asylum in North London in 1858, six were confined for
'masturbation'. Now there is no denying that it was during the

eighteenth century that fears were fuelled about the harmful effects of the solitary vice, first in *Onania or the heinous sin of self pollution* (1710) and then in the *Onanism of Tissot*, translated into English in 1766. Yet their condemnations of the practice are significantly different from those of later authors. For the anonymous author of *Onania*, masturbation was evil principally as a vice and a sin, and its consequences were essentially physical. Habitués would lose their appetite, grow weak, pale of complexion, sleepless and exhausted. Men would experience 'priapisms', stranguries, fainting fits; women would suffer from 'the whites'. Not least, masturbation would spur other vices, such as fornication. Tissot envisioned a similar dire train of consequences. Of a masturbating man, he wrote:

> The relaxation which these excesses occasion, disorders the functions of all the organs... Digestion, concoction, perspiration, and other evacuations, are no longer performed as they ought to be: hence arises a sensible diminution of the powers of the memory, and even of the understanding: the sight is hereby clouded; all kinds of gout and rheumatism; weakness in the back, and consumptions, arise from the same cause [etc.][49]

And of self-abusing women:

> Their stages are very irregular, their symptoms capricious, and their periods incertain; which after much difficulty the disorder is surmounted, the patient still remains rather in a languishing state, than upon the mending hand.[50]

And he quotes the autodiagnosis of a self-confessed masturbator in much the same vein:

> I feel my heat sensibly diminish, my senses are greatly blunted, the fire of my imagination greatly decreased, the sensation of my existence not near so quick.[51]

Ebenezer Sibly, equally hostile to self-abuse, likewise viewed its evil consequences as essentially somatic. He too presented case studies:

> A youth, apparently under age, applied to me for the cure of a disorder, which, he said, had deprived him of the power of erection... I brought him to confess what I above suspected, that he had so much addicted himself to this shameful and destructive vice, that the seminal vessels were completely relaxed; the erectories, the nerves, and glans, of the penis, had entirely lost their tone: an involuntary discharge of the semen, without irritation, or turgidity of the parts, had long taken place, and brought on a want of appetite as impoverished state of the blood, and an universal lassitude of the body.[52]

But perhaps the conclusive proof that masturbation was not regarded by Georgian physicians as precipitating insanity is the fact that contemporary psychiatric texts do not seem even to mention it; self-abuse is absent from the writings of Arnold, Harper, Crichton, Black, Haslam, Hallaran, Knight, and their colleagues. Their taxonomies of insanity, their casebooks and discussions of asylum populations, give no evidence that patients were being confined for masturbating, or were diagnosed to be suffering from onanism-caused madness. Thus eighteenth-century discussions of masturbation suggest that the links in the contemporary mind between sexual excitation and insanity were oblique and tenuous. Even so, anxiety over its prevalence and its habit-forming qualities, and thus the difficulty of eradicating it, indicate – as with alcoholism – that in many areas of attitudes and action Georgian opinion was discovering that the secret processes of the self went deeper, and were more deviously dangerous, than medicine had previously acknowledged.

The mid-Georgian understanding of mind-body interactions – Tristram Shandy graphically called them the relations between a man's jerkin and its lining – was thus intricate, contested and in flux. Eminent practitioners admitted their ignorance of the precise economy of influence:

> How mind acts upon matter, will, in all probability, ever remain a secret... It is sufficient for us to know that there is established a reciprocal influence betwixt the mental and corporeal parts, and that whatever disorders the one likewise hurts the other.[53]

Why this ignorance? The division of intellectual labour between philosophers of the mind and physicians of the body was often blamed for blocking progress. As John Gregory complained, most who had 'study'd the Philosophy of the Human Mind', had been 'little acquainted with the structure of the Human Body', while for their part physicians had 'been so generally inattentive to the peculiar laws of the Mind and their influence on the Body'. Not surprisingly, therefore, when a new discourse about insanity emerged, it developed outside the traditions of both regular medicine and metaphysical philosophy.

MORAL MANAGEMENT

Indeed, out of these confusions, polemics and indecisions there developed a mental medicine eclectic through and through. Many mad-doctors proceeded in practice as if they thought insanity had a dual aetiology and a twin therapeutics. The Revd Dr Francis Willis' treatment of George III affords a good instance. Willis' speciality was to fix the attention of lunatics by the eye, to win control and submission. But alongside such 'psychological' tricks he also liberally deployed purges, blisters, mechanical restraint (strait-waistcoats) and physical coercion (or at least its threat).

Certainly by the mid-eighteenth century, the tide had turned against the whip. As William Pargeter insisted:

> I at once condemn this practice, as altogether erroneous, and not to be justified upon any principles or pretences whatsoever.[54]

Moreover, time-honoured routine therapeutics such as Bethlem's annual spring bloodletting were, it was increasingly agreed, far too ham-fisted for so mercurial a malady as madness; and the lancet was as destructive 'as a sword'. Above all, as Battie stressed, neglect and inhumanity were no longer an acceptable mixture. Discussing melancholics, Gregory wrote:

> Madness is, contrary to the opinion of some unthinking persons, as manageable as many other distempers, which are equally dreadful and obstinate, and yet are not looked upon as incurable;... such unhappy objects ought by no means to be abandoned, much less shut up in loathsome prisons as criminals or nuisances to the society.[55]

It was Battie who became the prime mover in changing public attitudes, by means of a new formulation of the nature of insanity itself. In his *Treatise on Madness* (1758), Battie argued that though the disease was multiform, it did not resist classification and thus thwart action. Indeed, it could be reduced to two main heads. On the one hand, 'Original Madness', which was essentially endogenous or congenital, or at least resulted from organic defect. This kind of madness was the doctor's bane, being 'not removable by any method which the science of Physick in its present imperfect state is able to suggest', and hence, 'never radically cured'. On the other hand, there was 'Consequential Madness', exogenous madness, acquired during a patient's lifetime, often through anxieties or calamity, and manifesting itself in Lockean delusions, the mismatch between expectations and experience. Like Locke, whom he admired, Battie thought 'deluded imagination' central to consequential madness and in principle capable of remedy.

Probably Battie's polarisation was more propaganda than taxonomy; more for public consumption than for science; yet it represents a turning point. Here was a leading and prestigious mad-doctor publicly embracing reasoned therapeutic optimism. Yet his statement also meant a thumbs-down for medication.

Madness seemed hardly responsive to drugs. Traditional remedies were harsh and indiscriminate. In so far as madness could be cured, it would not be through medicine, but through management, directed to the mind and character of the sufferer, engaging his attention, gaining his respect, breaking evil habits and associations. 'The Regimen in this is perhaps of more importance than in any distemper', Battie assured:

> It was the saying of a very eminent practitioner in such cases that management did much more than medicine; and repeated experience has convinced me that confinement alone is oftentimes sufficient, but always so necessary, that without it every method hitherto devised for the cure of Madness would be ineffectual.[56]

This text became almost canonical for the treatment of mental disturbance, with its confident combination of Lockian associationism ('deluded imagination is... an essential character of Madness'), management, and the *sine qua non* of confinement. Battie's work became pivotal. It proclaimed a message of real power: see madness as delusion, put sufferers into asylums for treatment, use strict, intelligent, humane management techniques – and you will maximise cures. Throughout his brief tract, the contrast with Bethlem was total. When John Monro in reply characterised the mad as typically suffering from ingrained constitutional malaises, he was in effect endorsing Battie's 'original madness', and behind that, Original Sin, while hardly noticing 'consequential madness'. Embracing 'consequential madness', Battie could, by contrast, be on the side of progress. Monro thought 'madness is a distemper of such a nature, that very little of real use can be said concerning it'; Battie's followers aimed to prove him wrong.

Perhaps time finally vindicated Monro, but his was not the voice the age wanted to hear. The Enlightenment had filled the English with a practical faith that applied reason and education would liberate the present from the age-old 'delusions' and that humanity required the improvement of the lot of unfortunates, among whom lunatics were increasingly seen as both a deserving and a hopeful case (as hopeful as savages, and more so than idiots). The this-worldly temper of the times was turning attention from the Christian cure of souls to the cure of 'minds diseased'. And Locke's doctrine of man's malleability and the formation of character by environment both encouraged expectations of 'reform' and also pointed to the asylum as the site where, by breaking the chains of adverse circumstances, minds could be reformed. The exposures of illegal confinement which galvanised the public in the 1760s, and the passing of the 1774 Madhouses Act, opened a new era in asylum history, characterised by more active notions of treatment, and a new humane impulse of public interest.

Crucially important was Battie's insistence that though 'Madness is frequently taken for one species of disorder', it was in fact an individual condition, unresponsive to universal 'cures':

> Madness therefore, like most other morbid cases, rejects all general methods, e.g. bleeding, blisters, caustics, rough cathartics, the gumms and faetid anti-hysterics, opium, mineral waters, cold bathing, and vomits.[57]

This stimulated new approaches to treating the mad. Let us draw a contrast. Back in the 1720s Nicholas Robinson could offer the following case of spleen:

> It is not long ago since a very learned and ingenious Gentleman, so far started from his Reason, as to believe that his Body was metamorphos'd into a Hobby-Horse, and nothing would serve his Turn, but that his Friend, who came to see him, must mount his Back and ride. I must confess, that all the Philosophy I was Master of, could not dispossess him of this Conceit; 'till, by the Application of generous Medicines, I restor'd the disconcerted Nerves to their regular Motions, and, by that Means, gave him a Sight of his Error.[58]

Robinson evidently had two strings to his bow: logic ('all the Philosophy I was Master of'), trying to syllogise his patient into sense; and, when that failed, 'generous Medicines'. By 1750, however, everyone agreed that trying to outwit madness by argument was hopeless – indeed it had its own Swiftian lunacy – while Battie and others were increasingly sceptical about druggings.

Replacing these, a fresh therapeutics rose to favour – partly thanks to Battie – espousing a new intensification of personal contact between physician and patient. The precise inflections of the madman's demeanour and disposition, attitudes and ideas, address and responses, had all to be digested and then handled in ways appropriate to the particular case – sometimes by soothing, sometimes by shocking, perhaps by rest, maybe by exertion. By nice calculation of means and ends, the physician had to achieve command, substituting his control for that of the disease controlling the lunatic.

These initiatives – which are at the same time novel, yet also seem in many ways like a secularised echo of the techniques commonly used earlier by thaumaturgical healers – are spectacularly exemplified by the techniques of two of the more charismatic mad-doctors of the second half of the century. First, the Revd Dr Francis Willis, 'Doctor Duplicate', a Church of England clergyman-turned-physician and owner of a unique asylum at Greatford in Lincolnshire. Willis' first priority was to establish mastery over his charges. Called in to treat George III in 1788, he was so bold as to use a battery of harsh expedients to assert his dominion, applying a strait-waistcoat and purges quite explicitly as persuasives and punishments. And yet he also equally boldly – most thought rashly – allowed the king a razor to shave himself, as a way of demonstrating confidence in his royal charge. Required by Parliamentary Committee to explain himself, Willis replied:

> It is necessary for a Physician, especially in such Cases, to be able to judge, at the Moment, whether he can confide in the Professions of his Patient; and I never was disappointed in my Opinion.[59]

The trump card in what Haslam later called 'this fascinating power which the mad-doctor is said to possess over the wayward lunatic' lay in his power to command by fixing patients with the eye. Interestingly it was Edmund Burke – himself expert on the mental terror of the Sublime – who quizzed Willis about his 'power... of instantaneously terrifying [the king] into obedience'. In response, Willis offered a demonstration:

> 'Place the candles between us, Mr. Burke,' replied the Doctor, in an equally authoritative tone – 'and I'll give you an answer. There, Sir! by the EYE! I should have looked at him thus, Sir' – thus Burke instantaneously averted his head, and, making no reply, evidently acknowledged this basiliskan authority.[60]

Thereby Willis demonstrated himself a true proto-Romantic contemporary of Lavater and Mesmer.

The claims of Willis and his sons to have 'cured' the king are, at best, not proven (indeed, if Macalpine and Hunter were right that George was suffering from the hereditary condition porphyria, such claims become untenable). What is beyond dispute, however, is that before the Willises' *coup* at Windsor, court physicians-in-ordinary such as Sir George Baker had disastrously failed to stamp their authority upon the chaos of the king's condition. By failing to quell his irritation and hyperactivity, they had perhaps exacerbated his sickness. The Willises took charge, mastered the monarch and, by compelling docility and submission, created a climate congenial to his restoration.

Paralleling Willis as what George Nesse Hill dubbed a 'medical artist', was his younger contemporary, Dr William Pargeter. He too placed his faith in an intensely dramaturgic interplay between mad-doctor and patients, as his case notes demonstrate:

> When I was a pupil at St Bartholomew's Hospital employed on the subject of Insanity, I was requested... to visit a poor man... disordered in his mind...The maniac was locked in a room, raving

and exceedingly turbulent. I took two men with me, and learning that he had no offensive weapons, I planted them at the door, with directions to be silent, and to keep out of sight, unless I should want their assistance. I then suddenly unlocked the door – rushed into the room and caught his eye in an instant. The business was then done – he became peacable in a moment – trembled with fear, and was as governable as it was possible for a furious madman to be.[61]

A second case reveals how Pargeter understood that every person required an individual touch. Called in to deal with a melancholy young lady,

> I was introduced to her room, and found her in a thoughtful posture, her elbow on the table, and resting her cheek upon her hand. She did not, for some time, seem to know that any body was in the room; at length she looked up, and the moment I caught her eye, for, till then I had been silent, I told her I was perfectly acquainted with the cause of her complaint, and conversed with her on those topics, I thought most suitable to her case, and at last persuaded her to come down to dinner with the rest of the family, and to drink two or three glasses of wine, and to join in the conversation of the table. I recommended an immediate change of residence – gave directions respecting diet – exercise – amusements – reading – conversation – and had soon the pleasing satisfaction to be informed of the lady's perfect recovery.[62]

For Pargeter, gaining supremacy involved not only the *coup d'état* of a *coup d'œil* but taking the personal and family histories as well.

Not every late eighteenth-century mad-doctor, of course, exercised charisma so theatrically. But common to all was the belief that madness was curable (Willis claimed a nine-out-of-ten recovery rate), and could be conquered through energetic person-to-person encounters. Especially revealing here is

Thomas Percival's commendation on the vital importance of keeping a 'regular journal', or detailed case-notes. In so elusive a disease, a settled strategy was crucial and no detail was to be missed:

> Though casual success may sometimes be the result of empirical practice, the *medicina mentis* can only be administered with steady efficacy by him, who, to a knowledge of the animal oeconomy, and of the physical causes which regulate or disturb its movements, unites an intimate acquaintance with the laws of association; the controul of fancy over judgment: the force of habit; the direction and comparative strength of opposite passions; and the reciprocal dependences and relations of the moral and intellectual powers of man.[63]

To counter the regrettable fact 'that the various diseases which are classed under the title of insanity, remain less understood than any others with which mankind are visited', Percival recommended that full particulars of each patient be recorded, including 'age, sex, occupation, mode of life, and if possible hereditary constitution'. Finally, he advised post mortems:

> When the event proves fatal, the brain, and other organs affected should be carefully examined, and the appearance on dissection minutely inserted in the journal.[64]

The contemporary term for this novel strategy of 'close encounters' was 'moral management' – 'moral' in the sense of addressing itself to the patient's mind (and not just to the body), establishing a consciousness-to-consciousness rapport; 'management' because – and here the parallel with industrial entrepreneurs suggests itself – the mad-doctor had to prove supremely energetic and resourceful, prolific in initiatives which would impose discipline and sanity. What made management possible was Locke's doctrine of the malleability of man or, as James Burgh put it, 'by management the human species may be

moulded into any conceivable shape'. Battie's dictum as to how
management would do more than medicine was the gospel for
what became a progressive movement. As Ferriar stressed, in
dealing with disturbance humanity must replace cruelty, and
mental treatment had to supplant physical:

> The management of the mind is an object of great consequence,
> in the treatment of insane persons, and has been much misun-
> derstood. It was formerly supposed that lunatics could only be
> worked upon by terror; shackles and whips, therefore, became
> part of the medical apparatus.[65]

No longer!

> A system of mildness and conciliation is now generally adopted,
> which, if it does not always facilitate the cure, at least tends to
> soften the destiny of the sufferer.[66]

The point about Ferriar's remarks is that their cadences were
already becoming choruses – they could have been uttered by
any of a dozen of his contemporaries. Already a mythology of the
bad old days was crystallising. Developing a similar philosophy of
moral discipline, William Pargeter used much the same terms:

> The chief reliance in the cure of insanity must be rather on
> management than medicine. The government of maniacs is an
> art, not to be acquired without long experience, and frequent
> and attentive observation. Although it has been of late years much
> advanced, it is still capable of improvement.[67]

Pargeter regarded management as involving a battle of wits, a
war of nerves:

> As maniacs are extremely subdolous, the phisician's first visit
> should be by surprise. He must employ every moment of his
> time by mildness or menaces, as circumstances direct, to gain an

ascendancy over them, and to obtain their favour and prepos-
session. If this opportunity be lost, it will be difficult, if not
impossible, to effect it afterwards; and more especially, if he should
betray any signs of timidity.[68]

By consequence, the mad-doctor needed all the acting skills of
Garrick, all the virtuosity of Machiavelli's prince:

> He should be well acquainted with the pathology of the disease
> – should possess great acumen – a discerning and penetrating eye
> – much humanity and courtesy – and even disposition, and com-
> mand of temper. He may be obliged at one moment, according
> to the exigency of the case, to be placid and accommodating in
> his manners, and the next, angry and absolute.[69]

To some degree the precise tactics of interventionist management were personal, differing from individual to individual.
But the newer ranks of mad-doctors also shared key strategies.
To a man, they condemned the dark ages of lazy approaches
to madness, those techniques – be they soporific draughts or
chains – whose horizon was merely custodial. They denounced
the barbarity both of neglect and of brutality, endorsing instead
what Ferriar called a 'system of mildness'. Except for occasional
tactical coups, *physical* punishments such as beatings were to be
avoided, as above all were casual violence and arbitrary fluctuations in treatment, for these mixed 'impolicy and impropriety',
confusing the patient and arousing his suspicions. Put yourself
in the patient's shoes:

> Sudden changes of situation, and sudden removal from friends
> and relatives, may be attended with fatal, rather than happy con-
> sequences. Suppose the mind to be deranged for a moment,
> and in that moment this violent and sudden change takes place,
> what more can be wanting, on the slightest appearance of
> recovery, than the soothing attentions and assiduous cares of
> affection? What can so soon calm the troubled spirit, or enliven

the gloomy imagination, just on the point, perhaps of regaining its powers.[70]

In a similar vein Joseph Mason Cox, proprietor of Fishponds, commended a kind of empathy with patients. No advantage lay in attempting to enter into the delusions of the insane. But it was crucial to gauge their progressive *needs* within a long-term strategy of normalisation. Sensitivity with strength was required:

> It cannot be too frequently repeated that, even in the medical management of maniacs, the physician should never forget that sympathetic tenderness which the sufferings of humanity claim; he should only take care that this be not so far indulged as to diminish the steadiness and presence of mind, for the furious madman as well as the miserable melancholic is frequently sensible to tender impressions, and gentleness of behaviour makes the approach of a physician be felt like that of guardian angel sent to afford ease and comfort.[71]

Mildness, of course, precluded violence. No 'moral manager' dismissed physical coercion and constraint entirely, but most argued that they were at best necessary evils, commonly overused and abused. 'Here', wrote Benjamin Faulkner about his own private madhouse, 'all unnecessary confinement is avoided'. Whereas but a century earlier Thomas Willis had urged 'threatenings, bonds, or strokes, as well as Physick', arguing that 'Furious Mad-men are sooner, and more certainly cured by punishments, and hard usage, in a strait room, than by Physick or Medicines', by contrast moral managers stressed how the target of treatment had to be the mind. William Pargeter thus criticised not merely 'chains and cords... and other galling manacles', but also 'beating... a practice formerly much in use in treating the insane'. Writing in the 1790s, he contended that:

> If maniacs are not to be subdued by management... beating will never effect it... and therefore, I at once condemn this practice,

as altogether erroneous, and not justified upon any principles or pretences whatsoever.[72]

Violence should be redundant. This was demonstrated in series of parables proving the power of mind over matter, the moral over the physical, sanity over madness. Maniacs might appear terrifying (hence Norris' contraption in Bedlam), but they would cave in before the mental resourcefulness and agility of the morally astute mad-doctor. William Perfect showed how:

> In the year 1776, the parish officers of Friendsbury applied to me for advice in the case of a maniacal patient confined in their work-house. This unhappy object had been very desperate and had committed many acts of outrage and violence; was naturally of strong, muscular shape, and rendered much stronger by his present complaint. He had overpowered almost everyone before they could properly secure him, which was now effected in a very extraordinary manner. He was fastened to the floor by means of a staple and iron ring, which was tied to a pair of fetters about his legs, and he was hand-cuffed. The place of his confinement was a large lower room, occasionally made use of for a kitchen, and which opened into the Street; there were wooden bars to the windows, through the spaces of which continual visitors were observing, pointing at, ridiculing, and irritating the poor maniac, who thus became a specimen of public sport and amusement.[73]

Violence and counterviolence had formed a vicious circle. Perfect broke it:

> My advice was to take off his shackles and secure him in a strong strait-waistcoat... it was also my advice to have a small hovel built for his solitary residence... and to prohibit all persons from going near enough to converse with him, but those who should be appointed to the charge of attending him. Proper attention being paid to his person and diet, in a few weeks the patient entirely recovered his

reason; and begging hard to be released from his confinement, after I had been again consulted, it was granted, when he quietly and regularly returned to his labour and employment; and I have not heard of his having had any relapse.[74]

All the same, the leading mad-doctors of George III's reign certainly did not espouse the doctrinaire liberalism of kindness for kindness' sake. Clinical experience showed that confinement and coercion were sometimes salutary. As Erasmus Darwin put it:

> Where maniacs are outrageous, there can be no doubt but coercion is necessary: which may be done by means of a strait waistcoat; which disarms them without hurting them.[75]

The crux was to judge what was appropriate in the particular case. Thus, Darwin argued, in some cases confinement worked, whereas

> in others there can be no doubt, but that confinement retards rather than promotes their cure; which is forwarded by change of ideas in consequence of change of place and of objects, as by travelling or sailing.[76]

Physical threats were a last resort. Moral fear, however, was constructive, and creating appropriate terror in a patient could be salutary for securing the calm obedience necessary for effective treatment. As Robert Darling Willis described the practice he learned from his father:

> If they are delirious, they are put into a strait-waistcoat in which they can neither hurt themselves nor others. It has the further advantage of inculcating salutary fear so that on later occasions the mere threat of it will make them control themselves...[77]

Fear could provide the initial leverage, a starting point:

The emotion of fear is the first and often the only one by which they can be governed. By working on it one removes their thoughts from the phantasms occupying them and brings them back to reality, even if this entails inflicting pain and suffering. It is fear too which teaches them to judge their actions rightly and learn the consequences. By such means is their attention brought back to their surroundings.[78]

Thus physical should lead to moral treatment; initially it secured obedience; in time, attention; and thereby concentrated the disordered mind. Moral managers who, with John Gregory, stressed the necessity of an 'intimate knowledge of the human heart' did not see their charges through sentimental Rousseauvian spectacles, maddened by society, everywhere in chains, but needing only example to be restored to innocence. Rather lunatics were confused souls, at war with themselves, devious, damaged; treatments had to be bold, assertive, and strictly tailored to individual needs. The metaphors of therapy were those of the battleground and the theatre. A struggle was on, rather as in a gladiatorial combat. And for success, inventiveness, imagination and panache were imperative. After establishing that two modes of therapy were available, 'moral' and 'medical', and stressing how 'management which is of the highest importance in the treatment of maniacs in almost every case, is indispensable, and has succeeded where more active means have failed', Joseph Mason Cox defined his art:

> The essence of management results from experience, address and the natural endowments of the practitioner, and turns principally on making impressions on the senses.[79]

There were no rigid rules:

> the methods must be regulated by the circumstances of the case. In some, recourse must be had to the most extreme measures, for the security of the party and the restraint of fury; in others, the

THE MAKING OF PSYCHIATRY

most opposite methods are indicated. The generality of maniacs
being artful, and their minds intensely fixed on the accomplish-
ments of any wild purpose conjured up by the disease, physicians
should be constantly on their guard: their grand object is to
procure the confidence of the patient or excite fear.

Even here, Cox argued, numerous techniques were available,
requiring exquisite individual judgement, but capable of producing effects like magic:

I have seen the most furious maniacs by being liberated from
their shackles by my direction, and under my own immediate
inspection, so attached and devoted to me as never again to
require coercion.[80]

Like any impresario, the manager must dictate terms. Even 'pious
frauds' were legitimate, to 'humour the insane idea'. Illustrating
this, Cox conjured up a remarkable, Prospero-like scenario of
cure via sensory disorientation:

It certainly is allowable to try the effect of certain deceptions,
contrived to make strong impressions on the senses, by means of
unexpected, unusual, striking, or apparently supernatural agents;
such as after waking the party from sleep, either suddenly or by
a gradual process, by imitated thunder or soft music, according to
the peculiarity of the case, combatting the erroneous deranged
notion, either by some pointed sentence, or signs executed
in phosphorus upon the wall of the bedchamber, or by some
tale, assertion, or reasoning by one in the character of an angel,
prophet, or devil.[81]

Hardly surprisingly, Cox concluded this phantasmagoria with
some sober advice: 'But the actor in this drama must possess
much skill, and be very perfect in his part'. This need for insight,
astuteness, heroic initiatives and god-like virtuosity became an
idée fixe around the turn of the century. It marked and capitalised

upon the new face-to-face intimacy, offered in small private
asylums, between the madman and the mad-doctor. In this con-
frontation, cure prospects clearly depended little upon formal
therapeutics or new modes of medication, but instead primarily
upon personal rapport. This (William Hallaran stressed) required
a real meeting of minds, in which it was not enough for the
superintendent to empathise with the patient, but he had also
to anticipate the impact of his own self-presentation upon his
charge. Both parties would be constantly involved in sizing each
other up; the quality of the encounter would make or mar the
therapeutic possibilities:

> To the patient [the mad-doctor] becomes a personage for minute
> observation... That share of deference and estimation to which
> he would aspire, and which are so essential to the nature of
> his undertaking, will be freely granted, or as obstinately denied,
> according to the method by which they may be exacted at the
> first interview.[82]

From his vantage point early in the nineteenth century, Hallaran
could look back and dismiss the heroics of Pargeter as stagy,
unlikely to deceive the patient and, not least, *infra dig.* for the
medical profession:

> The vulgar and too generally received opinion, as to the neces-
> sity of a Physician making his first approach... with the assumed
> aspect of unbridled authority, bespeaks a principle sufficient to
> deter men of character from attending to this important depart-
> ment of the medical profession.[83]

Madmen were no fools, and they were 'not to be subdued *ex
officio*, by measures of mere force'; and the gauche mad-doctor
would readily find himself treated 'with marked contempt'.
Such ineptitude had even been known to produce situations
in which

Right: 16 An engraving of William
Perfect, who housed lunatics in his
private asylum in West Malling in
Kent, 1795.

Below: 17 St Luke's Lunatic Asylum,
second hospital, in 1787. St Luke's
was among the first wave of English
public asylums and was founded by
public subscription in 1751. It sought
to destroy the common image of
madhouses caused by the horrors of
Bethlem by banning sightseeing and
admitting medical students.

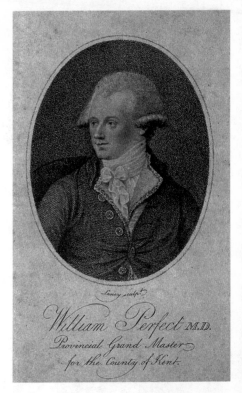

Laney sculpt.

William Perfect M.D.
Provincial Grand Master
for the County of Kent.

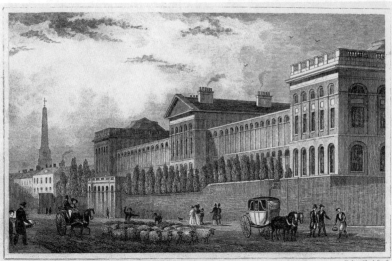

Drawn by Tho. H. Shepherd.
Pl. 135

Engraved by J. Gough.

LUNATIC HOSPITAL, ST. LUKE'S.

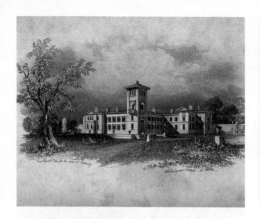

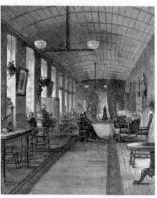

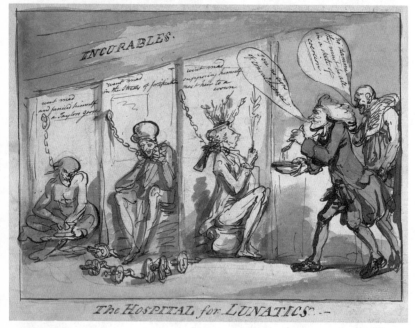

Clockwise from top left:

18 The Liverpool Lunatic Asylum opened in 1797 after the tireless campaigning of Dr James Currie.

19 Wards in Bethlem Hospital, *c.*1745.

20 Bethlem Hospital. The incurables are inspected by a member of the medical staff, with the patients represented by political figures. Drawing by Thomas Rowlandson, 1789.

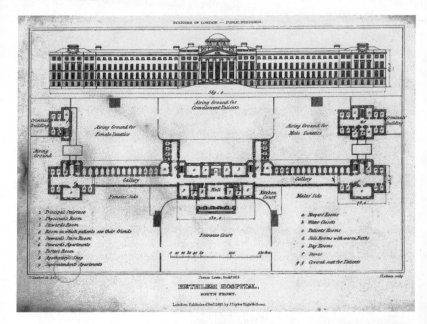

BETHLEM HOSPITAL,
SOUTH FRONT.

London Published Dec. 1 1823 by J. Taylor High Holborn.

Above: 21 Plan of Bethlem
Hospital with scale and a key,
1823. Though small in size,
the idea of 'Bedlam' loomed
large in eighteenth-century
society.

Right: 22 Statues of 'raving'
and 'melancholy' madness
on the gates of Bethlem
Hospital.

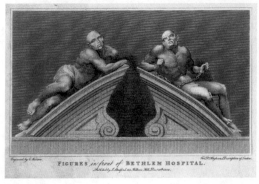

FIGURES *in front of* BETHLEM HOSPITAL.

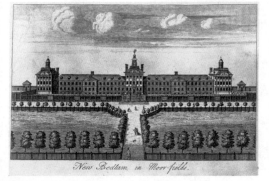

New Bedlam, in Moor-fields.

Left: 23 The hospital of Bethlem
seen from the north with people
walking in the foreground.
Visitors were welcomed
at Bethlem, and sightseers
could view inmates without
appointment. Such was the taste
for viewing the insane that Tom
Brown dryly remarked, 'Bedlam
is a pleasant place... and abounds
with amusements'.

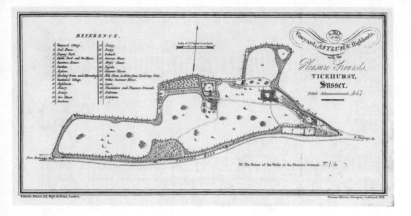

24 A map of the grounds of Ticehurst Hospital, 1827. Ticehurst House was one of the most opulent and respected private madhouses in the country, and contrasts with the revolting conditions in many other private and public madhouses. Its proprietor, the apothecary Samuel Newington, had been accepting individual lunatics for perhaps thirty years before the House proper opened in 1792.

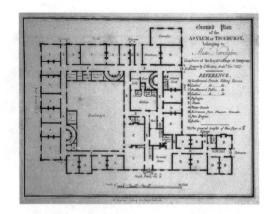

25 Architect's drawings of the ground floor of Ticehurst House.

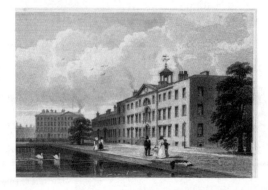

26 The Manchester Lunatic Hospital opened in 1766 with 'cells' for twenty-two inmates. Patients were expected to pay wherever possible for their keep, though they were to receive treatment *gratis*. The hospital flourished: by 1769 some 341 patients were admitted.

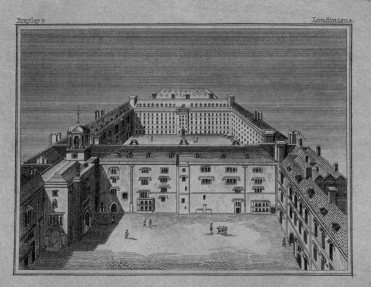

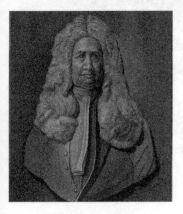

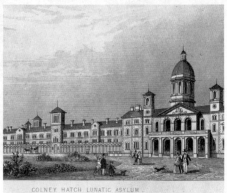

COLNEY HATCH LUNATIC ASYLUM.

Top: 27 Bridewell Hospital, London, in 1720. Bridewell was a house of correction managed by the same governors as Bethlem.

Above left: 28 Thomas Guy (1644–1724). A millionaire London bookseller, Thomas Guy made provision in his will for a wing of the hospital that bore his name to be provided for incurables, including lunatics.

Above right: 29 Colney Hatch Asylum, Middlesex.

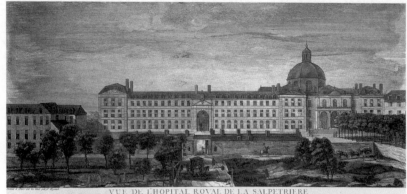

VUE DE L'HOPITAL ROYAL DE LA SALPETRIERE
du Hopital general hors de Paris a une petite promenade de la porte Saint Bernard

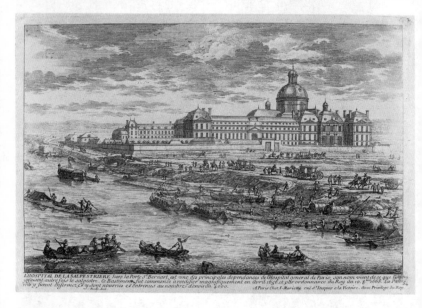

L'HOSPITAL DE LA SALPESTRIERE, hors la Porte S.t Bernard, est une des principales dependances de l'hospital general de Paris: son nom vient de ce que l'on y
qui on fait autres fois le salpestre. Ce Bastiment fut commence a rebastir magnifiquement en Avril 1656, et par ordonnance du Roy du 10.8.bre 1668. La Pauv.
vres y furent enfermes, et y sont nourries et entretenus au nombre d'environ 4000.   A Paris Chez I. Mariette, rue S.t Jacques a la Victoire, Avec Privilege du Roy

This page: 30, 31 The Salpêtrière in Paris, which housed mad people in the eighteenth century.

Opposite top left: 32 An etching of Samuel Tuke, one of the pioneering Tuke family of York. In 1813, Samuel wrote his *Description of the Retreat*, a glowing report of the York madhouse founded by his grandfather, showing that care for the mad could be both humane and effective.

Opposite top right: 33 A caricature of patients in a lunatic asylum, 1838. Inmates are drawing and scratching on the walls, poring over books and lamenting.

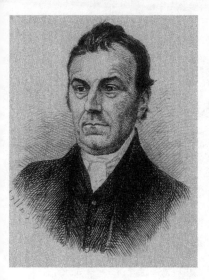
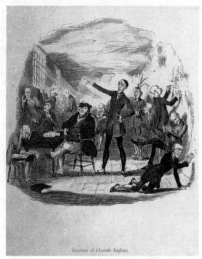
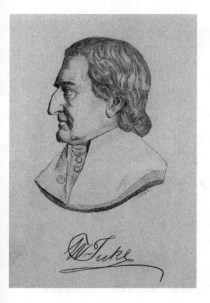
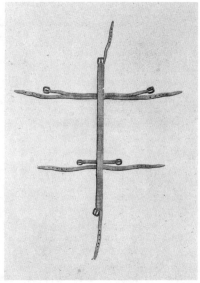

Above left: 34 William Tuke (1732–1822). Tuke was the founder of the York Retreat madhouse, a Quaker-led institution catering for the emotional needs of the insane through the much-celebrated 'moral therapy'.

Above right: 35 A leather restraining device used at York Asylum. The treatment of patients in this particular asylum was said to be brutal: JP Godfrey Higgins found cells whose stench made him instantly vomit, and discovered thirteen women cooped up for the day in a cell eight feet square.

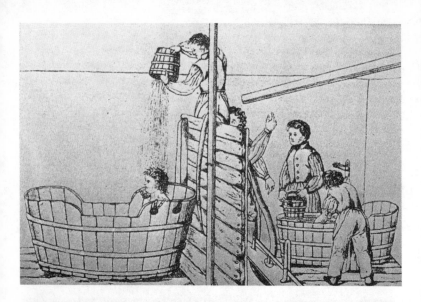

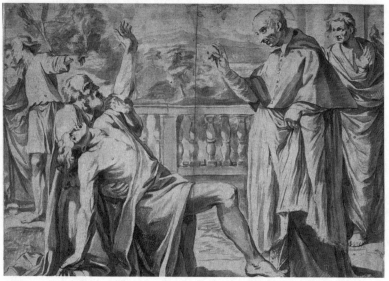

Top: 36 The douche, a method for calming the insane. John Wesley himself advocated the use of water-shock therapy in advising patients to sit under a great waterfall 'as long as the strength will bear'.

Above: 37 An epileptic man is restrained. Mad-doctor to George III Francis Willis performed case studies of convulsives, epileptics and defectives, emphasising the importance of the spinal column in neurogeography.

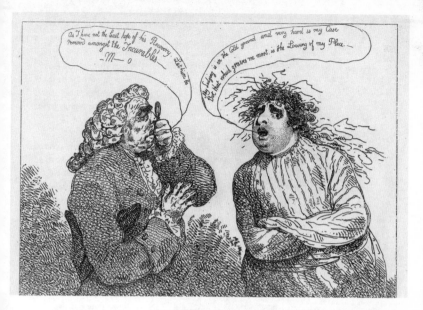

Above: 38 Dr Munro (physician to Bedlam) examining Dr Charles Fox, who is portrayed as a strait-jacketed and dishevelled patient. Etching by Thomas Rowlandson, 1784.

Right: 39 An unspecified method of coercion for violent lunatics, 1826.

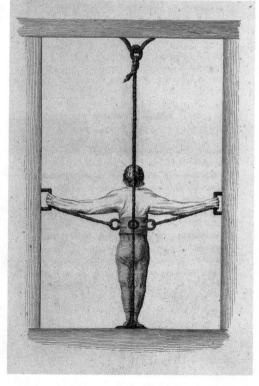

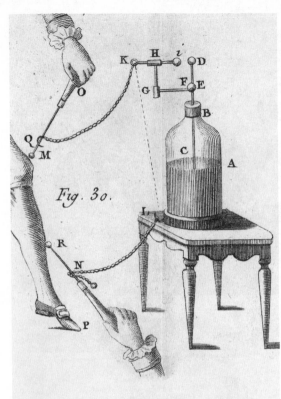

Fig. 30.

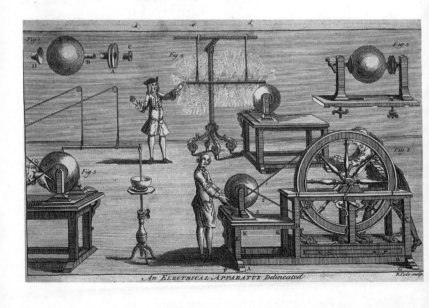

An ELECTRICAL APPARATUS Delineated.

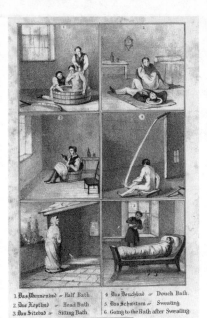

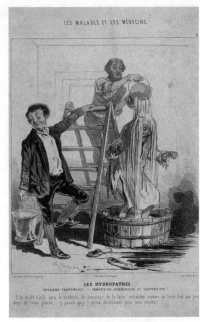

LES MALADES ET LES MÉDECINS.

LES HYDROPATHES.

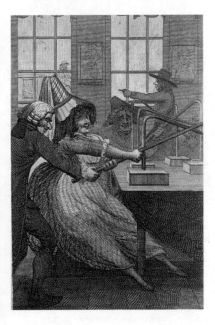

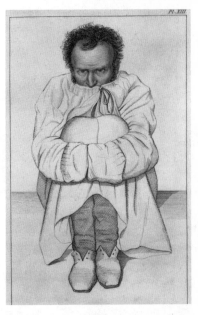

Above left: 44 A quack doctor assisting a voluptuous patient with group magnetic therapy *c.*1792.

Above right: 45 Engraving of a maniac in an asylum restrained in a straitjacket.

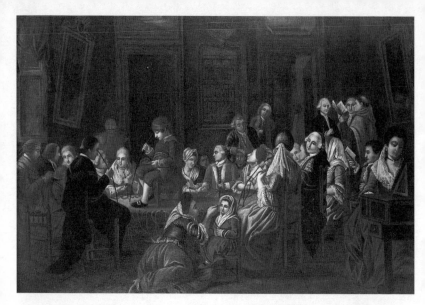

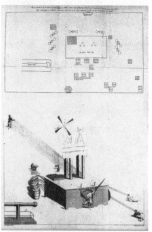

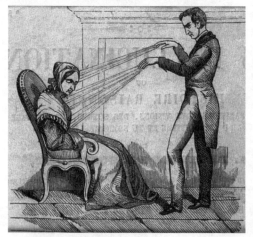

Top: 46 A group of mesmerised patients. Mesmerism was founded in the eighteenth century in France by Franz Anton Mesmer (1734–1815), and was supposedly effective in curing the mad through reducing the patient to a hypnotised state.

Above left: 47 In 1809 James Tilley Matthews petitioned for release from Bethlem, claiming his sanity; two eminent physicians, Drs Birkbeck and Clutterbuck, testified on his behalf. Bethlem's medical staff contested the case and John Haslam, apothecary to the hospital, publicised the affair in *Illustrations of Madness* (1810). Illustrated here is the 'airloom' that featured in the case.

Above right: 48 A practitioner of Mesmerism using animal magnetism on a woman who responds with convulsions.

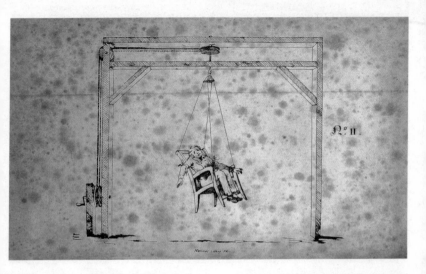

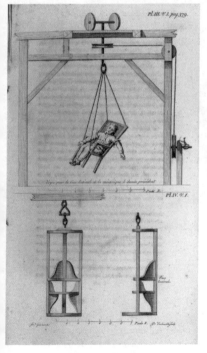

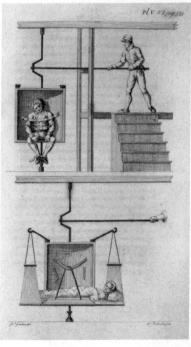

49, 50, 51 Rotary machines used to treat the mentally ill. The rotary machine, or swing-chair, rotated at around 100 times a minute, causing gushing of blood from the ears and nose and, ultimately, unconsciousness. Such a procedure was expected to have a surprisingly positive effect upon the mind.

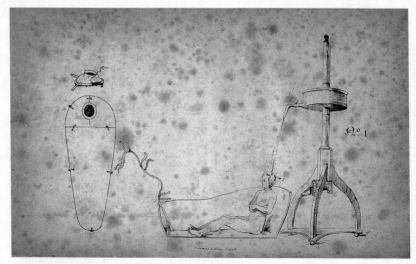

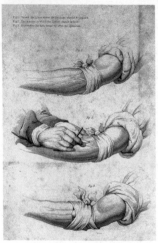

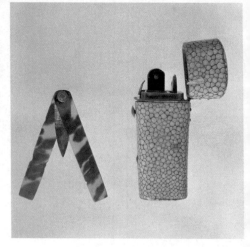

Top: 52 A variation on the ever-popular douche, 1828.

Above left: 53 Three diagrams illustrating how to bleed an arm.

Above right: 54 A lancet and case used for bloodletting. Popular in the early treatment of mad people, purification by bloodletting was, by the end of the eighteenth century, thought too ham-fisted for so mercurial a malady as madness. The lancet was said to be as destructive 'as a sword'.

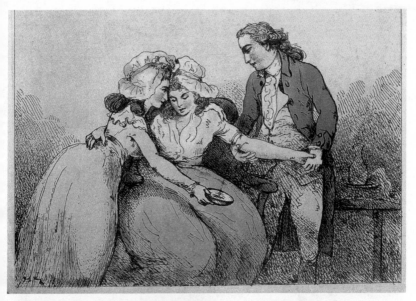

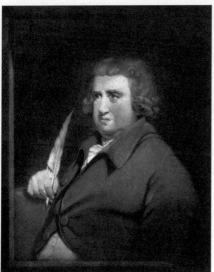

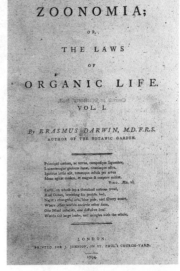

Top: 55 A surgeon bleeding the arm of a young woman. Mass bloodletting was an annual occurrence at Bethlem.

Above left: 56 Erasmus Darwin in 1797. An enthusiast of early psychiatry and the effective treatment of mad people, Darwin recommended such therapies as enormous doses of opium, restraint using the strait-waistcoat and the less-than-humane swing-chair.

Above right: 57 Erasmus Darwin's much-celebrated work, *Zoonomia*, 1794.

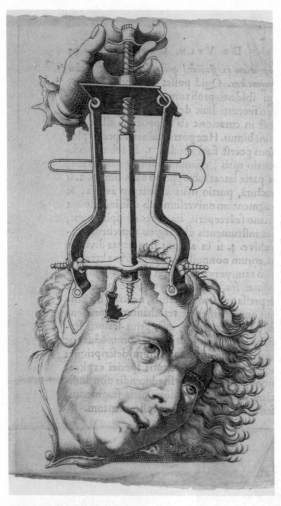

Left: 58 Removing the bone after the ancient surgical practice of trephination. This procedure was an attempt at healing the mind through supernatural means. Theory was that a malicious spirit had taken possession of the patient and was causing sickness, so opening the skull would allow the demon to escape.

Below left: 59 A surgeon extracting stones from a woman's head, *c.*1650.

Below right: 60 An itinerant surgeon extracting stones from a man's head.

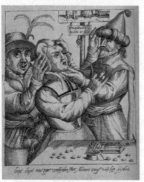

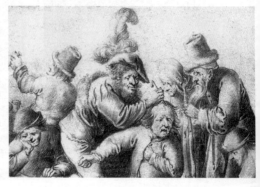

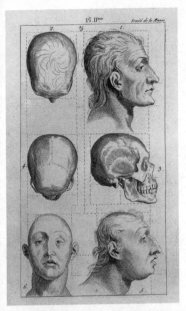

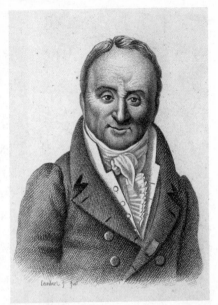

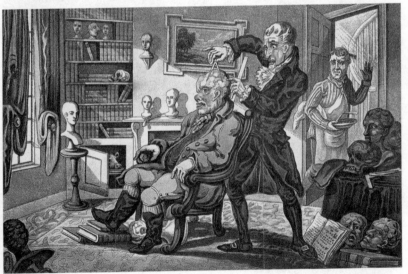

Top left: 61 Philippe Pinel's six pictures of crania and heads of the insane, *c.*1801. Pinel's revolution in the eighteenth century meant that the mad could be treated 'on medical rather than moral lines'.

Top right: 62 Philippe Pinel (1745–1826), pioneer of eighteenth-century psychiatry in revolutionary Paris.

Above: 63 Johann Caspar Spurzheim measuring the head of a patient.

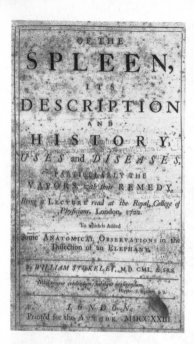

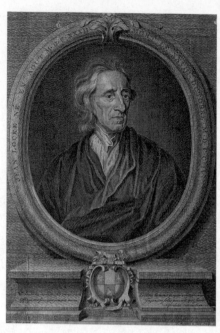

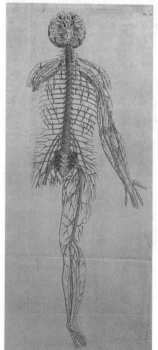

Clockwise from top left: 64 William Stukeley's *Of the Spleen, its Description and History, Uses and Diseases*. The eighteenth-century gout expert believed the spleen to be the source of disordered nerves and spirits.

65 John Locke in 1734. Locke propounded the theory that madness arose from false associations of ideas. He presented the mind as a *tabula rasa* subject to the influences of experience. Depending on how the mind processed experience, it might become filled with natural ideas and normal judgements, or it might end up cognitively and emotionally disorientated.

66 A drawing of the nervous system of the human body by Hermann Boerhaave, who presented the argument that nerves acted as hollow pipes, filled under pressure by a fluid composed of the subtlest of bodily particles. If these pipes became clogged by indulgence in 'heavy' diet and 'low' habits, the fluids grew sluggish, causing 'heaviness' and 'lowness'.

Opposite, top left: 67 Hermann Boerhaave's anatomy of the brain.

Opposite, top right: 68 George Cheyne in 1732. Author of *The English Malady*, Cheyne suggested that diet and digestion were responsible for melancholy.

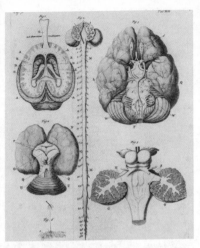

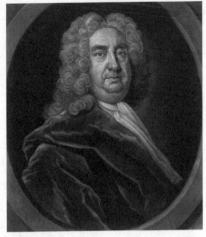

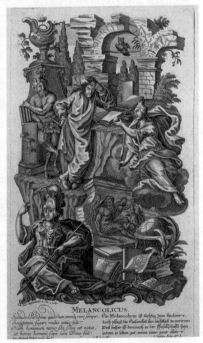

MELANCOLICUS.

A TREATISE

OF

MELANCHOLY.

CONTAINING THE
CAVSES THEREOF, AND
Reasons of the strange effects it worketh
in our minds and bodies: with the Phy-
sicke Cure, and spirituall consolation
for such as haue thereto adioyned
afflicted Conscience.

THE DIFFERENCE BE-
TWIXT IT, AND MELANCHOLY,
With diuers Philosophicall discourses
touching actions, and affections of
Soule, Spirit, and Body : the
particulars whereof are to
bee seene before the
BOOKE.

By T. BRIGHT Doctor of Phisicke.

Newly Corrected and amended.

LONDON.
Printed by *William Stansby*. 1613.

Above left: 69 A depressed scholar surrounded by mythological figures representing the melancholy temperament. The main image shows a scholar with a knife behind him and a goddess with an apple (fruit of knowledge) before him. In the bottom left-hand corner is Minerva, goddess of wisdom, and at the top an owl, one of her attributes. The price of wisdom is melancholy.

Above right: 70 Timothy Bright's *A Treatise on Melancholy*, published in 1586, was the first major tract on the subject, and was personally addressed to a fictitious sufferer called 'M'.

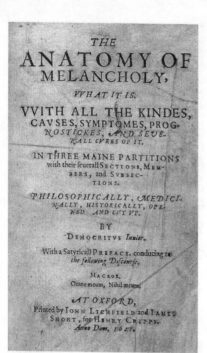

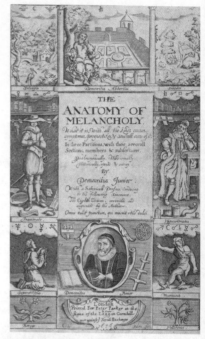

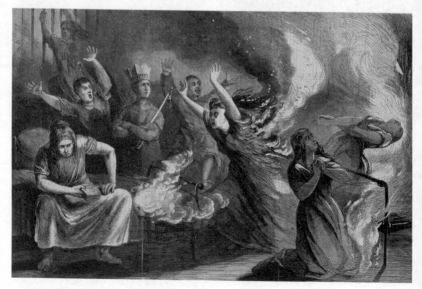

Top: 71, 72 Title page and frontispiece to Burton's *Anatomy of Melancholy* (1624).

Above: 73 A group of mentally ill patients dashing around a burning room. Wood engraving.

Right: 74 John Donaldson, a poor simpleton who lived in the eighteenth century and who made it a habit to walk before funeral processions in Edinburgh.

Below left: 75 Title page of Thomas Arnold's *Observations on the Nature, Kinds, Causes and Prevention of Insanity* (1782–86). Dr Thomas Arnold was a prominent physician and private madhouse-keeper, and had a rich case history of treatment of insane patients.

Below right: 76 Francis Willis (1718–1807). Willis was mad-doctor to the insane George III, who often complained that he 'beat me like a madman'. To contrast this alleged brutal treatment of the monarch, Willis' own madhouse in Greatford in Lincolnshire was described as an 'admirable system' and allowed patients to work as labourers, eat with their carers and dress as normal.

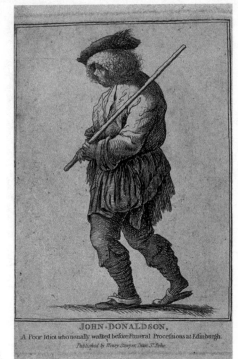

JOHN·DONALDSON,
A Poor Idiot who usually walked before Funeral Processions at Edinburgh.
Published by Henry Sawyer, Dean St Soho.

OBSERVATIONS
ON THE
NATURE, KINDS, CAUSES,
AND PREVENTION OF
INSANITY,
LUNACY,
OR
MADNESS.

BY THOMAS ARNOLD, M.D.

VOL. I.

CONTAINING
OBSERVATIONS ON THE NATURE, AND VARIOUS
KINDS OF INSANITY.

Ταράσσει τὰς ἀνθρώπως, ἳ τὰ πράγματα, ἀλλά
τὰ περὶ τῶν πραγμάτων δόγματα.
EPICTETI Enchirid. Cap. X.
*Men are not disturbed by things themselves; but by the
opinions which they form concerning them.*

And moody Madness laughing wild
Amid severest woe.   GRAY.

LEICESTER:

PRINTED BY G. IRELAND, FOR G. ROBINSON, IN PATER-
NOSTER-ROW, AND T. CADELL, IN THE STRAND,
LONDON. M.DCC.LXXXII.

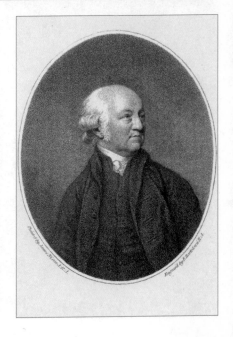

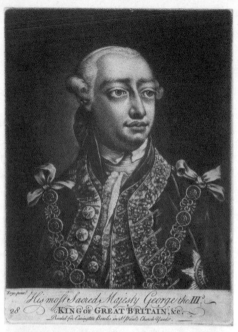

77 King George III. George was afflicted with porphyria, a maddening disease that affected his rule from 1765 onwards. His disease was made public to the extent that regular bulletins were published on his state of health.

His most Sacred Majesty George the III.
KING OF GREAT BRITAIN, &c.
Printed for Carington Bowles in St Paul's Church Yard.

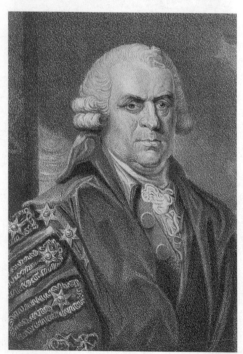

Left: **78** Sir George Baker in 1837. Baker was one of the first medical students of William Battie at St Luke's Asylum and became one of George III's mad-doctors.

Opposite page:

Top left: **79** Richard Warren, physician to George III.

Top right: **80** William Cowper in 1698. Cowper suffered mental illness in the 1760s, proved a spectacular failure at committing suicide by either drowning, stabbing or poison and finally recovered in Nathaniel Cotton's Collegium Insanorum at St Albans.

Below: **81** Tom Rakewell just before the onset of madness, from Hogarth's *Rake's Progress* series, 1735. Madness itself is symbolised by the outbreak of fire in the wainscoting.

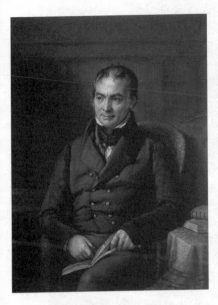

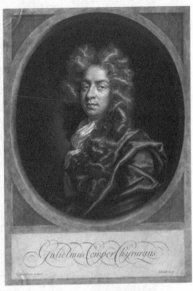

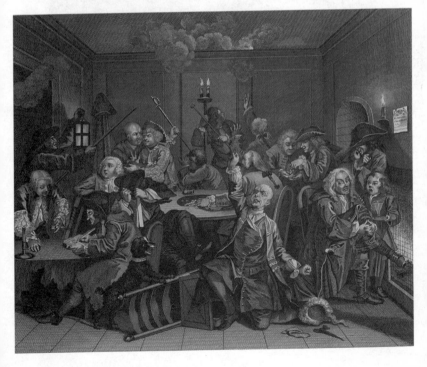

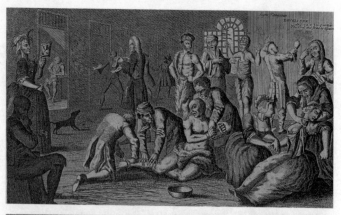

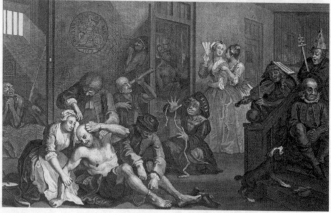

This page, top: 82 A half-naked asylum patient, his wrists chained, is restrained by orderlies and surrounded by a variety of other deranged individuals. The print (1735) is an obvious echo of Hogarth's *Rake's Progress* series, indicating the popularity of scenes out of Bedlam in the eighteenth century.

Above: 83 Plate VIII from Hogarth's *Rake's Progress* series, 1735. Now insane, Tom Rakewell sits on the floor of the gallery at Bethlem Hospital grasping at his head in the classic pose of the maniac. He is surrounded by other lunatics.

Opposite, clockwise from top left: 84 A 1722 tract entitled *Onania or the Heinous Sin of Self-Pollution* warned of the side-effects of masturbation.

85 Appliances for the treatment of masturbation by females. Female masturbators were said to experience uncertain periods, languishing, disorder and 'irregular stages'.

86 An eye-watering depiction of a four-pointed urethral ring for the treatment of masturbation. The side-effects of the habit were described in the eighteenth century as a loss of appetite, sleeplessness, gout, rheumatism, poor sight, caprice, memory loss and madness.

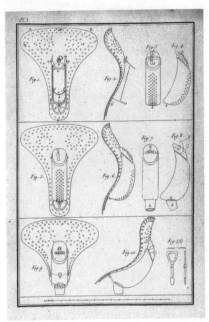

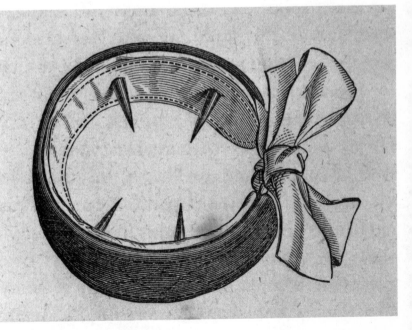

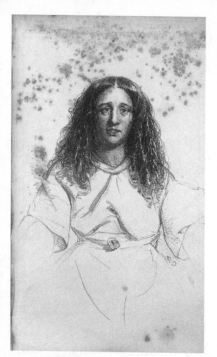

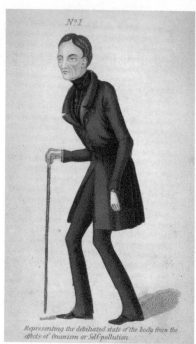

Representing the debilitated state of the body from the effects of Onanism or Self-pollution.

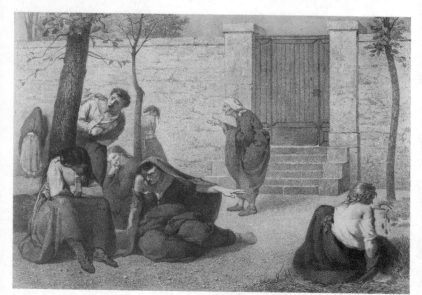

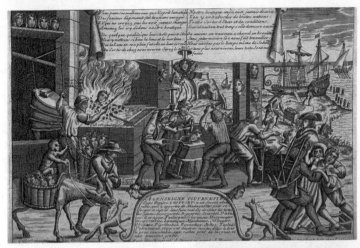

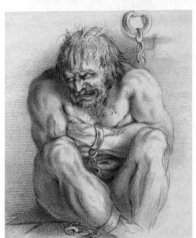

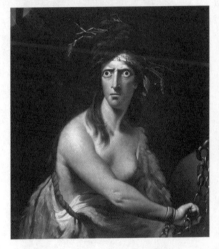

Opposite, clockwise from top left: 87 A female, aged twenty-three, who had been admitted to Bethlem Hospital 'labouring under an attack of mania', 1848.

88 An image representing the debilitated state of the body from the effects of masturbation, 1845.

89 Eight women representing the conditions of dementia, megalomania, acute mania, melancholia, idiocy, hallucination, erotic mania and paralysis in the gardens of the Salpêtrière Hospital, Paris, 1857.

This page, clockwise from top: 90 The heads of women are re-forged in a workshop by the sea, suggesting a brutal cure for the 'madness' of women.

91 A semi-naked woman with staring eyes and chained wrists representing madness, *c.*1775.

92 Representation of the expression of an insane patient, *c.*1806.

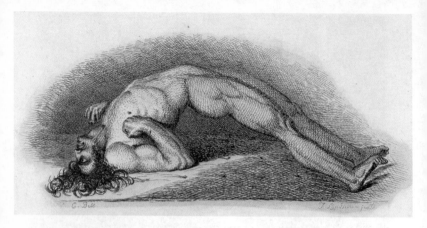

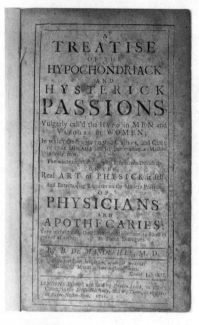

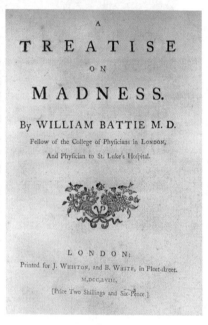

Top: 93 Representation of an insane patient in a convulsion, *c*.1806.

Above left: 94 Title page of Bernard Mandeville's *Treatise of the Hypochondriack and Hysterick Passions* (1711).

Above right: 95 William Battie's *A Treatise on Madness*, 1758.

the patient had really conceived the gentleman in attendance to be insane; so fixed was this idea established, that all confidence and submission were at an end, no other care remaining but that of having the Doctor properly secured, to prevent his offering violence to himself or others.[84]

In other words, crucial to the whole therapeutic strategy being adumbrated in Battie's shadow was the quality and intensity of doctor-patient contact, if the patient's mind were truly to be brought back from the mental underworld. For this – as was emphasised by Thomas Bakewell, the medically untrained keeper of Spring Vale Asylum in Staffordshire – there was no substitute for experience:

I confess that I am an empiric, whose opinions are entirely the result of assiduous observation; I have lived for a number of years among Lunatics; I have been in their company almost constantly from morning till night, and not unfrequently from night till morning. Besides the advantage of private practice for twenty years, and a knowledge of the practice of my grandfather and Uncle, who kept Mad Houses, in about an hundred and fifty cases, I have attended to every shade, of every variety, of this disorder, with the most anxious solicitude.[85]

Familiarity, practice, intimacy, sympathy – these, Bakewell stressed, were the key to mental rescue. Every patient was different, every problem almost – but not quite! – insoluble:

Female, single. Age, 25. Had been six months under the care of another keeper, when brought to me. I often said, that if ever the Devil was in woman, he was surely in this... her filth, her fury, disgusting language, and her almost constant nakedness for nearly two months, it being totally impossible to keep any clothes upon her, and it was scarcely possible to keep her from tearing her own flesh to pieces, as well as others; these altogether left her almost without the appearance of a human being: till I had her, I thought

I could manage any with the strait waistcoat; but her teeth bid defiance to every attempt to keep even that upon her.[86]

Eventually Bakewell cracked her mystery, which proved to be

a determined opposition to the wishes of those about her; and we had only to express the opposite of our wishes, and it was immediately done; as, Miss, you must not eat that food, it is for another person; and it was immediately taken and eaten up. Miss, you must not take that medicine, it is for such a lady, this is your's; and it was gone in an instant. Miss, you must lie still to-day; you must not get up, and wash you, and dress you very neatly; and up she got, and did all we bid her not to do. We therefore took care to bid her be sure to tear her clothes all to pieces, and she remained dressed. This was certainly a departure from my usual plan of treating my patients as rational beings; but it was a case of necessity... After this case, I shall never think any too bad for recovery.[87]

Pragmatism, flexibility, and individual care were paramount, medication subordinate. Not that the moral managers had any animus against medicines *per se*, merely against routine drugging given solely to deplete and pacify. Indeed, the surgeon-apothecary William Perfect, owner of a private madhouse in West Malling in Kent, was convinced that medicines should actively be used to good effect within the wider framework of management developed by the 'late learned and celebrated Dr William Battie'. Take the recovery of a gentleman,

aged fifty-eight... put under my care for insanity. The cause of his disorder was attributed to a sudden transition in his circumstances, which, from being easy and comfortable, were become doubtful and precarious; his complaints were great pain in the head, almost a continual noise in his ears, and, at intervals, a melancholy depression, or a frantic exaltation of spirits; he was inclined to be costive, his water was very highly coloured, he

passed whole nights without sleep, sometimes raved and was
convulsed, and his attention was invariably fixed to one object
namely, that he was ruined, lost, and undone! which was his
incessant exclamation both by night and day.[88]

Previous treatments had proved useless:

When I undertook the care of this person, he appeared very
impatient of contradiction.[89]

Vitally important, Perfect believed, was to remove the patient
from interference and hubbub and to gain total control over his
environment:

I therefore forbade all sorts of intercourse with his relations
and acquaintance... my curative plan... begun by... confining the
patient to a still, quiet, and almost totally darkened room: I never
suffered him to be spoken with, either by interrogation or reply,
nor permitted any one to visit him but such whose immediate
business it was to supply him with his aliment, which was light,
cooling and easy of digestion; at the same time his constant drink
was weak and diluting...[90]

To sedate his patient, Perfect used opium and camphor:

Till his nights became thoroughly still and composed, and his
days rendered so free from perturbation of spirits and hurry and
confusion of thoughts, that he talked rationally and just.[91]

Eventually the recovery established itself:

In this course I invariably persevered for nearly four months...
his reason now returned, his imagination grew stronger, his ideas
were more collected, and he spoke of things as they really were,
and of the primary cause of his mental infirmity, with philosophic
coolness, and resigned moderation... after having been with me

nearly five months, I restored him to his friends in that state of sanity, which he has happily preserved to the present period.[92]

Medicines thus helped, but only within a system in which the patient was given total rest, isolation and steady tranquillisation, and was treated 'with the affection of a parent'. But even Perfect's system of medication looked routine and crude to George Nesse Hill writing just a generation later.

Perfect's desire to protect patients from disturbance, to establish an uninterrupted rapport between doctor and patient, grew definitive of asylum practice. It too was the implementation of one of Battie's recommendations:

> The visits therefore of affecting friends as well as enemies, and the impertinent curiosity of those, who think it pastime to converse with madmen and to play upon their passions, ought strictly to be forbidden[93]

– one matter on which Monro could agree with Battie ('It is likewise a good general rule not to permit their friends to visit them').

Just as the moral managers were not hostile to drugs and surgical approaches – Perfect vindicated 'the free use of the lancet' – so neither did they disapprove of mechanical devices. Mere physical constraint was an evil. But the therapeutic technology being introduced in the late eighteenth century was not aimed merely at restraint or punishment. Water-shock therapies had, of course, been recommended for centuries, and electricity had come into vogue. These were now supplemented by the revolving swing-chair, capable of rotating a patient up to one hundred times a minute, which ultimately caused gushing of blood from ears and nose and unconsciousness. Such forms of apparatus found several advocates including Joseph Mason Cox, Erasmus Darwin and William Hallaran. Though incidentally relieving blood pressure, they were recommended essentially for their expected impact upon the mind. Traumatised by the disruption of his senses, the patient would, it was hoped, be shocked into sanity. Alternatively, the threat of future use could be an instrument of salutary fear. The depraved lunatic, deaf to kindness, would finally succumb before the terror of the swing-chair. Once again, it was not the technology but the generalship that mattered:

> The employment of such Herculean remedies requires the great-est caution and judgment, and should never be had recourse to but in the immediate presence of the physician...[94]

But the effects − it was claimed − could be miraculous:

> I have sometimes seen a patient almost deprived of his locomotive powers, by the protracted action of this remedy, who required the combined strength and address of several experienced attendants to place him in the swing, from whence he has been easily carried by a single person; the most profound sleep has followed, and this has been succeeded by convalescence and perfect recovery, without the assistance of any other means.[95]

MORAL THERAPY

Moral management constitutes the individualistic, heroic phase of early psychiatry − the analogy with disciplining a workforce in early industrialisation is not misplaced. Lunacy could be cured, but only via a strenuous battle of wits between mad-doctor and patient; it was psychomachy secularised. Madmen, like devils, were warped, wilful, wily. The mad-doctor must be a secular equivalent to the priest wrestling down demons. Above all, success depended upon personal qualities. The moral manag-ers were typically asylum proprietors. Yet they had little to say − contrast nineteenth-century loquacity! − about the power of institutions to reform and cure. Whereas many a nineteenth-century psychiatrist confidently expected the asylum itself to be therapeutic, it was the personality of the doctor himself which for the late eighteenth-century moral managers would prove

make-or-break. Men like Perfect, Willis and Cox ran respectable asylums, but bricks and mortar were decidedly secondary
to their heroic will.

This 'Herculean' phase proved short-lived. It was too personal to be permanent. Weberian bureaucratisation set in, and
the future was to lie with system rather than with charisma.
Personal dynamics were to become subject to routine in
institutional psychiatry. A crucial step in this modification was
the establishment of a new model asylum in the last decade of
the eighteenth century, embodying a different psychiatric slant.
This was the York Retreat.

There is no need to detail here the founding, or the 'mild'
economy, of the York Retreat: this has often been done admira-
bly elsewhere, most definitively by Anne Digby. It was launched
by a group of York Quakers, led by a tea merchant, William Tuke,
after a Quaker widow had died in strange circumstances in the
York Asylum. Opening in 1796, the Retreat was initially only for
Quakers of all ranks, from the opulent down to the subsidised
poor. It had a very favourable staff:patient ratio – about ten staff
waited on the charges, who originally numbered some thirty.
There was no resident physician. Members of the Tuke family
– first the patriarchal William and later his grandson, Samuel
– dominated its atmosphere and development.

Humanity, reason and kindness animated its philosophy. In its
early years in particular, minimal recourse was had to mechanical means of restraint. Similarly, medication was found wanting
and also discounted, particularly in the first decades. As with
the 'moral managers' just discussed, management was thought
paramount. As Samuel Tuke put it: 'The physician plainly perceived how much was to be done by moral and how little by
medical means'.

Yet management took on a very special connotation at the
Retreat. For little store was set by the theatrical talents or verbal
acrobatics of the doctor in breaking the will of, or outwitting,
the lunatics. Instead of Napoleonic generalship or the 'terrific
system', the Retreat emphasised community. On the outskirts

of York, it was designed to be dwelt in as a large private house. Its atmosphere was domestic, and it was run along paternal lines. The superintendent and his assistants were the 'family', and a spiritual bond was sought between staff and patients. 'There is much analogy', wrote Tuke, 'between the judicious treatment of children, and that of insane persons'.

Hence, patients were treated like children. They would be resocialised into the ways of Quaker fellowship through walking, talking, and taking tea with the superintendent and his family. ('All who attend, dress in their best clothes, and vie with each other in politeness and propriety.') Quakers from outside were encouraged to visit. Religious services were integral to the Retreat, as was silence. Its *Gemeinschaft* re-emphasised the traditional Quaker duty of being one's brother's keeper.

Above all, in this highly supportive atmosphere, patients would be expected to undergo moral reawakenings through the kindling of their own 'desire of esteem' and self-control, learning to 'restrain themselves'. Through a living round of kindness (backed by a modicum of fatherly fear: as much as would be exercised in a normal Quaker family), they would internalise order. Discipline would blossom into self-discipline. Patients would be nursed back into normalcy by smiles and frowns: as Samuel Tuke put it, even lunatics

> quickly perceive, or if not, they are informed on the first occasion, that their treatment depends in great measure, upon their conduct. Coercion thus flowing as a sort of necessary consequence, and being executed in a manner which marks the reluctance of the attendant, it seldom exasperates the violence of the patient, or produces that feverish and sometimes furious irritability, in which the maniacal character is completely developed: and under which all power of self-control is utterly lost.[96]

So therapy would put 'the patient as much in the manner of a rational being as the state of his mind will possibly allow'. Thus the Retreat underlined two key articles of the Quaker creed: the value of a spiritually close community or 'meeting', and every Friend's duty to lead a life of simple, rational self-control. It was the spiritual response of a minority religious group to the trials of the modern world.

What precisely was the Retreat's therapeutic orientation? Its regime was pragmatic, but its ultimate rationale was to restore normal conduct by example and imitation. No therapeutic bag of tricks was tried, nor did the Tukes attach much value to theorising about insanity. Although case notes were kept, there was no systematic exploration of patients' delusions as windows onto the mind or as keys to cure. The Tukes denied the value of entering into the hallucinations of the mad or trying to reason them out of their fantasies, expressly restricting themselves to treating symptoms and aiming to distract the distracted by work, amusement and diversions. They learnt as they went along. Medication was tried and found wanting. Whatever the ultimate cause of lunacy, moral therapy was more efficacious.

The kindness and humanity of the Retreat were universally admired. For the Swiss-American traveller Louis Simond, as for many others, it was a revelation:

> There is near York a retreat for lunatics, which appears admirably managed, and almost entirely by reason and kindness; it was instituted by the Quakers. Most of the patients move about at liberty, without noise and disorder, and by their demure and grave deportment shew they have not quite forgotten to what sect they belong... Some of the patients are allowed to go out of the premises, and even to town alone.[97]

Yet, like the moral managers, the Tukes also believed in the therapeutic power of fear ('of great importance in the management of the patients'). It was not a question of either kindness or fear. Tukean therapy was aimed at comprehensively restoring the entire moral self. For, as an early visitor, De la Rive, rightly perceived:

> They do not consider the patients as absolutely deprived of
> reason, that is to say, as inaccessible to the emotions of fear, hope,
> sentiment and honour. They consider them, rather it seems, as
> children... Their punishments and rewards must be immediate,
> because anything at a distance has no effect upon them. A new
> system of education must be adopted, to give a new course to
> their ideas: at first they must be subjected; afterwards encouraged,
> taught to work, and this work rendered agreeable to them by
> attractive means.[98]

Foucault has interpreted moral therapy as the imposition of
radical chains, a 'gigantic moral imprisonment'. The Retreat
could do away with manacles of iron, because it was enclosing
patients in manacles of mind; internalised control of patients'
consciences through creating guilt was so much more thorough,
silent, and far less scandalous. Foucault's judgement seems wilful,
not least in view of the fact that the Retreat clearly succeeded
in restoring so many of its patients to normal social life. Yet his
comment rightly draws attention to one point: the Retreat's
concern with self-mastery. The Retreat was opening up a new
psychiatric space.

   This new concern with the mind must not, however, be
appropriated by modern psychotherapies. The Tukes were not
interested in a 'talking cure', or in 'working through' problems.
Theirs was a psychiatry which operated not through peeling
off layers of consciousness or recovering the repressed, nor even
necessarily through a 'meeting of minds', but by making people
want to be good. In this respect, the Retreat perpetuated a
deep uncertainty running through the whole eighteenth century. Within the Humanist and Christian traditions, doctors and
preachers spoke directly to the mad – witness the therapeutics
of Richard Napier. Such practices certainly lasted into the eighteenth century, for as Dr George Baglivi stressed:

> I can scarce express what Influence the Physician's Words have
> upon the Patient's Life, and how much they sway the Fancy; for

a Physician that has his Tongue well hung, and is Master of the
Art of persuading, fastens, by the mere Force of Words, such a
Vertue upon his Remedies, and raises the Faith and Hopes of the
Patient to that Pitch, that sometimes he masters difficult Diseases
with the silliest Remedies:[99]

Timothy Rogers similarly thought the best way with melancholy lay in soothing talk.

Yet these techniques fell into disuse or disfavour. And particularly with the advent of the asylum, traditional talking cures
could give way to cure by silence, or at least by the therapeutic
manipulation of utterance: words not as shared experience or
a common language, but as strategic weapons. At his private
asylum, William Perfect, for example, claimed that the optimum
technique was to keep patients in individual cells, using depletive
medicines to quieten their Babel thoughts. Of one patient he
wrote: 'I never suffered him to be spoken with'; as a result, he
recovered so as to speak 'rational and just'.

Such 'shutting up' was not the hallmark of wantonly cruel,
benighted asylum practice but was a prized feature of enlightened, progressive therapies. At the Retreat, the Tukes aimed to
avoid dialogues of delusion:

> In regard to melancholics, conversation on the subject of their
> despondency, is found to be highly injudicious. The very opposite
> method is pursued. Every means is taken to seduce the mind
> from its favourite but unhappy musings, by bodily exercise, walks,
> conversation, reading, and other innocent recreations.[100]

William Hallaran at the Cork Asylum agreed:

> the less notice there can be taken even of the most obstinate
> fantasies of the insane, the less disposed will they be to retain
> them. So fully satisfied am I of this, that I never think of divert-
> ing them from their opinions, until they begin of themselves, to
> show surprise at their credulity.[101]

Thus earlier traditions had treated the voices of the mad as important; all too often dangerous (as with demonic possession); perhaps revelatory, as with the mad prophet or poet. Those became undercut. The resulting decline of dialogue between the doctor and the disturbed (now shut up in both senses) could, however, have deeply distressing, indeed disastrous, consequences for the sufferers. To glance forward in time, John Perceval was a patient in the 1830s in Brislington House and Ticehurst House – both liberal asylums – under the enlightened moral therapy regimes of physicians such as Edward Long Fox. Nevertheless he felt himself silenced, treated 'as if I were a piece of furniture, an image of wood, incapable of desire or will as well as judgement'.

Indeed, a kind of *folie à deux* was generated, a regime in which physician and patient refused to communicate with each other in normal speech. As Perceval put it:

I was not, however, once addressed by argument, expostulation, or persuasion. The persons round me consulted, directed, chose, ordered, and force was the unica and ultima ratio applied to me. If I were insane, in my resolution to be silent, because I was sure that neither of the doctors, or of my friends, would understand my motives, or give credit to facts they had not themselves experienced; they were surely no less insane who because of my silence forgot the use of their own tongues. [102]

It is difficult to gauge the precise significance of the Retreat, partly because we know too little about equivalent high-grade contemporary institutions like Ticehurst and Brislington House to be able to venture fair comparisons. But it was undoubtedly unique in the sense of banging the drum and demonstrating what could be done. Its legacy, however, proved ambiguous. For it helped to implant the idea that asylums were right for the mad, with all too little regard for the highly exceptional conditions attending the Retreat itself – its small size, its extraordinarily homogeneous community of Quakers, patients and staff, its support network of local Friends who ran informal halfway houses and paid visits etc. The nineteenth century put its faith in the asylum, but failed to pay enough attention to the unique conditions under which the asylum might actually repay such faith. Nineteenth-century medical professionals were able to take over the custodianship of the asylum, without being able to bring to it the qualities of the York Retreat (later drills and deple-tion proved poor substitutes for dedicated, supportive Quaker care). Perhaps it may have been better if the hopes raised by the Retreat had not been raised at all. With its own authenticated institution – the asylum – psychiatry gained roots and rationale. As the art of looking after asylums, psychiatry had gained a footing as an authentic material practice.

This chapter has traced the development of professional treatments for the disturbed in eighteenth-century England. I have argued that a cadre of specialist entrepreneurs of madness gradually arose, closely tied to the coming of the new, largely private lunatic asylums. Through their intimate, often individual exposure to patients, such mad-doctors developed a personal, intense experience of the encounter with madness. They drew upon medical traditions, in particular the new neuroanatomy, and upon the philosophy of human understanding stemming from Locke. But above all they took their cues from the practical problems and opportunities of treating those confined in the new asylums. A contemporary remarked that William Perfect had developed a 'practical science' of madhouse-keeping. That was precisely psychiatry's English matrix.

5

The Voice of the Mad

SILENCES

.M. Young suggested that the historian's job is to study his subject until he can hear the people speak. This book has eavesdropped on debates about madness in the eighteenth century, conducted among the public at large and, more specifically, among physicians and the emergent psychiatric profession, examining how they put thoughts into action and clothed actions in words. What we hear, of course, is discussion, dissent and dissonance, not unison. For John Wesley, writhing Methodist neophytes were having devils cast out of them; for his opponents, these converts had run clinically mad. The meanings of madness are thus manifold, equivocal, and hard to interpret, but at least a substantial body of discourse exists on which to form interpretations.

But can we ever hear mad themselves speaking – indeed, communicating their thoughts – down the ages? Today's medical historians are keen to recapture the 'patient's point of view', to discover from the grassroots how our forebears experienced and coped with sickness and medicine. In one particular respect, doing this had different implications in the case of the insane than with organic disease. For, by virtue of their unreason, the insane lost control of their affairs and so had relatively little direct say in managing their treatments: that was, indeed, precisely one of their complaints. By contrast, sufferers sick in body but sound of mind often, in earlier centuries, exercised notable sway over their medical attendants in negotiating their therapeutic regime. With the insane, we are seeing quite distinctive power relations.

Even so, it is important to get inside the heads of the mad. For one thing, their thought-worlds throw down a challenge, being at once so alien yet so uncannily familiar, like surrealist parodies of normality. For another, if we are to understand the treatment of the mad, we must not listen only to pillars of society, judges and psychiatrists: their charges must be allowed a right of reply. For instance, if we want to gauge whether 'moral therapy' at the York Retreat was indeed as humane to its patients as its advocates claimed, or whether (following Foucault) it was the racking of conscience, we should consult the people who experienced it. For many ex-patients' letters survive and most of them, as it happens, are warm in their gratitude for the kindly treatment experienced there. Of course, such answers then raise as many questions as they resolve, but examining what survives of the *vox insanorum* at least pitches the interpretative issues on to a higher plane.

The problem is that – especially before the nineteenth century – it is particularly difficult to resurrect the minds of the mad or to know how they regarded themselves, society at large, and particularly their keepers and physicians – because of the simple dearth of evidence. All too often they were mutes or muted, or we catch the depressed, disturbed and deranged only through the talk of others – their families, doctors, legal documents or asylum registers. These sources afford silhouettes – a miniature life history, a medical record, a cluster of symptoms. Such official records conceal as much as they reveal. Thus bulletins on George III's state of health in 1789 might admit that the king 'perspir'd through the night profusely', but the doctors' private diaries reveal that he was 'as incoherent as ever'. And, in any case, rarely do we find the inner state. Take, for instance, this in its own way quite circumstantial case in the 1670s, recorded by the Sussex vicar William Turner:

> Mr Francis Culham... a Chirurgion... complained of an alteration in his Health; and about Two Days after, became stupified in his Brain which gradually spread over his Body: to this Weakness in his Limbs succeeded; so that he was forced to take his Bed, and immediately grew not only speechless, but lost the use of his Reason. He lay a Month without eating any Food, or taking any other Sustenance, except a small quantity of Drink... At the expiration of this Month, he... did eat daily for some short time... then fasted another Week compleat... he afterwards did eat but once in Three Days; but then it was incredible, both in respect of the Quantity and Manner; for he would most greedily devour a whole Joynt of Meat at a Meal... But the Distemper he seemed to lie under after such extravagant Eating, was exceeding strange and remarkable: for he made a dreadful and horrid Noise, but inarticulate, and lay roaring and howling most part of the Day after, (as sometimes he did before he did eat) seeming to covet more Meat, even then when he had fed most plentifully.[1]

Culham had gone out of his mind – indeed, had turned brute:

> In this sad and deplorable Condition he continued, keeping his Bed continually, and refusing to take any internal Medicine: nor did he know either Wife or Children, Friends, or Visitants, or seem'd to take Notice of any other thing. He used several sorts of Tones and Cries, all lamentable enough, and lay (for the First Year) with his Eyes continually open, he would sometimes attempt to bite those that came near him. In this time he was once let Blood; and once Fluxed. About a Month before his

Recovery, he was twice let Blood; but how far that might sig-
nifie any thing is uncertain, seeing no effect appeared 'till the
Day of his Restauration, which was the Twelfth of May, 1676.
Only for Two Days before, he now and then wept, seeming to
have some sensible apprehension of his Wife and Children, by
holding them fast by the hand, when they stood near him; tho'
since his Recovery he remembers it not. But that Twelfth Day
of May, about Ten a Clock in the Morning, by the miraculous
Power and Mercy of God, his Understanding began to return;
whereupon he made Signs (by moving his Hands in a Writing
posture) for a Pen, Ink, and Paper; which being brought to him,
he wrote as followeth:

Lord, grant a Power from thy Divine Nature, I thought I saw
the Glorious appear to me. The Prayers of all good People I
desire.[2]

Within this pious tale we get a note, of course, of the devout
prayer which marks — we are told — his recovery; but what
thoughts, fears, pains gripped him? How did he feel about his
treatment? Unfortunately, nothing else about what Culham
thought, said, or did while in his alien condition is preserved.

The records of even the most bureaucratically conscientious
asylums during the eighteenth and early nineteenth centuries
are rarely more forthcoming. Here is a vignette from the early
years of the York Retreat:

Some years ago a man, about thirty-four years of age of almost
Herculean size and figure, was brought to the house. He had
been afflicted several times before; and so constantly, during the
present attack, had been kept chained, that his clothes were contrived to be taken off and put on by means of strings, without
removing his manacles. They were however taken off, when he
entered the Retreat, and he was ushered into the apartment,
where the superintendents were supping. He was calm; his attention appeared to be arrested by his new situation. He was desired

to join in the repast, during which he behaved with tolerable propriety. After it was concluded, the superintendent conducted him to his apartment, and told him the circumstances on which his treatment would depend; that it was his anxious wish to make every inhabitant in the house as comfortable as possible; and that he sincerely hoped the patient's conduct would render it unnecessary for him to have recourse to coercion.[3]

Kindness was met by kindness:

> The maniac was sensible of the kindness of his treatment. He promised to restrain himself, and he so completely succeeded, that, during his stay, no coercive means were ever employed towards him. This case affords a striking example of the efficacy of mild treatment.[4]

An exemplary success for the Retreat. But one would love to have this Hercules' own story, with all its hints of 'beauty and the beast'. It was, however, never taken down, for the business of the Retreat was not analysing insanity but restoring normality.

Moreover, in centuries when so many who went out of their senses were never brought before a magistrate or confined, we generally lack even one-sided or stereotyped case histories such as these. Instead we pick up mere snatches of disordered people struggling in the thickets of quotidian life. Early in the eighteenth century Dudley Ryder (himself peevish and melancholic: 'death was a little pleasant to me') records a friend in a black humour:

> When Mr Whatley came in he was extremely dejected and got into one of his melancholy fits. The poor man could not put on one pleasant look nor speak a word. He told me how he expected never to be happy and cheerful more. I did what I could to divert him out of this humour, but all in vain. I did know but reading over the Guardian wherein his case is exactly described might touch him and please him and therefore read

it, but he was unmoved at the description of himself, when I
mentioned Milton's poem upon melancholy and endeavoured
to change his melancholy into that agreeable one which Milton
there describes. But all in vain.[5]

Ryder's is an interesting – albeit, one suspects, totally maladroit!
– attempt to confront depression with itself: one wonders if such
tactics were common.

Whatley was a nobody, snapped by chance for posterity in a diary.
Sometimes, however, sufferers were figures of towering eminence,
yet even then we generally remain in tantalising ignorance. In 1716
Ryder noted in his diary, 'The Duke of Marlborough is very ill and
has lost much of his senses that he often falls into fits of crying.' He
drew the appropriate hackneyed moral:

> Methinks the frailty and mortality of human nature never
> appeared in a more moving and affecting light than in him. To
> see a man that was but just now the glory and pride of a nation,
> the hero of the world, of such vast abilities and knowledge and
> consequence sink almost below a rational creature, all his fine
> qualities disappear and fall away![6]

Yet next to nothing is known of Marlborough's mental decay
following his stroke.

Similarly, somewhat over a generation later, Pitt the Elder.
For long stretches in the 1760s Chatham lived as a semi-recluse,
unable to stomach company or disturbance, physically and mentally wrecked. 'Lord Chatham's state of health is certainly the
lowest dejection and debility that mind or body can be in', wrote
his brother-in-law, Grenille, in 1767:

> He sits all the day leaning on his hands, which he supports on the
> table; does not permit any person to remain in the room; knocks
> when he wants anything; and, having made his wants known,
> gives a signal without speaking to the person who answered his
> call to retire.[7]

Again, however, Chatham's inner anguish ('Junius' called him a 'lunatic') is lost to us. The same applies to Edmund Burke. Burke himself confessed to profound 'melancholy', and was often regarded – and not just by his foes – as teetering on the brink of insanity. Boswell recorded him 'foaming like Niagra'. and remarked that people 'represent him [Burke] as actually mad' Indeed Gibbon called him, not completely metaphorically, 'the most eloquent madman that I ever knew', and the diarist Wraxall portrayed as him quite out of control:

> His very features, and the undulating motions of his head... on some occasions seemed to approach towards alienation of mind. Even his friends could not always induce him to listen to reason and remonstrance, though they sometimes held him down in his seat, by the skirts of his coat, in order to prevent the ebullitions of his anger or indignation.[8]

Unfortunately, although Gillray caricatured him confined in a cell, nowhere did Burke himself explore his 'alienation of mind', feeling that it was a 'melancholy which is inexpressible'. Gillray himself subsequently went mad.

Indeed, we remain quite staggeringly ill-informed even about many of the most famous Georgian mad people. After Mary Lamb killed her mother she lived a further fifty-one years, alternating between spells in asylums and being cared for at home by her brother (Mary did the comedies and Charles the tragedies for the *Tales from Shakespeare*). Though Charles was a prolific correspondent, and prominent in the republic of letters, nothing survives to open up to us Mary's state of mind during that half century. The silence is quite deafening. Equally enigmatic is the descent into dejection ruining the later years of William Collins. A promising and feted mid-century poet, Collins' powers dried up, he became deeply melancholic and lethargic, and it seems that he spent some time in 1754 in MacDonald's madhouse in Chelsea, probably the worse for drink. No solid information survives on the twilight of his life. His madness did not give rise

to poetry, and his inner turmoil is lost to us. The water colour-
ist J.R. Cozens went out of his mind and came under Thomas
Monro's supervision, but his mental state is undocumented.

If frustratingly little survives about eminent mad people, at
large or confined to asylums, we remain equally ignorant of the
mental state of the Georgian century's throng of suicides (almost
all now routinely officially judged *non compos mentis*). From
the 'thresher poet' Stephen Duck up to the patrician Viscount
Castlereagh, the British earned their continental reputation as a
nation bent on self-destruction. But they hardly cultivated the
art of the suicide note, even after young Werther gave them the
model (Romanticism at last changed all that: *vide* the voluminous
journals of Benjamin Haydon, who killed himself in 1846). In
1700, the scholar and translator Thomas Creech hanged himself,
perhaps for love of Miss Philadelphia Pleydell (whose friends
advised her against him), perhaps because of his debts. Two tracts
were printed about his death, *A Step to Oxford, or a Mad Essay
on the Reverend Mr Thomas Creech Hanging Himself (as 'tis said)
for love. With the Character of his Mistress* (1700) and *Daphnis, or
a Pastoral Elegy upon the Unfortunate and Much-lamented Death of
Mr Thomas Creech* (1700); but Creech himself left no materials
to illuminate his state of mind. Though the Enlightenment saw
many philosophical vindications and moral dissuasives, few suicides – they included Robert Clive and John 'Estimate' Brown
– recorded the psychological pressures which drove them to
take their own lives.

Even the most famous mad person of the century remains
largely a closed book. George III – Shelley's 'old, mad, blind,
despised king' – suffered five distinct bouts of disturbance
between 1788 and his final descent into senility in 1809. Whether
he had a primary psychological disorder or not (Macalpine
and Hunter have argued that his delirium was secondary, a
consequence of the intense irritation caused by porphyria), he
certainly raved and hallucinated. Moreover, he was easily the
most closely observed mad person in English history, his condition being recorded in official bulletins and fiercely disputed

across the floor of the House, as well as featuring at length in the diaries of courtiers such as Robert Fulke Greville and Fanny Burney. We know how long he slept, down to the last quarter of an hour; when he was straitjacketed or blistered; and so forth. Yet we get no more than heavily censored snatches of what the king said. We catch George cursing the doctors ('I hate all the physicians, but most the Willises; they beat me like a madman' – it is not clear that the Willises did actually beat him, though they certainly used physical coercion). And guarded accounts come across of the king's delirious infatuation for Lady Pembroke; but the records are tantalisingly curtailed. On a famous occasion, George chased Fanny Burney round Windsor Park. When he caught up with her, Burney records, 'What a conversation followed... Everything that came uppermost in his mind he mentioned... What did he not say!'; unfortunately, however, Burney fails to tell us.

DELVING INTO DELUSIONS

This oblivion or erasure of the voices of the mad is no surprise. Embarrassment and diplomacy doubtless played their part. In any case, psychiatric theory advised that delusion was contagious and that it was foolish to reason with the mad. After all, their voices were just gabble and babble and, thankfully, not – as once thought – the suggestions of the Devil: why then record mere sound and fury, signifying nothing?

Sometimes, however, engagement with delusions was tried as a final attempt to unravel the chainmail of fantasies the mad protected themselves with. Erasmus Darwin found obsessions particularly tragic. For example:

> Miss —, a sensible and ingenious lady, about thirty, said she had seen an angel; who told her, that she need not eat, though all others were under the necessity of supporting their earthly exis-tence by food. After fruitless persuasions to take food, she starved herself to death. It was proposed to send an angel of an higher

order to tell her, that now she must begin to eat and drink again,
but it was not put into execution.[9]

The parlousness of such cases – particularly instances of religious
idées fixes which often proved fatal – meant that for Darwin it
was vital to grasp the 'maniacal idea' and to devise counter-
stratagems 'as it may not only acquaint us with the probable
designs of the patients... but also may some time lead to the
most effectual plan of cure'.

Neither Darwin nor his fellow physicians delved very far,
however, into aetiology of delusion. Indeed, it was not until the
nineteenth century that any British doctor even published a
detailed transcript of the utterances of a lunatic. In 1809 James
Tilley Matthews petitioned for release from Bethlem, claiming his
sanity; two eminent physicians, Drs Birkbeck and Clutterbuck, testified on his behalf. Bethlem's medical staff contested the case and
John Haslam, apothecary to the hospital, publicised the affair in
*Illustrations of Madness, exhibiting a singular case of insanity and no less
remarkable difference in medical opinion developing the nature of assailment and the manner of working events with a description of the experience
by bomb-bursting lobster-cracking and lengthening the brain, embellished
with a curious plate* (1810). Here Haslam told the Bedlamite's story,
following, he claimed, Matthews' own hand-written testimony.

Matthews was (ironically, like the Tukes!) a tea merchant who,
stirred by the French Revolution, migrated to Paris in 1793,
where he came under the influence of Mesmerism. Deploring
the outbreak of war between England and France, he launched
a peace mission, possibly on the basis of the Mesmeric doctrine of aethereal harmony. Following an audience with Lord
Liverpool, Matthews prepared to start negotiating with the
French. Meanwhile, however, the Jacobin seizure of power had
dire consequences for him. The Jacobins clearly distrusted his
Dantonesque politics and, in any case, were hostile to Mesmerism,
seeing it as *ancien régime* decadence.

Matthews felt himself coming under suspicion. As he put it
in a later letter to Lord Liverpool, 'I became equally the object

of intrigue... letters were fabricated, pretendedly found on the ramparts of Lisle, at St Omas, etc., discovering plots centred in me'. Luckily, 'it happens that I am not afraid soon by a whole Jacobin army!' Nevertheless, the Jacobins had him clapped in jail in 1793. Eventually released, he made his way back to England in March 1796, convinced that his destiny was to be Britain's saviour. For he alone was privy to a dastardly French plot for:

> surrendering to the French every secret of the British govern-
> ment, as for the republicanising Great Britain and Ireland, and
> particularly for disorganising the British navy, to create such a
> confusion therein, as to admit the French armaments to move
> without danger.[10]

The secret weapon the French would mobilise was Mesmerism. Teams of what Matthews termed 'magnetic spies' had infiltrated into England. They were stationing themselves in strategic positions 'near the Houses of Parliament, Admiralty, Treasury, etc.', armed with machines (intriguingly called 'airlooms') for generating and transmitting waves of animal magnetism. Thereby they would mesmerise the ministers, rendering them 'possessed' as under a 'spell', and like 'puppets'. As Matthews explained this 'event working' in a later document,

> In consequence of the numerous gangs established in this metrop-
> olis, all the persons holding high situations in the government are
> held impregnated. An expert of the gang, who is magnetically
> prepared, contrives to place himself near the person of a minister
> of state also impregnated, and is thus enabled to force any par-
> ticular thought into his mind and obtain his reflections on the
> thought so forced. Thus for instance, when the Secretary of War
> is at church, in the theatre, or sitting in his office and thinking on
> indifferent subjects; the expert magnetist would suddenly throw
> into his mind the subject of exchange of prisoners. The Secretary
> would, perhaps, wonder how he became possessed of such a sub-
> ject as it was by no means connected with his thoughts; he would

however turn the topic in his mind and conclude that such particular principle ought to form the basis of the negociation. The expert magnetist, having by watching and sucking, obtained his opinion, would immediately inform the French Minister of the sentiments of the English Secretary, and by such means become enabled to baffle him in the exchange.[11]

Above all, Pitt was especially subject to their influence, for (Matthews had heard it from the conspirators):

Mr Pitt was not half able to withstand magnetic fluid in its operative effect, but became actuated like a mere puppet by the expert magnetists employed in such villainies.[12]

It was, Matthews later claimed, through this hypnotic power of thought-control – using techniques Matthews called 'brain-sayings', 'event-workings' and 'dream-workings' to render English politicians 'automatons' – that the Mesmeric gangs brought about the British disasters at Walcheren and Buenos Aires. Similarly, these conspirators controlled James Hadfield when he fired at George III in his assassination attempt in 1800.

Because of his earlier associations with Mesmerism, Matthews was privy to all this; hence he became number one on the conspirators' hit-list. A 'gang of seven had been sent to wipe him out, enabled by their "science of assailment" to deploy drastic Mesmeric torture-at-a-distance which included such atrocities as "foot-curving, lethargy-making, spark-exploding, knee-nailing, burning out, eye-screwing, sight-screwing, roof-stringing, vital-tearing, fibre-ripping etc."'

These threats to his life explained the urgency with which, on his return, Matthews sent warning letters to the administration and to the Speaker of the House of Commons. In particular he wrote to Lord Liverpool reminding him of their past meeting, divulging the plots, and hinting at a reward. Grenville must have been silent or dismissive, for Matthews tried a follow-up letter on 6 December 1796 which opened:

I pronounce your Lordship to be in every sense of the word a most diabolical traitor. – After a long life of Political and real Iniquity, during which your Lordship by flattering and deceiving, and more than anyone contributing to deceive your King who believing your hypochritical [sic] Professions, has to the detriment of many of the Countries Friends loaded you with honours, and Emoluments, you have made yourself a principal in Schemes of Treason found upon the most extensive Intrigue.[13]

Matthews revealed that he was aware that Liverpool was actually colluding with revolutionary France and the Mesmeric conspirators, and knew 'you did actually affect the Murder of that Unfortunate Monarch', Louis XVI. Indeed, it had become clear to him that the British and French governments were in league to keep up the war and cause 'both nations to be assassinated', in order to 'deprive me of my existence' and 'sacrifice me to popular fury'.

Having discovered Liverpool's treachery, Matthews proceeded to the House of Commons gallery, where he accused the Ministry of 'perfidious venality'. Hauled before the Privy Council and examined, he was committed to Bethlem in January 1797 (his family's protests of his sanity were overruled by Lord Kenyon). Yet what did his committal do (Matthews later argued) but prove that the government was indeed controlled by a gang of Mesmeric assassins aiming to silence him? Still further proof of this was that soon after his detention, the gangs – now untroubled by his counter-efforts – were able to mesmerise the British navy and spark the Nore Mutiny.

Confined by his persecutors in Bethlem, Matthews despaired of the British government and appealed to the world, Napoleon-like, in a document beginning 'James, Absolute, Sole, Supreme, Sacred Omni-Imperious, Arch-Sovereign... Arch-Emperor', offering rewards beyond the dreams of avarice to any who would carry out his business.

Thus Haslam told Matthews' story, purportedly in his own words. His aim was simple. He wished to show Matthews condemning himself as a madman out of his own mouth. Haslam had no desire whatever to demonstrate that these visions of conspiracy and persecution may have had their own 'truth', literal or figurative. Neither did he – unlike later psychiatrists – aim to use *Verstehen* to 'decode' the 'real' meaning of Matthews' delusions, for instance by showing how his political paranoia might be read metaphorically to clarify the disorder of Matthews' psyche. Haslam's goal was much simpler: it was, as his title indicated, to 'illustrate' madness. A parallel may be drawn with another work about patients in that institution, *Sketches in Bedlam* (1823), which offered an old-style freak-show guided tour of its most notorious patients, making no attempts even to preserve their anonymity. The (anonymous) author coloured in their delusions, but only so as to turn them into Hogarthian tableaux. In this genre, the madman's voice was a source of mirth rather than insight.

Our reported-speech accounts of the mad are thus typically of little help for entering into their minds. Either we get just slivers of information, or – as with Haslam – the tone keeps its distance. The problems are similar with fictional accounts. I have noted above that literary depictions of Bethlem need to be taken with a pinch of salt, for conventional literary mad-folk, such as Ned Ward's Bedlamites, are either grotesque or sentimental. In turn, the Gothic vogue produced its own typologies of the mad person as monster in, say, Thomas Holcroft's *Anne St. Ives*, reaching their apogee in Bertha Mason in *Jane Eyre*. Charlotte Bronte's portrait of the first Mrs Rochester is utterly unsympathetic, a wild animal. Above all, she is never allowed to tell her own tale (a further century elapsed before Jean Rhys did). Moreover, the 'mad folk' of the Georgian novel throw no light on the mad in real life, precisely because the fictional hero or heroine manacled in the asylum typically is not mad at all.

More plausible, perhaps, are the fictional hypochondriacs and melancholics who mouth the lines in popular health-care manuals. These appear particularly in 'dialogues of comfort' against low spirits common in the late seventeenth century, though often the melancholic serves essentially as a stooge. Bernard Mandeville's

Treatise of the Hypochondriack and Hysterick Passions (1711) gives a family of polite society melancholics their own sad, soap-opera stories: a husband, Misomedon, who from idleness, dissipation, and *ennui* has sunken to become 'a crazy valetudinarian'; his wife Polytheca, who has turned vapourish through the self-drugging habit; and a teenage daughter sickening her way through puberty. Much in these thumbnail sketches rings true. Although our surviving first-hand evidence of profoundly insane people is slight, far richer materials survive from those who never underwent total alienation or breakdown, nor were confined, but suffered profound distress, depression and despair.

DISCUSSIONS OF DEPRESSION

Low spirits watermark the pages of so many Georgian lives. The causes were myriad. For some, the 'idiocy of rural life' spawned *ennui* and disgust. Elizabeth Montagu noted of her rusticated father:

> If the dire Hyp does haunt a solitary chimney corner, sure it will visit my Pappa, now it is sure to find him at home and alone.[14]

The remedies for such conditions were activity and sociability (in line with Burton's 'be not solitary, be not idle'). Noting that her father's 'physicians cannot prescribe him any cordial strong enough to keep up his spirits', she added, 'We think London would do it effectually, and I believe he will have recourse to it'. Horace Walpole knew a similar medicine against low spirits: '*Rx ccclxv days of London*'. In the same vein, Erasmus Darwin was constantly recommending activity to his morbid and languid patients. Retirement, in all senses, was almost a sure overture to hypochondriasis.

But with melancholy such a many-headed hydra, was this remedy more dangerous than the disease? For others got low through too much high-pressure living among the glitterati, rather as depicted by Mandeville or by Cheyne's *English Malady*

(1734). The hustle and bustle were more than Boswell's friend William Temple could stomach, and dissipation and trivial pursuits unsettled him totally. 'Mr Macgilivray passed some days with me', he lamented in his diary:

> a pleasing agreeable man, but such are my habits that any one in the house is a great interruption and oppresses my spirits. Long conversation distracts my head, and makes me quite unhappy. Must be content to live with and by myself. Though often wishing for conversation, yet always disappointed in the pleasure I expect from it. No enjoyment but from reading, air and exercise.[15]

Temple cajoled himself into a more disciplined regime, in accord with the non-naturals, which would cheer his spirits:

> After Wednesday (30th) shall give no voluntary dinners. Give myself entirely to my books and Papers.[16]

It was a rule hard to enforce:

> October 28th. This disagreeable restlessness intirely owing to want of books and a pursuit. Must subdue it.[17]

Some, like Erasmus Darwin, recommended travel for recuperating the spirits. Temple went on a jaunt to London and Cambridge; it made him worse:

> 29th. Astonishingly depressed in my Spirits. How shall I hold out till Wednesday or Thursday?... O what a foolish expedition is this![18]

Like many another contemporary melancholic and hypochondriac, Temple's troubles were compounded by dreams. Characteristically, he imputed these to organic causes, to late suppers:

Frightful dreams to-night owing, I suppose, to tasting a very small
slice of tongue, contrary to my usual custom of never touching
any thing after tea.[19]

Georgian melancholics were legion, and they do not fit into
a single mould. Yet certain 'types' do emerge. In late Stuart
times, for instance, there appears an uncommon bunching of
eminent melancholic intellectuals, plagued by rivalry, secre-
tiveness, and suspicion. Many thinkers – Robert Hooke, Isaac
Newton, John Locke, William Whiston, and so forth – were
tortured by morbid dispositions, doubts about both their souls
and their worldly worth, anxieties about health, intense soul-
searching and jealousy, coupled with vindictive tempers and
overbearing miens. Typical was John North, scholar, fellow and
finally Master of Trinity College, Cambridge. Born physically
feeble, as his brother Roger tells us, he continued delicate in
body, hounded by fear (not least, fear of the dark). Above all,
he developed 'fancies', especially of a hypochondriacal kind,
imagining – compare Richard Baxter! – that he was developing
the stone, or going blind, all of which consigned him to the
solitary life of *il penseroso*,

which, with his austere way of ordering himself drew upon him
a most deplorable sickness, and that proved the decadence of all
his powers of body and mind, and then by a slow and painful
graduation laid him down in the arms of everlasting rest.[20]

North's touchiness, perfectionism and morbid sensitivity meant
that he suffered crucifixion during his office as Master of Trinity,
feuding with dons and students alike. His brother's biography
is revealing in tone. It fully acknowledges that North's mental
perturbations were quite unbecoming, and mixes an old-style
moral censoriousness towards the condition with a measure of
excuse. Probably the conscience pangs, soul-scouring and self-
proving demanded by Puritan upbringings, intensified by the
sheer sociopolitical insecurity of that century of revolutions,

combined to induce the troubled states of so many ambitious late-Stuart public figures.

Another conspicuous profile of melancholy was that of the outsider or the downwardly socially mobile. Sylas Neville came from the ranks of distressed shabby gentlefolk, possessed of a scanty private income, just enough to support idleness but not enough to keep him from debt, insecurity and envy. Rather late in life he went to study medicine at Edinburgh University. Neville was hypercritical of his fellows, proud of his own independent opinions and censorious of the degeneracy of the times. His gloom, exacerbated by money worries, settled into self-pity and general misanthropy, expressing itself particularly in fears for his bodily health, especially after associating with prostitutes:

> My spirits very low; which they always are on seeing any of the children of Misfortune. I hope in God this will not tend to any opening I would not like...[21]

Neville also suffered, while a medical student, from the melancholy of anatomy. Cadavers made him brood on mortality:

> Fri. Dec. 6. We had a recent subject at Monro's Theatre today for the first time. It is the body of a woman. The melancholy nature of my present studies increases the lowness of my spirits. Indeed Dr Manning asked me concerning my spirits, saying that Physic was not the most proper study for one that had not good spirits.[22]

One suffering even more from social alienation was Thomas Hollis, an independent gentleman true to his family's long-standing 'republican' principles yet acutely pained by the isolation such a stance produced, so that he saw all men as his enemies. Below him, his servants were saucy, cunning, and ever on the cheat; above, the body politic was riddled with conspiracy. Loyalty was dead, tyranny and popery rampant. Hounded by his foes, perpetually spied upon, Hollis was the persecuted innocent.

In cases such as those of Hollis, Matthews and Burke, where (one asks) does political ideology stop and personal paranoia begin? After all, much of what one might call Hollis' hallucinatory paranoia was but the ale-house scaremongering of orthodox backwoods politics writ large. Matthews was locked up in Bethlem for his scenario of Jacobin conspiracy; for his, Burke became a public hero.

Two further manifestations of melancholy seem particularly common. One is the melancholy of sensibility. As noted above in Chapter Two, disorders of the nerves arising from exquisite feelings commonly found excuse, exposure and acclaim, particularly after Cheyne formulated the idea of *The English Malady* (1734). Graveyard poetry equated bruised, brooding moodiness with the person of parts, destined to suffer because too delicate for this rude, tragic scene of life. In this climate, the pleasures of melancholy became a major poetic trope. Particularly significantly, sensibility afforded a mode of melancholy in which ladies *par excellence* could participate. The classical stereotypes of madness – the maniac, the melancholic – were through and through male. As mad poet, mad genius, malcontent or jester, men had monopolised madness. But at long last, sensibility feminised disorder and created modes of disturbance which women could not merely share, but shape. Thus in her yearning, heartache years while a governess in Ireland, the frustrated Mary Wollstonecraft suffered 'spasms and disordered nerves', 'constant nervous fever', a melancholy misery, accompanied by violent pains in her side, difficulties in breathing, trembling fits, a rising in the throat (*globus hystericus*) and faintness. We have not a single testimony penned by an eighteenth-century woman who went utterly out of her mind; but the melancholy of sensibility, shading into hysteria and couched in the language of 'nerves', became a common role through which women established a self – but one which ultimately affirmed gender stereotypes.

Lastly, religious melancholy must be mentioned. Religion still formed the prime language of the inner self and the great prick of conscience, and it should be no surprise that many of those disturbed in thought and feeling were crucified by some sort of religious crisis (not of faith *per se*, as with the Victorians, but of worth). Since, however, religious melancholy shades into religious madness, which I shall consider shortly, I shall defer my discussion of it.

Numerically at least, we have far more access to the minds of melancholics than to those of mad people. Many anguished Georgians, men and women, set down copious accounts in letters, diaries and autobiographies of their brittle, fickle moods, terror of dying, self-doubts, dreams and nightmares – and they did so with acute self-perception and analytic insight. Plenty of spiritual diaries, especially those of Protestant Dissenters in the shadows of Bunyan and Baxter, record guilt, unworthiness, a dread of perdition, a disgust for the filthiness of the flesh and for carnal temptations – sometimes resolved through spiritual crisis, cataclysmic but purifying, opening into new certainty and joy. Often these crises were repeated. Men of the world, for their part, in their secular language likewise chronicled the strain of establishing a place in the sun and of finding a satisfying identity within the fashionable whirlpool which placed such high premiums upon polish and aplomb. Early in his career as a man of letters David Hume underwent a deep crisis, expressed in physical collapse (we might popularly call it a nervous breakdown), when confronted with integrating the intense and radical introspection of his vocation as philosopher with getting into the swim as a poised, self-possessed social success – a crisis doubtless objectified in his speculations on the elusive rope of sand which was personal identity.

Deep introspection doubled with melancholy in many leading literary figures in the age of sensibility. Edward Young's phrase 'the stranger within thee' captures both the profound uncertainty felt by many mid-Georgian writers about their personal authorial voice, and their uncertain relation to their audience. In Thomas Gray's case, the well of loneliness of a career spent largely as a Cambridge don, exacerbated by his secretive homosexual leanings, consolidated a chronic gloom. By contrast, Coleridge's melancholy, oozing self-pity ('No one on earth has ever *loved* me'), was always far more dramatic, occasionally threatening catastrophe. Wretchedly torn in his private life between desire and duty, and struggling to sustain his reputation as a precocious genius, Coleridge turned to opium for stimulus and relief; only to find himself racked by nightmares, guilt and almost unbearable physical and mental agonies. Thus, in November 1794, he explained to Southey his shattering confusion of terror and pleasure:

> There is a feverish distemperature of the Brain, during which some horrible phantom threatens our Eyes in every corner, until emboldened by Terror we rush on it – and then – why then we return, the Heart indignant at it's own palpitation! Even so will the greater part of our mental Miseries vanish before an Effort. Whatever of mind we will to do, we can do! What then palsies the Will? The Joy of Grief! A mysterious Pleasure broods with dusky Wing over the tumultuous Mind –[23]

Coleridge frequently pictured himself in extremis, 'my body diseased and fevered by my imagination'. 'Since I last wrote you', he opened a letter to his friend Edwards in March 1796,

> I have been tottering on the edge of madness – my mind overbalanced on the contra side of Happiness... Such has been my situation for this last fortnight – I have been obliged to take Laudanum almost every night.[24]

But, acute self-analyst as he was, he recognised that he was not in fact likely to go irrevocably mad: 'There is little danger', he consoled Southey,

> of my being confined – Advice offered with respect from a Brother – affected coldness, an assumed alienation – mixed with involuntary bursts of Anguish and disappointed Affection – questions concerning the mode in which I would have it mentioned

to my aged Mother – these are the daggers, which are plunged
into my Peace! Enough![25]

For Coleridge had a grasp – both intuitive and philosophical
– of a strong transcendental self; and not least he knew how to
turn madness into performance – indeed, into art.

Exactly how plumbing the lower depths might become a nose-
dive into insanity proper was, of course, much debated. Coleridge
displayed a 'Romantic' faith in the sinews of the self: be the storms
never so great, the self-conscious mind could remain at the helm,
preventing the shipwreck of the soul. Others, however, had been
less sanguine. The Augustans had earlier sternly warned how the
ego could be quite crazy precisely when convincing itself that it
was most supremely sane: Swift's heroes, such as the narrator of
The Tale of the Tub and Lemuel Gulliver, are terrifying, self-blind
fools in that way. For humanists such as Pope, the 'thin partitions'
between sanity and unreason had to be kept absolute. That is why
the great mid-century melancholic, Samuel Johnson, was so terrified, recognising how easily imagination, having seized the mind,
created the illusion that reason remained at the helm.

SPEAKING INSANITY

The turmoils of Georgian melancholics are well recorded. By
contrast, we encounter grave interpretative problems when
addressing that small body of testimony written by those whose
mental alienation went far beyond, losing all grasp of the bor-
derlines between reason and irrationality, reality and fantasy,
objective and the subjective. Much of our difficulty is that such
people were generally more socially obscure or isolated than
Johnson or Boswell, Hume, Gray or Cheyne, and so it is infinitely harder to anchor them in 'normal' contexts.

Take, for instance, Goodwin Wharton as a prime example of
one whose writings suggest a person adrift from public reality,
yet whose condition defies evaluation because of the absence of
independent testimony about it from his peers.

In the late seventeenth-century public eye, Goodwin Wharton, born in 1653, seemed an ordinary enough middleweight politician, enjoying a position commensurate with being the younger son of a titled, land-owning family. Certainly he never commanded the moral stature of his father Philip, Lord Wharton, often styled 'the good' – that austere, unwavering paragon of Dissenting and Whiggish righteousness. Neither could he match his elder brother Tom as a politician, nor his younger brother Henry, a soldier who died young campaigning in Ireland.

Yet Goodwin was no nonentity. Sitting as an MP from 1690 to his death in 1704, he was a vocal supporter of William III, an energetic Whig and a ferret in search of Jacobite plotters. Rising to become a Lord of the Admiralty, he saw active service in the Channel before suffering a stroke in 1698. By then he was a substantial squire, a JP and Knight of the Shire. Though never marrying, in his later years he kept up a society mistress, Lady Elizabeth Gerard, and an illegitimate son, Hezekiah Knowles, came to light in his will. All in all, his public profile looked conventional enough.

The small circle who knew Goodwin at closer quarters may have found him a man of stranger mettle. From his twenties he fancied himself as a projector and entrepreneur. He invented a new patent fire-engine, pursued alchemical experiments, seeking 'the powder of projection', and sank a fortune – some his, some his father's, some other people's – in wreck-salvaging, diving for doubloons in sunken Armada galleons. His family clearly found him hard to handle. Secretive, suspicious and brooding, he was long alienated from his father, stepmother and elder brother, family tensions being exacerbated by his mounting debts and his failure to hook an heiress.

Who even suspected that behind this conventional exterior lay a truly extraordinary inner self? – one, it appears, shared with only one other human being, though a wide range of spirits, demons and angels grew to know it intimately. We know, however, for we are fortunate to possess a window on to his soul, since from 1686 onwards he penned a monumental autobiography. Written in a

microscopic hand, its margins festooned with alchemical, astrological and occult symbols, Wharton's autobiography stands alongside
John Perceval's *Narrative of the Treatment Received by a Gentleman
During a State of Mental Derangement* or Daniel Schreber's *Memoirs
of my Nervous Illness*, as a testament of a mind enmeshed in the
thickets of delusion. Unlike Perceval and Schreber, however, who
wrote to come to grips with their condition or to vindicate their
sanity, Wharton never even entertained the slightest conjecture
that he might be mad. Rather, he wrote his memoirs for the
edification of his son Peregrine, painting his own life as 'full of
such unusual and unhappy circumstances', and suggesting how his
son should learn from it. Probably no such person existed.

In Wharton's self-portrait, the conventional and the abnormal
jar against each other right from the beginning. He sets out by
informing the reader – his 'son' – that he will record little of
his childhood, it being so ordinary. Yet from the opening page
he is explaining how he became introspective, 'secretly inclined',
'addicted to reading and writing', given over to 'musings and
prayings', and aspiring towards personal communion with the
angels. Even so, women always found him irresistible; panting
suitors queued up, one even died for love of him; yet he rejected
them all, saving himself for better things: beware siren seduc-
tresses, he warns Peregrine.

Not least, amidst the moils and toils besetting him, his family
wronged him: he suffered endless 'injuries' and was treated 'like
a slave', coming under their 'remedilesse lash'. His own piety
and purity notwithstanding, his relatives shamelessly cheated,
exploited and abused him. His father – a man, according to
Goodwin's recent biographer, 'easier to honour than to obey,
easier to obey than to love, and easier to love than to please'
– bullied him into surrendering to his favourite elder brother
the estate, Wooburn, bequeathed him by his mother. His stepmother then tried to lure him into bed, and when he rebuffed
her she wreaked revenge by turning his father against him.
His sister-in-law, Tom's wife Anne, then seduced him before
rejecting him in wanton cruelty. Later still, after her death, Tom

remarried and finally produced an heir, thus robbing Goodwin of his expectations of inheriting the family property. 'Neither loved nor respected at home', he grew up 'under a heavy load of groans'.

Early manhood saw no improvement. So disastrous were his diving and alchemical losses that he had to go into hiding from his creditors. Soon he had to lie low politically as well. Briefly sitting in the Commons at the height of the Exclusion Crisis of 1680, Wharton launched an extraordinary harangue against Charles II's brother James, then heir to the throne, and spent the next years in dread of reprisal. Through these dark times, all he had to fall back upon was an unshakable assurance of his own virtue and of God's righteousness. The early pages of the autobiography witness Wharton's pervasive conviction of 'divine deliverance' and 'particular providence'. In his teens he had been miraculously saved from drowning at sea, and he shortly began seeing God in dreams and hearing a divine voice which, countering 'afflictions outward', gave him 'spiritual directions', 'inwardly'. Soon he found himself entrusted with supernatural powers. A friend fell mortally sick and was at death's door; Wharton prayed; he recovered. A blackguard maliciously challenged him to a duel. Wharton prayed; his foe fell mortally sick. No wonder that from an early age he grew to nurture the conviction of greatness thrust upon him: God would make him 'greater in his service than either Moses or Aaron'.

But how? This became clearer when in 1683, seeking someone to put him in touch with the angels, Wharton was directed to a certain Mary Parish, a London healer, cunning-woman and medium – some probably called her a witch. The first service Mary Parish actually performed for him, however, was to make him a 'play piece', a gambling charm, to guarantee success at the tables. It did not work, in fact, but in the course of making it, testing it, and probing its failure, Mary Parish began spinning out her life story to him and, rather like Scheherazade, she was to weave a narrative of fact, fiction, romance, delusion or what you will which captivated Wharton for the next twenty years.

A Catholic in her early fifties, she had been married three times and vilely abused by each of her husbands; she had had scores of children – fourteen had died in the Plague of 1665 alone; she had been in and out of debtors' prisons. Yet she was a profound adept in alchemy, expert in tracking buried treasure and, above all, in tune with spirits, below and above. Through her, Wharton saw how he could realise his frustrated drive for wealth, power and holiness.

Mary Parish was familiar with the fairies. In better days, she had personally descended into their lowland kingdom (which was monarchical in government and Papist in religion) and become party to the secrets of the 'Lowlanders', creatures about half human size, combining human attributes (they were mortal, though enjoying extreme longevity) and supernatural (they had the power to fly, pass through walls, and make themselves invisible by popping a magic pea into their mouth). Though now – following a tragic contretemps – excluded from their realms, Mary Parish still kept track of their dealings through the services of spiritual go-betweens, such as George Whitmore, the ghost of an executed highwayman; Mr Ahab, the spirit of a Jewish alchemist; and a friendly fairy, Father Friar.

Wharton – who could neither hear nor see these intermediaries – ached to meet the fairies; all the more so because Mary Parish assured him that through the Lowlanders' good offices, they would locate and liberate untold stores of buried treasure. Moreover, Mary soon hinted that Penelope, the Queen of the Fairies, had taken quite a fancy to him.

So a meeting was arranged. Mary was informed by the spirit George that the Queen would pay Wharton a nocturnal call in his chamber; he must wait up in bed for her. To his chagrin, however, the first couple of rendezvous proved abortive – on one occasion the Queen fell sick, on another the King did. At last she did get through, only to find that this time Wharton had fallen asleep and, with regal courtesy, she declined to wake him and stole away unnoticed.

So the plans changed. Mary Parish and Wharton, shadowed by George as scout, would visit the fairy kingdom. The main entrance to this was on Hounslow Heath, accessible to humans only for a few minutes at New Moon. They journeyed down at New Moon in May 1683, only to be told the meeting was off: the Queen was sick. Down they came again in June, but now the King was ill again. Once more they rode down in July, but now the encounter had to be abandoned because the King, an old debauchee named Byron, had just expired. Month after month they travelled down; month after month the best laid plans were frustrated by last-minute hitches – bad weather, unforeseen state visits, Mary's illnesses and, not least, the Queen's menstrual periods, for the Lowlanders observed strict Mosaic purity laws, requiring ritual purification during menstruation.

Yet it is an ill wind that blows nobody good, and in the course of these agonising trips Mary Parish and Wharton, aided by trusty spirits (still invisible to Wharton), located priceless treasure hoards at adjacent sites beneath a clump of trees on Hounslow Heath, in a haunted house nearby (which they subsequently rented), and at Northend in Buckinghamshire, near where Mary had grown up. These riches they set about recovering through spells and rituals. Once again, however, easier said, easier planned, than done. Sharp frosts, curious wayfarers, a rampaging cow – all successively wrecked operations at the crucial moment; not least it transpired that evil spirits were guarding the hoards, which in turn would require exacting and costly exorcism. Meanwhile other projects, especially alchemical experiments designed to transform mercury into gold, were put in motion, supported by the capital of that inveterate opportunist plotter, Major Wildman.

In the course of all this the footing of the relationship changed, turning from business to friendship, and then to emotional partnership; finally it became sexual. Though now in her fifties, Mary Parish conceived immediately at their first lovemaking, the first of 106 conceptions she enjoyed by Wharton right up to the time of her death at the age of seventy-two. A deep and enduring bond had been struck. In each other's eyes and also in God's (so the spirits told Mary) they were truly man and wife, though they never went through a legal marriage ceremony, which would have constituted an abominable misalliance in the eyes of the Whartons.

Their union was only occasionally threatened by the fact that after her husband's death Queen Penelope herself vowed to marry Wharton, make him her King, and have him to sire an heir; she even used Mary as her matchmaker. This sign of fairy favour cannot have surprised Wharton, for he knew that all women fell at his feet. But there was a sound eugenic reason, too, for the Queen's choice. The Lowlanders were cold creatures. Though long-lived, they were sluggish breeders. Penelope was childless, her kingdom heirless. Naturally she would grab the opportunity to mate with a lusty Uplander, for they were far more potent.

Indeed, so hot was Penelope's passion that she could not wait for their nuptials. She fell into the habit of slipping invisibly into Wharton's chamber as he lay asleep, riding him through the night, and hastening away before cock-crow. Wharton had no direct awareness of this succubus experience, this rape, yet he now found himself unaccountably aching and exhausted when he awoke in the morning. It took the spirit George and Mary Parish to reveal to him the cause of his symptoms; indeed, so great had been Penelope's predatory ecstasy that she drew in the very marrow from his bones and almost 'sucked my life and nature from me'.

Penelope was probably wise to take her chances when she could, because each time she travelled up in state to London finally to make the acquaintance of her husband-to-be on a lawful occasion, yet more obstacles supervened. Not least, furious machinations arose from rival suitors for her hand, such as the fairy Duke of Hungary, and from her double-dealing younger sister Ursula (she was only fifty, whereas the Queen was 350), who had developed an itch for Wharton herself. On one occasion, Queen Penelope lodged underground at Moorfields

– a mere stone's throw from Bedlam! – to be near the seat of the fairy Pope who would marry the royal pair, only to find that all the tunnel exits had been mined by her enemy, the Duke of Hungary. The ensuing damage took months to repair, and spelt still more interminable delays. At another time, the royal carriage was involved in a street accident with a careless carter at Knightsbridge; numbed with shock, she slipped into a tavern for a soothing drink, became fuddled, took a nap, awoke menstruating, and headed back to Hounslow. Wharton followed all this aghast, as the spirit George told it to Mary and Mary relayed it to him. Beside himself with frustration, Wharton urged pursuit; he would overtake and abduct her. But as George reminded him, such desperate measures would be useless; by now Penelope had popped her magic pea in her mouth, and rendered herself invisible.

Such 'troubles and delays' stretched Wharton to breaking point: so near and yet so far. Months of heroic effort and expenditure had yielded not a penny of treasure, nor even his promised wife. 'Being thus disappointed in every thing', small wonder he exploded occasionally in fits of rage, cursing the feckless fairies for their infidelities – a rage, as Mary sternly rebuked him, which must prove totally counterproductive, for it drove the spirits away; the reminder brought Wharton contritely to heel.

The nub of Wharton's problem was that – despite endless fairy promises – no spirit had yet either appeared or spoken directly to him. George, for instance, conducted his dealings with Mary privately, in a separate room; at best Wharton caught fragmentary and garbled snatches of their conversations. When distant from Mary, as when visiting his father cap-in-hand to wheedle further loans, Wharton felt totally cut off from the spirit powers which should be his lifeline.

It was fortunate then, and in the nick of time, that Mary Parish started being visited not just by exasperating fairies but by angels, unambiguous signs of divine favour. Fairies were alluring, but who could trust a race who in immorality and skulduggery were a fit match for the Uplands court of the Merrie Monarch himself? Angels by contrast were God's servants, regulars in the holy war against Anti-Christ depicted by Wharton's Protestant indoctrination. From his childhood Wharton had been reaching out to meet the angels.

To the end of his days Wharton never directly encountered the Lowlanders, but the advent of the angels did indeed herald better things. Soon angelic marks of heavenly blessing began to appear. Of course, Wharton did not at first experience these personally; he still relied on Mary's witness:

> She, being awake in the night (but I was asleep), sees a great light round my head, and a sort of white fire as it were on the bed; and then heard these words spoke loud and intelligibly:

> Be patient Wharton, and a croune
> Thou shalt weare with great renoune.[26]

Before long, promises were flowing thick and fast from the angel trio, Gabriel, Uriel and Ahab, and sure enough Goodwin himself began to have first-hand experiences, at first in dreams and then awake – hearing sonorous noises, seeing bright and flashing lights, and finally receiving personal messages. Typically these came to him as he lay in bed, half asleep; often they were preceded by the ringing of a bell somewhere outside his room, and a voice would come from beyond his door. Sadly, the syllables themselves were frequently hard to distinguish (all he could pick up of one message was 'I have no more to say now'), and Wharton typically had to consult Mary Parish who would offer him, via her spirit interlocutor, a full transcript and elucidation.

Unlike most of his contemporaries when they heard disembodied voices, Wharton did not harbour sharp suspicions that they were surely the suggestion of the Devil – though he certainly did not doubt the power of His Satanic Majesty to thwart his treasure-hunting and matrimonial plans. Neither did it occur to him that the lights and voices were part of elaborate 'theatricals' staged for his benefit by Mary Parish. That is why when, rarely, such suspicions crossed his mind, they proved so devastating. One day, kneeling at prayer in the candlelight and hearing himself addressed by Gabriel from somewhere behind his shoulder, he glanced up and glimpsed Mary's lips moving to the words. Shattered, he accused her of fabricating the divine message. Her response was outrage: Wharton's distrust was offensive to the angel. Riddled with guilt, he begged forgiveness. There was now, he wrote, 'no remedie but prayer'.

Episodes such as this must have made Wharton trebly grateful that he eventually ceased to be dependent upon such outer voices speaking from beyond his door. He began at last to be able to pick up an inner voice as well. For a spell, he regularly enjoyed an intense experience of divine indwelling. Angels would instruct him to lie expectant on his bed at a stipulated hour, tuned to receive divine communications. These would generally come in the form of doggerel rhymes, verse being the elevated prophetic tongue. And, he comforted himself, there was no risk of mistaking mere imagination or Satanic suggestion for the true divine inner voice, for the heavenly revelations were 'all infallible'.

Now it was, in the dark days of James II's tyranny, about the time of Monmouth's rebellion, when his brothers fell under deep suspicion, his father found it prudent to travel abroad for his health, and Goodwin himself was checked out by government spies, that his destiny as the Lord's anointed came gradually to be unfolded. Already he had been awarded by Queen Penelope his diadem as King of the Lowlanders. Now God revealed his human calling: he would be made priest, prophet, and saviour. 'You, my son, should be King of Kings, and Solar King of the world'; 'I should see the Lord in Glory', glossed Wharton, 'I should save much people'.

From time to time tokens of his translation started to appear around the little altar Mary Parish had fitted out in her room: a sceptre, a scroll, an oak branch as a symbol of his strength, a heart-shaped relic the size of a walnut which bled real blood. Angelic voices told him he had been renamed Hezekia (Mary became Lucretia), that he would be 'such a king, as was never before nor since Christ', and that his glory would be to rebuild the walls of Jerusalem. The godly messages kept up their doggerel promises of glory just around the corner:

Hezekia thou art my true and well beloved son
On Wednesday next this business shall be done
And so to thee it shall be said
That thou no more shall be dismaid
Without thy woman thou shalt surely know
The things above, and things below.[27]

These same voices also warned him of necessary delays while his purification rituals were completed. God's pledge to him had been the delivery of a 'first covenant'; at the second, His business would reach perfection. Divine trials were no problem to Wharton. After all, he had had much fairy prevarication to accept, and he knew the tribulations that Abraham, Moses and Job had undergone for the Lord. When the angels started mentioning martyrdom, that was a cross he was glad to bear, now that he had been proclaimed God's 'only son'.

Thus fortified, new horizons of prosperity opened out. The prospects of growing rich beyond the dreams of avarice brightened as Mary Parish managed to bump into the spirit of Cardinal Wolsey, who had his fingers on fabulous buried treasure stashed away in the cellars of various London houses (mainly in pubs, which unfortunately resulted in her frequently returning home much the worse for brandy). In principle the Cardinal was happy to release the hoards, though in practice he proved fractious and petulant: the predictable delays ensued, and when some of the wealth was at last transferred to the Wharton household, it arrived in trunks securely padlocked under strict instructions not to be opened except upon spiritual command.

Moreover, Wharton's own future now seemed about to blossom forth in directions personal, sexual and imperial. To a prophet king, attending patriarchally to the need to populate his kingdoms with blessed stock, lying only with Mary Parish could hardly suffice. He may have been perturbed by his lack of visible offspring by her. It was all very well that she conceived regularly, often having multiple conceptions (at one time she was carrying thirty-eight of his children); but she commonly lost them, or they died just after birth, and in any case he was never allowed to see them – not even Peregrine, the dedicatee of the auto-biography. He may also have been worried for his health. For Mary did not come to lie with him every night, and he found that a few days' enforced abstinence resulted in the discomfort of 'an unimaginable quantity of seed'. To solve these problems, he launched himself upon brief encounters – he bedded Mary's friend, Mrs Wilder (or rather she bedded him, since she leapt upon him even before he had finished propositioning her), and then on a trip to Bath his landlady too (and she too, like the original wife of Bath, was beside herself with desire) But both episodes left him poxed – leading to anguished scenes with the outraged Mary – and resulted in an alienation from her which cut Wharton to the quick, after which reconciliation was slow.

Racked by sexual torments, he prayed for heavenly guidance. The divine answer came back loud and clear with instructions even conveniently numerically tabulated:

1. Swear not at all
2. Fuck (every weeke) where you used to do

– here Wharton interjects, 'at this broad word (as we call it) my thought stuck, as if I had not rightly understood it; upon which, it was repeated and then was added' –

3. That is, give to her her due

and then 'thinking suddenly on the unruly rising of the flesh, it was added'

4. Throw water on yourself, so shall the Lord prosper you.[28]

Pondering the heavenly precepts, or rather the divine vernacular, Wharton explained that on reflection God's use of the broad expression seemed proper: 'the God of nature, I hope, may be allowed to speake plainly of all things whatever... I hope I need not plead for God further; who dare accuse or censure him?'.

Goodwin's problem remained to decide where exactly his service, was due. Clearly with Mary – and surely also with Queen Penelope, his other lawful (Lowland) wife, if ever he were to meet her. But also with those other great ladies spiritual voices told him it was his mission to lie with as King of Kings. First there was James II's spouse, Mary of Modena – who, providentially, was childless like Penelope. Obviously God intended Wharton to give her an heir – at which point, he presumed, James II, overwhelmed by gratitude, would abdicate, Wharton would replace him, and he would reconvert the court to Protestantism. When Mary ignored his advances, like Malvolio he took it as a come-on, proof of just how smitten she was.

Of course, James speedily fell (sweet punishment!), to be succeeded by William of Orange. Wharton soon discovered that the Dutchman's wife, Queen Mary, was also providentially infatuated with him; he paid her court, even vouchsafing her copies of his prophetic writings. And when she fell desperately ill with smallpox, he seized his chance. Commandeering spiritual aid, he would cure her, and, melting with gratitude, she would admit him. Unaccountably, however, she died. But when William himself perished soon after (yet another divine blow, to smite him for his failure to advance Wharton), Goodwin knew his day at last had come, for while yet a princess, Anne, now Queen Anne, had long been eyeing him up. Once more death intervened, though this time it was Wharton's.

Yet as the saga of Wharton's amours unfolded, his life had been undergoing great changes. The Protestant wind that in 1688 won William of Orange the English crown also blew Wharton out of hiding on to the public stage. Up to his thirty-seventh year he had lived under a cloud, in debt and obscurity, focusing his energies on the intensest of inner lives, on Paradise within.

Now, as part of the Wharton dynasty, he was expected to play his part in public affairs. His family secured him a Commons seat in 1690, and from then on his life became one of parliamentary sittings, manoeuvrings, committee work, vetting finances and organising military supplies, all these engrossing more and more of his attention over his remaining fifteen years.

Wharton's autobiography gives no sign that he regarded his spiritual life as hermetically sealed from his public duties. Far from it: the two were utterly intertwined. After all, his divine mission was to become an earthly potentate and, initially at least, he automatically expected fairy help and divine prompting when about to embark upon his Commons speeches (in fact no voices came, and their silence schooled him to fall back upon his own rhetorical resources, at which he proved not unsuccessful). Very gradually, however, Wharton seems to have looked less to communications from the Lowlanders and spirits. Perhaps he grew disenchanted. Delays were one thing, blunders another. Thus during the siege of Mons in 1691, Wharton, like many others, laid a bet on the outcome. It was odds on that Mons would fall to the French. But the angels told him it would hold out. Wharton staked his £100. Not only, however, did Mons fall, but Wharton discovered that it had already capitulated when the angels slipped him their tip. Whatever had happened? He quizzed George and Mary, but answer came there none. By this time, however, Wharton had grown stoical about these matters.

Indeed, during his last decade the intensity of his involvement with the spirit world probably diminished. He must have felt less of a fugitive. He gained a taste at least of power; on the death of his father in 1696 he had stopped being hounded by creditors; and from 1695 he got himself a society mistress, Lady Elizabeth Gerard. And the springs of anxiety which had caused his cup of troubles to overflow dried up. His father's death removed a source of constant censure; the deaths of Henry and William took away rival siblings; the death of his stepmother removed a temptress and predator. And Mary Parish remained, steady as a rock. She at least kept communing with the fairies to the end of her days, kept up the fruitless treasure hunts. And when she died, Wharton gave 'the best of women' a fine burial at St Giles-in-the-Fields. But, for all her promises, she did not appear to him translated into a spirit. And so Wharton's spiritual life ended. The span of her death to his own occupies only one page out of 500 in the autobiography.

What do we make of all this? Of all the thousands of hours Wharton and Mary spent haggling with the Lowlanders or straining for angelic voices? What is the meaning of the Byzantine poli-tickings in the smoke-filled Lowlander corridors of power which occupy hundreds of thousands of words in Wharton's text, and who knows how many more pages of his initial jottings later destroyed? How do we interpret the bizarre Lear-like scenes on Hounslow Heath, with a nobleman's son and his hag-like medium command-ing clumps of trees, strewing them with parchments and witch-hazel sprigs, and ordering the ground to open? How do we understand the autobiographer whose voices assured him that he was irresistible to women, and was called to be the saviour of men?

Above all, can we even tell whether Wharton's journal records nothing but events occurring only in his own head (or jointly between his and Mary Parish's), or whether some at least of the events recorded had some sort of everyday objective truth as well? We can in fact establish, at some points, a certain minimal reality about the events Wharton describes. His relations with his family and with late-Stuart politics can be corroborated from external sources. Mary Parish was indeed a real person, not just a figment of Wharton's imagination. No papers of hers survive, however, and her voice exists only as mediated through Wharton, so there is no confirmation from that side, and we can resurrect her – and what we might call her psychiatric distur-bance – only through Wharton. For most of the events Wharton recorded, such as the treasure hunts on Hounslow Heath, there is no independent proof: they may have transpired simply between her crystal and his mind.

Wharton thus becomes a fascinating but extraordinarily elusive figure. It would be easy, of course – with the aid of

Freud, Jung, or any other heroes of dynamic psychiatry – to set Wharton on the couch, and to offer a speculative psycho-analytical account of his neuroses, perhaps paralleling Freud's interpretation of the fantasies of Wharton's near-contemporary, Christoph Haizmann. Wharton's succubus experiences, and his fantasies of universal fertility and so forth, seem tailor-made for Freud's sexual aetiologies. But such a hermeneutics would run the risk of standing outside time, and would tell us nothing about the shifting dynamics of normal and abnormal consciousness in the late-Stuart period.

Another tack might therefore be tried. Instead of diagnosing his neuroses, we could normalise Wharton's brilliant career by contextualising it within the common cultures of the age. Certainly it was quite normal within the seventeenth-century *Lebenswelt* to believe in fairies, though by Wharton's time such beliefs were mainly the preserve of the lower orders – the likes of Mary Parish – and had become rare among the gentry. Likewise, those enculturated in a Puritan family such as Wharton's would have found it sufficiently 'normal' that God would appear directly to them by visions and through voices. Indeed, for seventeenth-century Christians the idea that the personal Christian God would not have private contact with 'saints' would have been deeply disturbing and certainly divine silence would have been a cause for despair. Yet Wharton resists being 'normalised' in these ways. If people believed in fairies, few (one imagines) seriously believed that they were about to marry the fairy queen. If Christians heard divine voices, few expected to be the new Messiah. If men had macho fantasies, few thought that all the queens of England were smitten with them. In the terms of contemporary philosophy, Wharton clearly suffered from misassociation of ideas.

Interpretation so far is easy. Beyond, there are huge problems if we try to insert Wharton within a history of madness, precisely because his story remains hermetically sealed; despite Wharton's political career, his autobiography finds little point of contact with public reason, with the rebukes of the normal, and none with medical therapeutics or the regime of madhouses. Unlike his contemporary, James Carkesse, Wharton was never called upon to defend his consciousness at the bar of the outside world. This fact is of real historical significance. It shows that in the late seventeenth century it was still possible – as Wharton's writings prove – even for a public figure to lead an imaginative life of exotic uniqueness without check. No brother, no arm of the state, and no doctor stepped in to cure, or secure, him. The encroachment of mad-doctors and madhouses throughout the next century made later Whartons increasingly unlikely. Were there any later equivalents who did not at some point, voluntarily or not, come under some kind of psychiatric gaze?

We possess extensive writings by a handful of other late Stuart and Georgian people – almost all are males – whose days were riddled with insanity. At some stage all underwent custody and treatment; all were writing after the event, either to explain – to themselves and to the world – their insanity and subsequent recovery, or to vindicate themselves from the accusation that they ever had been crazy. George Trosse in the mid-seventeenth century was taken off by friends (raving so badly that he needed to be tied down) to a special house for lunatics; James Carkesse was locked up in a Finsbury madhouse and then in Bethlem; Alexander Cruden was confined on at least three occasions in madhouses in Bethnal Green and Chelsea; William Cowper recovered while lodged in Nathaniel Cotton's Collegium Insanorum at St Albans; Samuel Bruckshaw was confined, against his will, in a private madhouse at Ashton-under-Lyne; William Belcher spent thirteen years in a Hackney madhouse; Urbane Metcalf, like James Tilley Matthews, was a resident of Bethlem; and John Perceval – to look forward into the 1830s – was placed by his family in two highly prestigious private madhouses: Brislington House, near Bristol, and Ticehurst House in Sussex. Being so few in number, they are necessarily unrepresentative. Their *apologiae* are the works of highly literate people. Hence such narratives pose intractable problems for the evaluation of the inner experience of madness. A few connecting threads may, however, very tentatively be drawn out.

One fundamental division marks these writings. Certain authors – Alexander Cruden, Samuel Bruckshaw and (if more ambiguously) William Belcher – staunchly denied their insanity. Others, such as Cowper and Perceval, confessed that at some stage they had come to recognise their mental delusions. They therefore wrote to prove that they were now sane once more. Whereas the former clutch of authors wrote to assert their rights, indict crimes committed against them, and obtain justice, the others aimed to put the record straight with themselves – as well, in some cases, as aspiring to serve other unfortunates through sharing their own harrowing experiences. In general, the former class of apologists wrote within a secular frame of reference, the latter within a religious. This turns out to be a distinction of great significance.

In what remains of this chapter, I shall explore these writings. First I shall gauge what they reveal about the consciousness of Georgian 'mad people' (that is, both those admitting they were mad, and those regarded as mad though claiming to be sane); then I shall see what they tell us ('from below') about the experience of receiving Georgian psychiatry.

PROVING YOURSELF SANE

For people judged insane but trying to prove their sanity, the very act of putting pen to paper, 'composing' a testament, was clearly significant in itself – evidence, surely, of 'composure'. For instance, Samuel Bruckshaw set out in enormous detail the facts of his sequestration, in a circumstantial narrative which he expected would carry intellectual conviction simply as a full record of the facts. In documenting the events leading to his confinement, names, statements, dates, times etc. were all minutely registered, as in a legal indictment. He was particularly punctilious about recording the testimony of everyone who declared him sane.

Bruckshaw was a Stamford merchant. In 1770 he had a succession of brushes with neighbours, fellow-tradesmen and town officials, which can now be reconstructed only from his own account. Bruckshaw thought he was being cheated and then persecuted through 'conspiracy'. He records that he was then carried off by two surgeons under the instructions of a town cabal, restrained and driven into Lancashire to Wilson's, a private madhouse at Scout Mill, Ashton-under-Lyne. There he was confined for 284 days in, he claimed, oppressive conditions, being poorly fed, denied exercise, kept as a 'prisoner' in a poky, cold attic, and abused by loutish and cynical keepers, who made no pretence even of treatment. Most of his attempts to communicate with his friends by letter were intercepted, though finally he was released through the good offices of his brother, but not before his business had collapsed. One of the aims of his vindications – *The Case, Petition and Address of Samuel Bruckshaw, who Suffered a Most Severe Imprisonment for Very Nearly the Whole Year* (1774) and *One More Proof of the Iniquitous Abuse of Private Madhouses* (1774) – was to seek redress for his financial ruin. It may be no accident that these were published while the bill for regulating private madhouses was before Parliament.

All to no avail. Indeed, Bruckshaw's publications may have been counterproductive, rather as Haslam clearly believed that the best way to demonstrate James Tilley Matthews' insanity was simply to let his story be heard. Bruckshaw presented himself as a lily-white innocent, a sacrificial lamb, slaughtered by the fiendish burghers of Stamford whose persecuting spirit knew no bounds. Little reading between the lines is needed to suggest that he was (to say the least) fractious, suspicious and litigious; moreover, while in confinement he heard disembodied voices.

Bruckshaw's testimony echoes that of an earlier, more substantial figure, Alexander Cruden. Cruden (1700-71), a Presbyterian, famous as the compiler of the still-standard Biblical concordance, published in 1739 his *The London-Citizen Exceedingly Injured: or a British Inquisition Display'd in an Account of the Unparallel'd Case of a Citizen of London, Bookseller to the late Queen, who was... sent...*

to a Private Madhouse (1739). In it, he told how he had been gratuitously locked up, though perfectly sane, by tormentors in Wright's private madhouse at Bethnal Green in 1738. It is not totally clear from Cruden's vivid, angry, but incoherent account what motives he thought his neighbours had for persecuting him. Although he accuses them of mercenariness, there are hints that he believed the malice originated with his landlady, whose lecherous designs on him he had righteously rebuffed. Like Bruckshaw, Cruden composed his book as a legal document, referring to himself in the third person ('the prisoner'), indicating the perfidy of his oppressors, and rationalising with elaborate apologies all his own peculiarities (for example, why, at one point, he had set his room alight). Cruden incriminated Dr James Monro, physician to Bethlem, who prescribed physic for him without even troubling to visit him. He was also able to provide an ultimate vindication of his case, for he escaped from the madhouse and succeeded in presenting himself before the Lord Mayor of London, who granted his freedom.

Cruden was incarcerated on at least two further occasions, writing up his escapades as *The Adventures of Alexander the Corrector* (3 parts, 1754-55). These later works contrasted in tone with the earlier *The London Citizen Exceedingly Injured*. Whereas the earlier publication was earnest and legalistic, seeking private justice in the particular case, by the 1750s Cruden had assumed a very different persona, as a public hero (an 'Alexander') and deliverer, a scourge divinely sent to whip the wicked, a defender of the exploited, a 'Corrector of the People Under God'. In portraying himself as an avenging angel, the later Cruden was nothing if not egotistical (megalomaniac might be today's diagnostic term). He struts like a Swiftian mad-hero come to life – like the narrator of *A Tale of a Tub*, a windbag inflated within his own canting self-righteousness. The performance lurches towards self-parody – he sought a knighthood and government office. But there is no let-up in his professions of his own holiness and sanity, or his indictments of the madness of the persecuting world.

Cruden's scenario of the innocent abroad in a persecuting world (that classic theme of Georgian fiction) is resumed in William Belcher's *Address to Humanity: Containing a Letter to Dr Monro, A Receipt to Make a Lunatic and Seize his Estate, and a Sketch of a True Smiling Hyena* (1796). Belcher had been locked up in a private asylum in Hackney between 1778 and 1795, when he was released partly because of a good word from Thomas Monro. Belcher continually claimed to have been pronounced insane by a jury which had never seen him, kept in filth and squalor, straitjacketed, force-fed and taunted while under lock and key. His wrongful confinement, he alleges, was aimed at the seizure of his estate. Particularly noteworthy in Belcher's account is his explicit statement that 'the trade of lunacy' is 'an approved receipt to make a lunatic' (is this his way of saying that, if he now appears peculiar, he was at least perfectly sane when detained?). It may be significant that in a later work, *Intellectual Electricity* (1798), Belcher glories in the aura of madness, developing a 'gay science' which travesties contemporary metaphysics, contradicting himself as he proceeds, confessing that he does not understand what he is saying, and creating philosophical mayhem in the persona of a thinking man's buffoon.

Thus, for a certain genre of 'mad writers', the crucial task was to demonstrate their own sanity. But to prove one's reason through writing was no easy task – witness the plight of the Bedlam poet, James Carkesse, discussed above in Chapter Two. Carkesse chose to express himself in verse, to prove his wits; but in doing so, he risked writing himself into the stereotype of the mad poet and witty fool. His attempt was not altogether successful, as is suggested even by the title of his book of verse. *Lucida intervalla*. Carkesse might contend:

> The Truth on't is, my Brains well fixt condition
> Apollo better knows, that his Physitian:
> 'Tis Quacks disease, not mine, my Poetry
> By the blind Moon-Calf, took for Lunacy.[29]

Dr Allen's response was a version of Catch 22: 'till he left off making Verses, he was not fit to be discharg'd'.

DIVINE MADNESS

For certain other 'mad' authors, however, vindicating rationality was not what counted. These are the writers who admit that they have struggled in the eddies of insanity, but claim to have regained the bank of health. Reason is less crucial within this genre because, without exception, such authors cast their spiritual shipwrecks in the language of religion. For them, the dramas of temptation, sin, divine mercy and faith determined mental and spiritual well-being.

George Trosse offers a good example from the mid-seventeenth century. A young Royalist debauchee (as he recalls his rebellious, misspent youth), Trosse found himself encouraged, apparently by God's voice, to a series of temptations to sin, beginning with minor mundane truculence, transgressions and profanities. Eventually an inner voice commanded him to cut off his hair. When it dawned on Trosse that the next command would be to cut his own throat, he recognised that what he had taken for God's voice was actually Satan's. Thus ensnared into sin by the Tempter, taunted by demons, he fell into raving madness, 'wild and outragious'. When his friends tried to restrain him, he lashed out, mistaking them for yet further devils. The astonishing force of Trosse's experience lies in its superposition of the spiritual world of torturing demons onto the mundane realities of his friends restraining, yet helping, him. As for Perceval later, Trosse regarded his 'treatment' as an extension of the torment, until finally his 'hell within' yielded to a sense of the mercy of God. Spiritual and physical struggles were all of a piece. When he was wrestling with the Devil, it took an exceedingly strong man to pinion him down.

His autobiography, *The Life of the Reverend Mr George Trosse*, was written well over a generation after his recovery and published posthumously. Does it accurately render Trosse's contemporary experiences? It reads basically as a composed, pious recension, a thanksgiving for the successful conclusion of the psychomachy – Trosse's temptation, fall and readmission to grace abounding. It seems a warning to fellow youthful debauchees. What is significant in Trosse's tale is that the Devil is still a literal combatant; the experience of Satanic possession is madness.

Numerous later sufferers fell into derangements precipitated by religious crisis. Many (outside sectarian autobiography) are noteworthy for the diminished role granted to Satan. No longer is the crisis one of literal possession by the Devil. Instead the sufferer experiences the torments of alienation from God, feelings of guilt, abandonment and annihilation. Nevertheless, Satan often remains a presence. A telling example is offered by the life of the poet William Cowper, which we can reconstruct partly from an autobiographical *apologia pro vita sua* composed in middle age, and partly from profuse letters and other memorials from his later life.

Cowper was a young man-about-town in the 1760s. His crisis was sparked in 1763, when an uncle obtained him the prospect of employment as a clerk to the House of Lords, in succession to the existing incumbent. When that man promptly died, however, Cowper was overwhelmed by guilt at having willed his death. Mentally paralysed, he found the prospects of being interviewed, or judged, for the office unbearable. He panicked. To evade 'judgment', he attempted suicide by drowning, stabbing and poison. These 'temptations' of Satan failed (we might interpret them nowadays as 'gestures'), whereupon Cowper decided that one route only lay ahead: to escape from the burden of responsibility into 'the chastisement of madness':

> I now began to look upon madness as the only chance remaining.
> I had a strong kind of foreboding that it would one day fare with
> me, and I had wished for it earnestly and looked forward to it
> with impatient expectation.[30]

He grew deranged, pacing up and down, saying 'There never was so abandoned a wretch; so great a sinner', but was rescued from his 'dismay of soul' by his clergyman brother, and carried off to the respectable asylum run by Dr Nathaniel Cotton in St Albans.

Precisely why Cowper reacted so catastrophically, collapsing into self-hatred, is somewhat unclear. He had, however, been brought up a Calvinist. His mother had died while he was a child, and he may have felt both 'abandoned' by her and to blame for her death. His father was distant and indifferent – a model for Cowper's image of God the Father? – and an early experience possibly led him to suspect that his father would welcome his suicide. From early youth Cowper assumed that he was one of the reprobate, predestined to his fate. The House of Lords interviewing panel was probably a foretaste of God's wrath.

If religious dread prompted his collapse into unremitting 'expectation of punishment', religious hope sped his recovery. One day in the asylum, under the 'chastisement' of lunacy, he experienced a providence:

> But the happy period which was to shake off my fetters and afford me a clear opening of the free mercy of God in Christ Jesus was now arrived. I flung myself in a chair near the window, and seeing a Bible there, ventured once more to apply to it for comfort and instruction. The first verse I saw, was the 25th of the 3rd of Romans: 'Whom God sent forth to be a propitiation through faith in his blood, to declare his righteousness for the remission of sins that are past, through the forebearance of God.'
>
> Immediately I received strength to believe and the full beams of the Sun of righteousness shone upon me. I saw the sufficiency of the atonement he had made, my pardon sealed in his blood, and justification.[31]

Assured at last that he was not a foredoomed wretch, the worst of sinners, Cowper was released from his sense of perdition. He turned evangelistic. His *Memoir*, composed fairly soon after his recovery, was an act of thanksgiving to the God of mercy.

It proved premature, however, for recovery was not permanent. Though he led a sheltered life, busying himself with writing as a form of occupational therapy, Cowper lapsed into doubt, torment and breakdown on three further occasions, each bout triggered by an indelible sense of religious guilt and pollution, overshadowed by the implacable rod of divine wrath, a sentence of doom captured in his 'Lines Written during a Period of Insanity':

> Hatred and vengeance, my external portion,
> Scarce can endure delay of execution,
> Wait, with impatient readiness, to seize my
>   Soul in a moment.
> Damn'd below Judas: more abhorr'd than he was,
> Who for a few pence sold his holy Master.
> Twice betrayed Jesus me, the last delinquent,
>   Deems me the profanest.[32]

The experience of being a defenceless creature – a stricken deer – caught in an infinitely cruel and arbitrary religious trap precipitated Cowper's final collapse and possible suicide. Almost as in Greek tragedy, madness was torment by the gods.

Samuel Johnson, the Augustan, and the castaway Cowper, the man of sensibility, offer two facets of the religious melancholy and madness of mid-Georgian Anglicanism. Both buckled under a terrifying faith which heaped crushing burdens upon the believer. In both, personal redemptive love from a Divine Father had been cast in doubt through indoctrination which saw God as Majesty, distant, awesome. Cowper felt isolated, separate, alien, persecuted, cursed. Encountering the torments of men such as Cowper, no wonder MacDonald and others have lamented the demise of Providentialist faith in the age of the Enlightenment. For the rationalisation of religion had removed that experience of personal psychomachy which had ultimately eased the individual's personal burden of responsibility. Reasonable religion rebuked unreason as sinful, yet yoked the individual to the sternest duties.

Among the votaries of New Dissent, however, there survived traditions of holy madness, of visions and speaking in tongues. This is exemplified in the fullest text penned by one who had gone through the purifying fires of madness, and had come to terms with his condition, John Perceval's *Narrative of the Treatment Received by a Gentleman, During a State of Mental Derangement* (1838-40). Son of the assassinated Prime Minister, Spencer Perceval, John spent a dissipated youth, first in the army and then at Oxford University, until falling in with the sect known as the Irvingites, or the Glasgow Row Heresy. They believed in an elect marked by direct divine communication. The Holy Ghost spoke personally through the medium of born-again Christians in tongues which sounded mere gibberish to the unregenerate (as Perceval puts it, 'with sounds like these: "*Hola mi hastos, Hola me hastos, disca capita crustos bustos*"').

Soon Perceval was personally having Pentecostal ecstasies. However, he came to experience his possession as being less by God than by tormenting demons. He grew desperate (partly due to having earlier been infected with syphilis) and his brother had him confined in Brislington House in 1831. Initially, Perceval recalls, he believed that he had been removed there to receive and communicate the new gospel better. Only subsequently did he discover that he was in an asylum; only later still did he accept that he was indeed mad. Acceptance of religious madness did not, however, destroy Perceval's faith but merely modified his grasp of his vocation. He came to view madness as a divine trial. Torment by demons was part of the Higher Purpose.

Certain points stand out from these narratives of religious madness. The first is that during the eighteenth century, the only belief-system within which people could acknowledge themselves as mad was a religious one. Within secular values, insanity – though not 'nerves' or melancholy – was wholly negative, meaningless; unreason betokened utter personal and social nothingness. Being out of one's mind, however, had its place within Christian values as a potentially positive phase of spirituality, a response to the experiences of temptation, torment and trial. One may agree with *philosophes* such as Erasmus Darwin that Christianity's imperious demands were responsible for unhinging some; but those people it drove mad saw rationales for their state, and sometimes pointers to recovery. Not till the Romantic odyssey of the ego was there a secular equivalent to this ideology of insanity as spiritual pilgrimage.

Further, it seems that those Georgians who believed in the Christian spirit-world to the letter, and heeded the injunctions of scriptural Christianity, ran greater risks than their predecessors of being disqualified as mad and even confined. Thus it clearly mattered in the age of the Enlightenment to be tenacious of one's reason. We know from Johnson how strongly he believed it his duty – a Christian's duty – to safeguard his rationality, and a flourishing genre of moral and religious advice books likewise expounded rules for self-command. Georgian madmen give little sign of experiencing madness as a blessed condition, or even as release. With few exceptions such as Kit Smart and William Blake ('under direction from Messengers from God'), no one relished insanity, or expected to ascend through it to new peaks of insight, illumination, holiness or genius. Insanity became an object of dread and moral reprobation.

EXPERIENCING MADNESS

Finally, I shall pose a different question to this body of mad people's writings: what do they tell us of how attitudes towards, and treatment of, madness were experienced by sufferers themselves? Again we must remember how unrepresentative a sample we have (no illiterates, no women, hardly anyone from the lower orders). We must therefore tread tentatively. Nevertheless, some patterns emerge which corroborate certain interpretations outlined earlier.

It is first noteworthy that of the three seventeenth-century texts, one, Goodwin Wharton's autobiography, chronicles the

life of a man who, though in the protracted grip of a comprehensive delusional system, never fell under supervision from
family, doctors or magistrates. No writs *De Lunatico Inquirendo*
were taken out against him, nor attempts made to incarcerate
him. In later generations there were frequent Chancery suits
for people of Wharton's standing, and private asylum treatment
for mad gentlefolk was common by the eighteenth century.
Wharton's is conspicuous in being the only diary of a madman
in which the subject remained free all his life to build his own
castles in the air.

The other two seventeenth-century examples are equally
revealing. George Trosse's madness was handled purely privately;
he was taken up by friends and deposited in a physician's house.
The main 'psychiatry' used on him lay in Gospel-reading. This
finds a later echo, perhaps, in Cowper's account of his confinement in Cotton's Collegium Insanorum in 1763-64. Cowper
found his treatment humane. He mentions, however, nothing
by way of 'psychiatry'; according to his own account, what triggered his recovery was the chance reading of a biblical verse.

James Carkesse's account of Bethlem and the Finsbury
madhouse is also illuminating. He makes passing reference to ill-
treatment, confirming the popular image of brutal Bethlem; but
that was not his main concern. He was interested not in the physical but in the metaphysical nature of the madhouse. He dwells
upon the moral and existential paradox that his incarceration
marks the topsy-turvy world: he who is sane is confined by the
crazy, above all Dr Allen ('Dr Mad Quack'). Thus Carkesse's barbs
against the asylum are not those of a Benthamite reformer *avant
la lettre*, but those of a railer against the human tragicomedy.

Looking forward, the eighteenth-century texts are different
because they come to be dominated by one exceedingly tangible
presence: notably, the madhouse, a totally secular institution. For
Cruden, Bruckshaw, Belcher and Metcalf, writing about madness becomes writing about life in the madhouse. The accounts
these authors give are collectively noteworthy for two features.
First, as patients they are basically confined to their own room.

They give few clues of any kind of communal asylum life. They rarely mention other patients. Second, there is almost no indication – even of a hostile nature – that they were receiving any regular treatment. The therapy thought appropriate for them was sequestration.

Detention was the greatest complaint of Cruden, Bruckshaw and Belcher. Their testimony confirms the view that many Georgian madhouse proprietors did little more than provide a place of security. The fury of Cruden and Bruckshaw was not directed against the 'abuses of psychiatry', against the asylum as a total institution in Goffmann's sense, against the 'manufacture of madness' as conceived by Szasz. Though protesting about his treatment by Dr Monro, Cruden did not primarily perceive himself to be a victim of 'psychiatry', but rather above all a victim of injustice, through the infringement of his constitutional rights as a freeborn Englishman. Protagonists such as Cruden saw themselves not as sufferers made more sick by inappropriate treatment, but as John Bulls, unlawfully detained. They experienced themselves not as patients but as prisoners; their superiors were not doctors but captors. The protest was less against the nonperson stigma of madness than against larceny of liberties. Whereas by the late 1830s Perceval wrote his narrative as a tract of 'anti-psychiatry', a century earlier Cruden used the libertarian rhetoric we associate with John Wilkes in his significantly titled

The London Citizen Exceedingly Injured
or
A British Inquisition Display'd In an account of the Unparallel'd Case
of a Citizen of London, Bookseller to the late Queen, who was in a
most unjust and arbitrary Manner sent on the 23rd March last by one
Robert Wightman, a mere Stranger, to a Private Madhouse[33]

The Georgian asylum was criticised by its vocal inmates not principally in terms of psychiatric regime but of individual rights. Surely this reflected the realities; for patients did not experience relentless surveillance and regimentation. Rather, asylum life shared the common coinage of all other Hanoverian institutions – prisons, bridewells, the army. It was the world of Old Corruption, where the fabric was honeycombed with venality, peculation, petty oppressions, neglect, chicanery, bullying, profiteering, cruelties, and nepotism.

This is all illustrated in a text hitherto hardly mentioned, Urbane Metcalf's *The Interior of Bethlehem Hospital* (1818). Metcalf himself had been an inmate between 1804 and 1806, and in 1817 (he admitted that he had been intermittently mad, thinking himself heir to the throne of Denmark). The great evils of Bethlem in his view consisted in exploitation and abuse of power. Supineness from above – he particularly deplored the absences of the physician Thomas Monro – left the 'cruel, unjust and drunken' attendants to commit whatever abuses, peculation, and neglect they wished. Some went absent; others gave their time to private patients; many profiteered out of food and supplies. Lunatics were easily exploited, both by staff and by their peers. Beatings went on, and deaths were hushed up. Protection was in reality exploitation. Bethlem institutionalised the abuse of power:

> The institution in itself is an honor to humanity, and purged of the villains who oppress its unfortunate inmates would reflect a lustre on the individuals who support it by their fortunes. Our country has been famed throughout the world for the splendour of her charitable institutions; remedy their abuses, her fame will be just; at present, however laudable the intentions of its supporters may be, the unfortunate who are compelled to claim their protection finds virtuous establishments prostituted to vicious purposes by wretches whose least crime is a total abuse of humanity.[34]

A couple of decades later, in the 1830s, the account which John Perceval gave of his stay in two of the most opulent, liberal and respected asylums in England, Brislington House and Ticehurst

House, is extremely revealing because of the contrast with what had come before. Unlike Cruden or Bruckshaw, Perceval's protest was not against unlawful confinement; after all, he eventually came to admit that he had been disordered. Nor was it against neglect, arbitrary cruelty, or want of treatment. The evil was the treatment itself, 'moral therapy', the 'progressive' 'humane' psychiatry which had come to the fore by the 1830s. Even the name 'asylum' was a 'travesty', he insisted, 'for to call that, or any like that, an asylum, is cruel mockery and revolting duplicity'. Perceval was indeed in no doubt about Dr Edward Long Fox's goals at Brislington, referring time and again to his 'system of treatment'. But he experienced what he sarcastically dubbed 'wholesome restraint', simply as a 'brutal and tyrannical control over my will'. Far from being humane, the treatment was inhumanity itself: 'In truth the humanity is that of the patients, not that of the system and of its agents'.

Fox's psychiatric paternalism amounted – as Perceval experienced it – to a round of unwanted and unwarranted intrusions whose effects were defacing, negating his will, personality and identity. The treatment was never explained to him; he was not consulted. His word was never trusted, yet the doctors and staff lied to him ('my senses were all mocked and deceived' by this 'system of dupery'). He was denied pen and paper; his letters were opened ('by what rights can a doctor presume to pry into the secrets of a patient's conscience, who is not only a perfect stranger to him, but also a gentleman?'). All in all, he complained, he was treated 'as if I were a piece of furniture, an image of wood, incapable of desire or will as well as judgement':

> Men acted as though my body, and soul were fairly given up to
> their control, to work their mischief and folly upon. My silence,
> I suppose, gave consent. I mean, that I was never told such things
> we are going to do; we think it advisable to administer such and
> such medicine, in this or that manner: I was never asked – Do
> you want anything? do you wish for, prefer any thing? have you
> any objection to this or that? I was fastened down in bed; a

meagre diet was ordered for me; this and medicine forced down
my throat or in the contrary direction; my will, my wishes, my
repugnances, my habits, my delicacy, my inclinations, my neces-
sities, were not consulted, I may say, thought of. I did not find
the respect paid usually to a child.[35]

For Perceval, this grind of treatment *de haut en bas* was a disgrace,
'designed to insult', exacerbated because he was denied his rank
as a gentleman and treated as a nobody, not least by the insolent
Quaker staff who failed to acknowledge themselves his inferiors.
But worse than that, the regime was mercenary – 'their end is to
make money not to make whole'. All in all, it was not rational
but actually insane, a 'burlesque' run by one who was 'the dupe
of his own system'. Therapeutic will comprised instrusions and
impositions. 'If he resists the treatment', wrote Perceval, 'he is
then a madman'. But who wouldn't resist? 'They kept drenching
my body to take away the evil which their system was continually exciting'.

Tie an active limbed, active minded, actively imagining young
man in bed, hand and foot, for a fortnight, drench him with
medicines, slops, clysters; when reduced to the extremes of nervous debility his derangement is successfully confirmed... Do all
in your power to crush any germ of self-respect that may yet
remain or rise up in his bosom; manacle him as you would a
felon; expose him to ridicule and give him no opportunity of
retirement or self reflection; and what are you to expect? And
whose agents are you? Those of God or Satan? And what can
you reasonably dare to expect?[36]

In short, concluded Perceval, 'I will be bold to say that the
greatest part of the violence that occurs in lunatic asylums is to
be attributed to the conduct of those who are dealing with the
disease, not the disease itself'.

The patient was in the classic Catch 22 situation. He was
expected to submit to degradation, and 'if to resent neglect,

insult and ruffian-like violence is a proof of madness', then he was insane. 'You never can tell if the patient's eccentricities are the symptoms of his disorder or the result of antipathy to the new circumstances in which you have placed him'. Little is wanting from Perceval's narrative as an account of the manufacture of madness.

After Perceval, the history of mad people's writing is a crescendo of reaction to, and protest against, the dominating presence of the asylum. In such writings as those of Richard Paternoster or Louisa Lowe, madness almost ceased to have its own integral, self-contained history; it was essentially defined by, and had been appropriated by, the madhouse system and its techniques of psychiatric care. One truth which mad people's writing bears out beyond ambiguity is the rising presence of the asylum and of psychological medicine as the framework which increasingly defined and mastered madness.

Conclusion

There are many prominent moments in the treatment of the mad around the turn of the nineteenth century, any of which could be invoked to demonstrate, in one way or another, that old beliefs and practices had played themselves out (or alternatively come to maturity) and that a new era was dawning. The closing of Old Bethlem in 1815 and its removal from Moorfields to a new building at St George's Fields (for which designs had been submitted by one of the inmates, James Tilley Matthews) would be hard to match as a symbolic closure of the old regime. A more momentous pivotal point from the old to the new was surely the hearings of the House of Commons Committee of 1815, which brought to light and preserved for posterity a nonpareil moral and physical panorama of the Georgian madhouse world and its *misérables*. The calling of that Committee signalled that madness truly was Parliament's concern (a pity no reforms of any consequence followed it for more than a decade). Not least of course, all such exemplary events were occurring against the backdrop of the mental alienation and ultimate dementia of the monarch who 'gloried in the name of Briton', the king's treatment then as now generating fierce controversy (here was the most archaic therapeutic brutality, here a king was being cured).

As illuminating a turning point as any, I believe, comes from an incident in the career of Thomas Bakewell, proprietor of Spring Vale Asylum in Staffordshire. Struggling with a formidably perverse young woman – the case is given in detail in Chapter Four – Bakewell records in his *Domestic Guide in Cases of Insanity*, 'Good heavens! When I look back upon the trouble and anxiety I underwent with this creature, I wonder I ever got through it'. Cases of such severity, Bakewell confessed, would all but convince you that madness could be so hideous, so wilful, such a negation of all that was human, as to be beyond hope. But not quite.

Eventually he rumbled her ruses, overcame her resistance, and restored her to normality. Bakewell's vignette, of course, forms part of a tale. Yet it is also an all-too-rare snatch of the mad-doctor himself 'unbuttoned'. If we rarely hear the 'voice of the mad', we pick up from the sources, if that is possible, even less of the daily thoughts and table-talk of those in charge of them. The historical record effectively masks the minds of madhouse-keepers behind prospectuses, parliamentary answers and clinical case notes: the trade seems to have silenced the doctors hardly less than their patients.

Bakewell's vignette reveals a most significant phenomenon, presumably fairly common by the close of the eighteenth century but perhaps hardly known previously. Here is an intelligent and humane middle-class Midlander devoting his energies – his life, in fact – to the daunting and (as Bakewell himself stresses) quite exhausting business of restoring a houseful of mad people to some semblance of well-being. Almost two centuries earlier, Robert Burton had confined himself in an Oxford college to writing about – indeed, celebrating – the world's madness in all its tragicomedy; but there is no evidence that he ever came face to face with a living lunatic. Burton's contemporary, Richard Napier, certainly treated thousands of strange people brought to him for relief. But the bulk of his patients typically turned up for a single consultation, were offered their prescription and advice, and went away again, never to return. We have no reason to believe that Napier, for all the wise and humane spiritual healing which MacDonald has shown he dispensed, ever saw a patient day by day through the entire course of an episode of mental alienation, still less attempted to manage or cure such a case. By the close of the eighteenth century, Thomas Bakewell and a score of other superintendents and doctors were making it their business – their *savoir pouvoir* – to live among mad people as part of a healing regime.

Of course, some did so deploying a brutality which shocks us; of course, all made a living out of it and a few a fat one; and of course, the element of repressive control, individual and social, that such practices involved has been properly exposed by modern critics. All that is true. Nevertheless, historically speaking, the appearance of a score or two of professionals, daily gaining experience of insanity at close quarters, having to gauge and steer the precarious dialectic between madness and management and in many cases distilling their experiences into print forms a crucial juncture. Historians often point to the 'brutal' treatment meted out by Francis Willis to King George III as proof of eighteenth-century benightedness. What may be truly significant about this incident, however, is that a man with a lifetime's experience in handling the insane could be summoned from the depths of the Lincolnshire countryside; indeed that he should actually prove so confident at managing a king! If Queen Anne had gone out of her mind, could a Willis then have been found?

In some ways, of course, this secular 'empirical psychiatry' of the age of Bakewell, Willis and others may not have been worlds apart from the 'spiritual healing' of earlier exorcists and ministers of grace within Christian thaumaturgy. But exorcism had not generally been a full-time occupation which stayed in the family for generations, as madhouse-keeping became for the Finches, Coxes, Arnolds, Newingtons etc.; nor did thaumaturgical healers watch over their charges sometimes for years on end in special institutions. Exorcists were principally preoccupied with heresy or the Devil, not with the people with the Devil in them. In this light, the eighteenth century has a good claim to have generated the practices from which subsequent practical psychiatry developed.

Above all, careful attention to the life work of practitioners such as William Battie, Thomas Arnold, Thomas Bakewell, William Perfect, Joseph Mason Cox and so forth should make us hesitate before rehashing cliché judgements on the treatment of the mad during the eighteenth century. I hope this book has amply demonstrated, for one thing, that Leigh's verdict that eighteenth-century English psychiatric writings were either tedious or second-hand simply does not hold water. Without resorting to silly priority games, it can be pointed out that Battie's *Treatise on Madness* (1758) contains (albeit in a rather schematic and theoretical guise) the key ideas of Tukean moral therapy. Indeed, notwithstanding Foucault's denial that the eighteenth century had a 'psychology', it is hard to see what other historical label would be better for the Lockian heritage in England, so powerful an influence on so many managers of the mad, from Battie through to the Tukes. English treatises on depression in the generation of Mandeville and Cheyne, and works on mental alienation in the half century between Bathe and Crichton, reveal a fertile and innovative mixture of insightful advocacy – and criticism – of the emergent theoretical practice of what was to become psychiatry.

I hope, furthermore, that the view, summed up by Scull, of the Georgian madhouse as a world of 'shit, straw and stench' has been shown to be at best partially true, and taken over from nineteenth-century reformist sloganising. Neither is it clear that, as MacDonald puts it, 'the eighteenth century was a disaster for the insane – at least any more than any other era inevitably must be'. It depended – as in previous centuries – on who you were, and where you were, and who was treating you. Going out of his mind certainly proved disastrous for William Cowper, but we have it from his own memoirs that being under medical care in a madhouse was a true cordial to his spirits. For pauper mad people, the Georgian madhouse was hell; but as yet we know too little about how they were treated previously to be able to say with confidence whether it was a worse, or just a different, hell. In terms of its capacity for being a systematically and routinely soul-destroying, repressive institution, the eighteenth-century madhouse was but a portent of things to come.

Several substantive points of revaluation emerge from the evidence I have scrutinised in the course of this book. For one thing, it is historically misleading to posit some sort of 'episte-mological rupture' around 1800, involving a radical switch from handling the mad like animals to treating them as people, from physical therapy to moral therapy, or from scandal to reform. Much of what the nineteenth century claimed for its own had been established in the previous era. Both in rhetoric and in reality, 'moral' forms of therapy were well tried and tested long before the close of the eighteenth century. It would not even be outrageous to suggest that the heyday of a *de facto* kind of moral therapy lay in the eighteenth century, in a small 'cot-tage asylum' such as the one run by Nathaniel Cotton in St Albans. Perhaps it was the championing of schemes of moral therapy, and their application to ever larger asylums as part of the nineteenth-century reform movement, which inadvertently traduced their essentials. A big madhouse, pronounced Harper, is 'big with ignorance and absurdity'.

Moreover, a serious distortion of what actually happened during the 'long eighteenth century' can result if we look at it through eyes principally trained on the star role of the public asylum after 1800. Because of the intensity of today's debates about the future of mental hospitals within state psychiatry, the history of psychiatry as it has recently been written has been monopolised by assessments of the history of the asylums. *Decarceration* and *Museums of Madness* have thus gone together. From this 'institutionalisation' viewpoint, it is easy to assume that because it was the nineteenth century which saw the gigantic and systematic expansion of the asylum system, it follows that

in the eighteenth century either no developments of any consequence occurred or, as Foucault has claimed, the mad were
rounded up indiscriminately with the bad as part of a strategy of
social policing. There is something neat about supposing that the
age of institutionalisation was preceded by the age of neglect.

It is crucial, however, to contest this vision, which perpetuates the all-too-common myth that public-spirited action was
the prerogative of the nineteenth century. Pre-industrial society
developed and deployed within the social infrastructure its own
expedients and appropriate institutions for handling the mad
(as also the sick and other problem people requiring care and
control). MacDonald has lamented the decay of therapeutic
eclecticism, but in its own way the Georgian age practised its
own lively therapeutic eclecticism in treating the disturbed, using
a variety of sites and techniques, medical, moral and managerial.
As I suggested above, particularly in Chapter Three, community
concern and parochial financial and personal support are not
hard to find. Many possibilities were tried including domiciliary
care, boarding out in the community, sending the insane to stay
with a clergyman or physician, placing them in private asylums,
applying to Bethlem or, particularly if violent, securing them in
houses of correction. Better-off patients often lived with their
own personal attendant. The spread of private asylums clearly
gave families and overseers of the poor an extra option. Georgian
society had a flexible repertoire of techniques – some market-
based, others community-based – for handling social problems,
and it would be as gratuitous to assume that all lunatics not in
asylums were utterly neglected as it would be to infer that lunatics were put into madhouses only for the most callous motives.
To think that is to presuppose that the chorus of Georgian
concern was simply hypocritical from beginning to end.

Among the mad poor, the era of relatively informal arrangements presumably came to an end essentially through the
establishment of a comprehensive workhouse system under the
New Poor Law of 1834, and then through the universalisation
of county asylums after 1845. But the continuation of relatively

informal ways of handling the mentally abnormal among the better-off – not least through the practice of 'single patient' boarding and the subsequent rise of 'nursing homes' – is an important phenomenon which would repay study. Of course problems became colossal in the nineteenth century, not least because of staggering population growth; and of course the Victorians, matching those crises with a necessary zeal, responded with tidy administrative solutions, setting great store by efficiency, economy and expertise. It is vital, however, not to be blinded to the 'interstitial' settlements typical earlier – which, by a peculiar irony, perhaps bear some resemblance to the arrangements for the mentally ill ('community care') which our own society is currently favouring.

Foucault was way off the mark, I have contended, to talk of the eighteenth century – at least in England – as a time marked by a 'great confinement'. In two other respects, however, his insights are particularly valuable. He stressed, for one thing, that what he was writing – indeed, what must be written – was a history of reason or rationality, as a necessary condition for a history of madness or irrationality. History cannot understand the constitution of madness without first understanding what constituted it as madness – without, in other words, accepting how the progress of the subject, Reason, presupposes its own negation. The point is crucial, not merely because it reminds us of the authentically Hegelian dialectical movement of subject and alienation, but because it also more specifically forces us to recognise that the rise of psychiatry is so much more than simply the emergence of yet another professional elite. Its preconditions include issues of how 'normal people' – the 'moral majority' – think of their own being and their characteristic attributes and values. Foucault himself made much play of how the sway after 1650 of an expansive, aggressive, ambitious type of Rationality invalidated and marginalised modes of being – being poor, being odd, being mad – which had hitherto possessed voices and truths of their own. The new Rationality saw being poor, being bad and being mad all as equivalents, modes of Unreason.

Foucault's general insight must be welcomed, but I have argued that his account of how Reason stigmatised those beyond the bourgeois work ethic seems off-beam for England. Much more relevant for the constitution of English madness were surely the processes of naturalisation ('demystification') and secularisation gathering pace from the latter half of the seventeenth century. These ideological drives supplanted the religious fundamental-ist doctrine that all men were mad in sin – indeed, all equally vulnerable to diabolical possession. By consequence, it became easier to construe insanity as a distinct condition of specific people with various physical or mental defects, and not least to believe – in the absence of Original Sin – that such madness was remediable. These became rationales for selective confinement. In Foucault's interpretation, sequestrating the mad was basically an act of anathematisation and quarantine. But the ideology and expectations typically found in England, from Bethlem to the ritziest asylum, principally endorsed curability – incidentally explaining why separate institutions for incurables were set up. As reason became more important than faith, and as culture became more central than Christianity, the elite increasingly looked upon disturbance not as destiny but as a problem – one which could be solved. That entailed taking more intervention-ist steps to manage the mad, but doing so not simply in the crudest and cheapest way possible – the gaol – but in ways which reflected in various measure the progressive self-image of Enlightened society.

In this respect, Foucault's liberal deployment of the abstrac-tion Unreason may be extremely misleading. For it suggests something final (Being), which misrepresents the much more dynamic English Enlightenment perception of reasoning as a process. It would be better, following Locke, to think of the mad characterised as the 'unreasonable', having a capacity – like chil-dren – to mature into 'reasonability'. Foucault's divide between 'Reason' and 'Unreason' proposes a frozen absoluteness which ill catches the common English empiricist view that Rationality was Becoming and that mental disorder was something which came and went by degree, being subject to fits of intensification and remission, and which – if caught early enough and well treated – was possibly as amenable to relief or cure as any disease. Above all, to the eighteenth-century English mind, the distinction between sanity and madness seemed one not of kind but of degree, and a whole range of symptoms and dispositions (hypochondria, hysteria, depression, the spleen) linked the two.

If Foucault is broadly correct to argue that madness and its treatment can be understood only in its dialectical relations with rationality and normality, he is also right to emphasise that, during the eighteenth century, the mad were silenced. Whether or not there ever had been any true dialogue (as Foucault implies) between society at large and living mad people (as distinct from literary representations of madness) is a separate and debatable point. But it is certainly true that the utterances of 'mad people' were commonly heeded in earlier centuries, not least because the mad were seen as the mouthpieces through whom Otherworldly Powers would speak.

All the indications, however, are that during the eighteenth century it was believed important for enhancing cure prospects to minimise mad talk. Attending to the delusions of the mad would only confirm them in their system. Hypochondriacs would inevitably talk themselves into further ills; talking about themselves would make hysterics grow overexcited and detrimentally secure the attention their morbid vanity craved. To the Enlightenment anthropological imagination, it was no longer true (as had once been thought) that early man and his myths contained the coded essence of true religion – these myths turned out to be, after all, just silly and superstitious. So, by parallel, madness also now had nothing authentic to say. The case was slightly different, however, with the mad. For their delusions were seen not as silly but as dangerous, the products of uncontrollable or twisted imaginations. Diversion or suppression were in order as preventives of utter chaos.

Strategies of control devised to contain and quieten the mad were central to that body of thinking, writing and practice, gelling in the latter half of the eighteenth century and the early part of the nineteenth – which, without serious anachronism, we can call the emergence of English psychiatry. Often drawing upon a neuroanatomy of nervous overexcitation – or of course, in the case of depression, underexcitation – they aimed, commonly by medical means, to deplete or stimulate the system and bring it into order. And they particularly stressed the need to achieve mental mastery – by physical control, by diversion, by the winning of moral authority, by tactical manoeuvres, by building up trust, indeed by a whole battery of measures.

Such techniques placed emergent psychiatry in a position of immense potential power yet also one of great vulnerability, and thereby mapped out the dilemmas of psychiatry for the coming century. The root of the matter lay in the ambivalence of psychiatry's object, the sense of self or psyche.

The great upheavals of early modern times had produced profound difficulties for conceptualising the nature of personal identity and consciousness, and grasping their relations to the world in which people lived. Belief in a transcendental (Christian) soul was generally retained in eighteenth-century discourse, but it ceased to be the medium through which daily life was conducted. Moreover, as traditional humoralism waned, its associated language for mapping a self on to the body went by the wayside. Thus the links in the chain between mind and body grew less tangible; the more it was analysed, the more intractable the mind/body problem became. And many features of late Enlightenment thought made it attractive to refined elites to nurture ways of talking about personality in which the mark of true distinction lay in the cultivation of 'mind', 'soul' or 'sensibility', viewed as distinct from the grossly corporeal. The age of the 'march of mind' was dawning; mind over matter was to become the new watchword.

Above all, budding Romanticism gave coherent expression to that new sense of self as something inner, private and potent, the product of Bildung, which had been emerging during the eighteenth century. It despised the merely material, reaffirmed the

spirit, reinstated the imagination, and within Coleridgean philosophy formulated a superior metaphysic of the 'Understanding'
as a kind of occult faculty. For that set of values, madness could
be recuperated within the literary and cultural vision.

Thus in the transition from Enlightenment to Romanticism,
literate culture espoused a new mystique of mind, regarded as a *je
ne sais quoi*, present within – if ill formulated by – metaphysics. This
played its part in the outlook of emergent psychiatry. On the one
hand, somewhat paralleling Lavaterian physiognomy, it underwrote psychiatry's claims to possess the power to see into minds.
At the individual level, practitioners such as William Pargeter,
Joseph Mason Cox and William Hallaran prided themselves on
their ability to pierce the smokescreen of sanity which the mad
so often put up. As witnesses in court, early nineteenth-century
psychiatrists vaunted their ability to seize upon the slightest clue
which, dextrously unravelled, would reveal an entire delusional
system. At the collective level, alienists increasingly claimed that
they, and probably they alone, could perceive the epidemic of
madness infiltrating civilisation. John Ferriar wrote of 'latent
insanity'; John Reid of 'atoms, or specks of insanity', pervading society (the implication being that they formed essentially
minute particles, visible only to the expert microscopic gaze), and
James Cowles Prichard was soon to devise the category of 'moral
insanity', a terrifying personality perversion, detectable initially
only from the most indirect hints. The moral manager or the
alienist was set fair to become the new clairvoyant.

But therein lay the rub. For in the 'disenchanted' world, magic
had been discredited. The ontological base of old occultist science had been undermined by the naturalising epistemological
scepticism which had made the world safe for the Enlightenment.
The new psychiatry possessed practical techniques of control,
closely linked with the asylum. But could it achieve a common
postulate, an agreed theory of consciousness and of mind/body
relations – in short, could it achieve scientific authority and public
credence? In the event it found itself stymied in its attempts to
resolve such dilemmas. Disciplines such as phrenology, aiming

to set the theory of mind upon physical foundations, met with hostility and scepticism. Yet purely mentalist formulations were put under abiding pressure from the medical profession, whose overlordship of psychiatry necessarily hinged ultimately on the establishment of a physical stratum. Could psychiatry ever become anything but modern charlatanry?

The resolution in England was *ad hoc*; it lay in the intimate association between psychiatry and the asylum, as the best sheet anchor the practice possessed. But that linkage undoubtedly proved as much a bane as a blessing. For the confinement of psychiatry within huge public pauper institutions – and its identification with the notoriety inseparable from the role of moral gaoler – restricted its appeal, hindered the development of a prestigious office practice and created the cold climate surrounding the various dynamic psychiatries in the present century. The Victorian era became the golden age of depression, nervous disorder and breakdown – witness the psychic health of the Victorian intellectuals such as John Stuart Mill and Thomas Carlyle – without generating a commensurate rise of fashionable, influential psychiatric practice. Psychiatry continued to lie in the lap of the laity, and lastingly suffered immense difficulty in establishing its credentials as a cast-iron, *bona fide* science.

Notes

CHAPTER ONE: ORIENTATIONS

1   Parkinson, *Madhouses*, 160.

2   Woods and Carlson, 'The Psychiatry of Philippe Pinel', 18. Compare Mora, 'The Psychiatrist's Approach'; idem., 'The History of Psychiatry'; idem., 'Historical and Theoretical Trends in Psychiatry'.

3   King-Hele, *Doctor of Revolution*, 35.

4   Foucault, *Madness and Civilization*, 74-75.

5   Quoted in Craig, *The Legacy of Swift*, 20.

6   E. Reynolds, *Life and Times*, 154.

7   Ibid.

8   Ferriar, *Medical Histories*, ii, 12.

9   Quoted in MacDonald, *Mystical Bedlam*, 169.

10   Shakespeare, *A Midsummer Night's Dream* V.

11   Boswell, *Life of Johnson*, iv, 31. See also Balderston, 'Johnson's Vile Melancholy'; Porter, 'The Hunger of Imagination'; and compare Johnson's comment in *Rasselas* (113-14): 'All power of fancy over reason is a degree of insanity; but while this power is such as we can controul and repress, it is not visible to others, not considered as any deprivation of the mental faculties; it is not pronounced madness but when it comes ungovernable, and apparently influences speech or action.'

12   Toynbee (ed.), *The Letters of Horace Walpole*, x, 219 (9 April 1778). Cf. earlier, vol. ix (1777), 48: 'I rejoice you have got your nephew again, and Lady Lucy, and that she is so much better than you expected. I trust Lord Orford's agreement with his grandfather's creditors, which he had just signed is good. The law will probably think so. In my private opinion, he has been mad these twenty years and more. On his coming of age, I obtained a fortune of one hundred and fifty-two thousand pounds for him: he would not look at her. Had I remained

charged with his affairs six months longer on his last illness, he
would have been five thousand a year richer than the day he fell ill.
My reward was, not see him for three years.'

13   Toynbee (ed.), *The Letters of Horace Walpole*, x, 219 (9 April 1778). Cf.
earlier, vol. ix (1777), 48:

14   Beddoes, *Hygeia*, iii, Tenth Essay, 40.

15   Darwin, *Temple of Nature*, Canto iv, 139.

16   Clifford, *Dr Campbell's Diary*, 45.

17   Latham and Matthews (eds), *The Diary of Samuel Pepys*, vi, 324.

18   Ibid., ix, 203.

19   Ibid., vii, 171. Cf. ibid., v, 59: 'The Court are mad for a Dutch war'.

20   Toynbee (ed.), *The Letters of Horace Walpole*, iii, 438. See also Lytes,
Methodism Mocked.

21   Johnson (ed.), *Letters from Lady Mary Wortley Montagu*, 506-07.

22   Ibid., 410.

23   Lindsay, *William Blake*, 208.

24   Quoted in Byrd, *Visits to Bedlam*, 30.

25   Burton, *Anatomy of Melancholy*, 638. For the monster theme see
Porter, 'Madmen and Monsters'.

26   Wesley, *Primitive Physick*; see Rousseau, 'John Wesley's Primitive
Physick'.

CHAPTER TWO: CULTURES OF MADNESS

1   Black, *Dissertation on Insanity*, quoted in Hunter and Macalpine, *Three
Hundred Years*, 646.

2   Ward, *London Spy*, 48-50.

3   Ibid., 50.

4   Fitzgerald, 'Bedlam', 1-4.

5   Ibid., 10-11.

6   Pargeter, *Observations on Maniacal Disorders*, 2-3.

7   Quoted in Byrd, *Visits to Bedlam*, 63.

8   Faulkner, *Observations on... Insanity*, 4.

9   Cheyne, *The English Malady*, 183-4.

10   Blackmore, *A Treatise of the Spleen and Vapours*, 162-3. See Jobe,
'Medical Theories of Melancholia'.

11   Blackmore, *A Treatise of the Spleen and Vapours*, 163; Jackson,
Melancholia and Depression, 289 f.

12   Thomas Willis, *Practice of Physick*, 201.

13   Robinson, *A New System of the Spleen*, 399.

14   Purcell, *Treatise on Vapours*, 103-4.

15   Willis, *Practice of Physick*, 69, 71; Boss, 'The Seventeenth Century
Transformation of the Hysteric Affection'; Rousseau, 'Nerves, Spirits
and Fibres'.

16   Willis, *Practice of Physick*.

17   Blackmore, *Treatise of the Spleen and Vapours*, 96.

18   Blackmore, *Treatise of the Spleen and Vapours*, 97.

19   Ibid.

20   Ibid., 100; see also 101, 50, 54.

21   Arbuthnot, *Essay Concerning the Nature of Aliments*, 374-75.

22   Purcell, *A Treatise of Vapours, or, Hysterick Fits*, 1, 7-8.

23   Ibid., 24.

24   Ibid.

25   Ibid., 164. See, for context, Temkin, *The Falling Sickness*.

26   Quoted in Hunter and Macalpine, *Three Hundred Years*, 190.

27   Robinson, *A New System of the Spleen*, 344-45.

28   Ibid.

29   Cheyne, *The Natural Method of Cureing*, 78.

30   Ibid., 90.

31   Ibid. For similar arguments see Beddoes, *Hygeia*, ii, 95ff.

32   Robinson, *New System of the Spleen*, 401-02, 406.

33   *The Ladies Dispensatory*, 88. Among the recommendations were a 'Grand Hypo-chondriac Elixir, and an anti-hysteric syrop'.

34   Dewhurst (ed.), *Willis's Oxford Casebook*, 126–7.

35   Cheyne, *The English Malady* 260-62.

36   Blackmore, *Treatise of the Spleen and Vapours*, 97-99.

37   Baxter, *Reliquiae Baxterianae*, Pt.1, 10.

38   Ibid., 3, 173. See his advice in *The Signs and Causes of Melancholy*, 254, not to believe melancholy people who think 'it is only their soul that is afflicted... I have seen Abundance cured by Physick.'

39   Grew, *Cosmologia Sacra*, 60-61.

40   For interpretation see Reed, 'This Tasteless Tranquillity'.

41   McAdam Jr (ed.), *Samuel Johnson: Diaries, Prayers and Annals*, 77; Golden, *The Self Observed*, 68 f. This section draws heavily upon Porter, 'The Hunger of Imagination'.

42   McAdam, Jr (ed.), *Samuel Johnson: Diaries, Prayers and Annals*, 257; cf. 26.

43   Ibid., 146-47.

44   Johnson, *Rasselas*, 694.

45   Bate and Straus (eds), *Samuel Johnson, The Rambler*, ii, 142; cf. ii, 146.

46   Quoted in MacDonald, 'Religion, Social Change and Psychological Healing', 118.

47   Burton, *Anatomy of Melancholy*, 157.

48   Whitefield, *Journals*, 266-67.

49   Ibid.

50   Wesley, *Journal of John Wesley*, i, 363.

51   Ibid., i, 412.

52   Ibid.

53   Ibid., ii, 461.

54   Ibid., ii, 100.

55   Ibid.

56   Ibid., i, 551.

57   Ibid., i, 190. This is precisely the kind of case which was grist to the mill of all those blaming religious excesses for madness.

58   Ibid.

59   Ibid., i, 210.

60   Ibid., i, 416. Cf. vol. ii, 489 – Wesley knew he was treading on difficult ground: 'The danger was to regard extraordinary circumstances too much, such as outcries, convulsions, visions, trances, as if these were essential to the inward work, so that it could not go on without

them.' All the same, the hand of God was clear, and its providential purposes crucial: '1. God suddenly and strongly convinced many that they were lost sinners; the natural consequence whereof were sudden outcries, and strong bodily convulsions: 2. To strengthen and encourage them that believed, and to make his work more apparent, he favoured several of them with divine dreams, others with trances and visions: 3. In some of these instances, after a time, nature mixed with grace: 4. Satan likewise mimicked this work of God, in order to discredit the whole work.'

61   Ibid., ii, 225.

62   Ibid.

63   Darwin, *Zoonomia*, ii, 379. Likewise Hobbes had accused Presbyterian ministers of bringing 'young men to despair'. Quoted in Hill, *World Turned Upside Down*, 139.

64   Darwin, *Zoonomia*, ibid.

65   Ibid.

66   Blackmore, *Treatise of the Spleen and Vapours*, 158. Cf. the comments of Richard Baxter: 'Melancholy Persons are commonly exceeding fearful... Their Fantasie most erreth in aggravating their Sin, or Dangers or Unhappiness... They are still addicted to Excess of Sadness, some weeping they know not why, and some thinking it ought to be so; and if they should. Smile or speak merrily, their Hearts smite them for it, as if they had done amiss... They are continual Self-Accusers... They never read or hear of any miserable Instance, but they are thinking that this is their Case... And yet they think that never any one was as they are... They are utterly unable to rejoyce in anything: They cannot apprehend, believe or think of any thing that is comfortable to them... They are still displeased and discontented with themselves;... They are much averse to the Labours of their Callings, and given to Idleness, either to lie in Beds, or to sit unprofitably by themselves. Their Thoughts are most upon themselves;... They are endless in their Scruples... Hence it comes to pass that they are greatly addicted to Superstition... They have lost the Power of Governing their Thoughts by Reason; so that if you convince them that they should cast out their Self-perplexing unprofitable Thoughts, and turn their Thoughts to other Subjects, or be vacant, they are notable to obey you.' (*Signs and Causes of Melancholy*, 5-19).

67   Bate, Bullitt and Powell (eds), *Samuel Johnson: The Idler and Adventurer*, 468.

68   McAdam, Jr (ed.), *Samuel Johnson, Diaries, Prayers and Annals*, 38.

69   Brack Jr, *Journal Narrative Relative to Doctor Johnson's Last Illness* (unpaginated).

70   Quoted in Byrd, *Visits to Bedlam*, 108. For some parallels, see Baker, 'Mad Grimshaw'.

71   Walpole, *Memoirs of the Reign of George II*, iii, 8. Cf. Lytes, *Methodism Mocked*.

72   Wesley, *Journal*, iii, 267.

73   Burrows, *Commentaries*, 33; Compare Oliver, *Prophets and Millennialists*; Garrett, *Respectable Folly*. Dr John Ferriar developed the medical notion of 'Daemonoi' in *Medical Histories*, 111.

74   Trotter, *A View of the Nervous Temperament*, xv.

75   Brown, *Estimate of the Manners*, 88.

76   Rowley, *A Treatise of Female Nervous, Hysterical, Hypochondriacal, Bilious, Convulsive Diseases*, 253-54. Compare Sekora, *Luxury* for background.

77   Rowley, *A Treatise*.

78   Cheyne, *The English Malady*, i-v.

79   Mandeville, *A Treatise of the Hypochondriack and Hysterick Passions*, 150-51.

80   Cheyne, *The Natural Method of Cureing*, 82-83.

81   Quoted in Rousseau, 'Psychology', 207.

82   Mayer, *Outsiders*, 18-21; Babb, *Elizabethan Malady*.

83   Quoted in DePorte, *Nightmares and Hobbyhorses*, 128.

84   Boswell, *Life of Johnson*, ii, 421.

85   Johnson, 'Review of Soame Jenyns'. For discussion see Byrd, *Visits to Bedlam*, 111.

86   Golden, *William Cowper*, 45.

87   Byrd, *Visits to Bedlam*, 90. Samuel Richardson's reactions are comparable. See ibid., 89: 'A more affecting scene my eyes never beheld; and surely madam, any one inclined to proud of human nature, and to value themselves above others, cannot go to a place that will more effectually convince them of their folly: For there we see man destitute of every mark of reason and wisdom, and levelled to the brute creation, if not beneath it; and all the remains of good sense or education serve only to make the unhappy person appear more deplorable!'

88   Mackenzie, *Man of Feeling*, 79.

89   Toynbee and Whibley (eds), *Correspondence of Thomas Gray*, 27 May 1742, iii.

90   Ibid. Cf. Sells, *Thomas Gray*, 75 f.

91   Ricks (ed.), *Laurence Sterne: Tristram Shandy*, 500; Tuveson, 'Locke and Sterne'; Abrams, *The Mirror and the Lamp*; idem, *Natural Supernaturalism*; Rousseau, 'Science and the Discovery of the Imagination'; Powell, *Fuseli's 'The Nightmare'*; Rousseau, 'Science'; Engell, *The Creative Imagination*. For a French parallel to Sterne, see Diderot, *Rameau's Nephew*.

92   Byrd, *Visits to Bedlam*, 123.

93   Carkesse, *Lucida Intervalla*, 39.

94   Ibid., 32.

95   Ibid., 24.

96   Keynes (ed.), *William Blake: Complete Writings*, 772.

97   Carlson, Wollcock and Noel (eds), *Benjamin Rush's Lectures on the Mind*, 603.

98   Conolly, *Indications of Insanity*, 148-49.

99   Arnold, *Observations on... Insanity*, ii, 263.

100   Conolly, *Indications of Insanity*, 154-55. See also Hoeldtke, 'The History of Associationism'; Abrams, *The Mirror and the Lamp*; Rousseau, 'Science and the Discovery of the Imagination'; Kallich, *The Association of Ideas and Critical Theory*.

101   Quoted in DePorte, *Nightmares and Hobbyhorses*, 72.

102   Ibid.

103   Quoted in Becker, *The Mad Genius Controversy*, 26.

104   Blackmore, *A Treatise of the Spleen and Vapours*, 259.

105   Fielding, *Amelia*, Bk 3, ch. 7.

106   Brimley Johnson (ed.), *Letters from Lady Mary Wortley Montagu*, 465.

107   Feder, *Madness in Literature*, 175 f.; cf. Gilbert and Gubarr, *Madwoman in the Attic*.

108   Wardle, *Collected Letters of Mary Wollstonecraft*, 151.

CHAPTER THREE: CONFINEMENT AND ITS RATIONALES

1   Quoted in Hunter and Macalpine, *Three Hundred Years*, 435.

2   Ibid., 374-75.

3   Ibid., 375.

4   Blackstone, quoted in Hunter and Macalpine, *Three Hundred Years*, 437.

5   Ibid.

6   Paget Toynbee (ed.), *The Letters of Horace Walpole*, iv, 373 (a letter to Sir Horace Mann of 20 April 1760). For Ferrers see Walker, *Crime and Insanity in England*, i, 60f.

7   Hunter and Macalpine, *Three Hundred Years*, 571. He continues: 'The jury must... decide, whether the prisoner, when he did the act, was under the uncontrollable dominion of insanity, and was impelled to it by a morbid delusion; or whether it was the act of a man, who, though occasionally mad... was yet not actuated by the disease...'.

8   Howard, *The State of the Prisons*, 160; see more generally DeLacy, *Prison Reform in Lancashire*.

9   Quoted in Hunter and Macalpine, *Three Hundred Years*, 277. The writer went on to suggest penalties for wrongful confinement and safeguards for the sane: 'None shall be esteemed mad, or used as such, until their Case be publickly try'd by such Judges as the Legislature shall appoint; and that if they are by them found and determined to be truly mad, and then there shall be publick Notice given to their Relations (if any they have, else they should be the Care of the Publick) to take care of them; Trustees should be appointed and they shall be obliged under a proper penalty, to give notice to these Judges every Half-year by three regular Physicians of the College, if within the Bills of Mortality, or if the Country by the best Physician in the Neighbourhood and the Minister of the Parish, and a Gentleman of note or a Justice of the Peace, and they may be accordingly continued or discharg'd.'

10   Defoe, *An Essay Upon Projects* (1697), quoted in Hunter and Macalpine, *Three Hundred Years*, 265-66.

11   Bagley (ed.), *The Great Diurnal of Nicholas Blundell*, ii, 208. 31 August 1717.

12   Fenwick (ed.), *Ned Ward: The London Spy*, 51.

13   Quoted in Masters, *Bedlam*, 15.

14   Quoted in Masters, *Bedlam*, 14.

15   Quoted in O'Donoghue, *The Story of Bethlem Hospital*, 282-83.

16   Saussure, *A Foreign View of England*, 92-93.

17   Hunter and Macalpine, *Three Hundred Years*, 306.

18   Ibid.
19   J. Strype, quoted in ibid., 309. Note that Defoe, generally highly
      critical of madhouses, approved of Bethlem: 'The orders for the
      government of the hospital of Bethlem are exceedingly good, and
      a remarkable instance of the good disposition of the gentlemen
      concerned in it.' (Defoe, *Tour Through the Whole Island of Great Britain*,
      329).
20   See Hunter and Macalpine, *Three Hundred Years*, 331.
21   Wesley, *Journal*, iii, 124.
22   For the following, see Currie, *Medical Reports*, ii, 32–34. In some
      towns, a lunatic asylum grew out of a general infirmary; in others
      not. Thus at Leicester the Infirmary governors invited their physician,
      Dr Thomas Arnold, to organise an asylum in an adjoining build-
      ing to provide facilities till then available only in his own private
      madhouse. It opened two years later for ten patients at eight shillings
      a week for 'board and medicines'. For Arnold, see Carpenter, 'The
      Private Lunatic Asylums of Leicestershire'. At Gloucester Sir George
      Onesiphorus Paul tried to do the same, was obstructed by the local
      doctors, and failed.
23   Currie, ibid.
24   Digby, 'Changes in the Asylum'; idem, *From York Lunatic Asylum*, 4f.
25   For Paul, see Hunter and Macalpine, *Three Hundred Years*, 624. See
      also Digby, 'Moral Treatment at the York Retreat'.
26   Aikin, *Thoughts on Hospitals*, 67.
27   Ibid.
28   Currie, *Medical Reports*, ii, Appendix II, 23– 24.
29   Fallowes, quoted in Hunter and Macalpine, *Three Hundred Years*, 295.
30   Ibid.
31   Quoted in Hunter and Macalpine, *Three Hundred Years*, 472; see
      Parry-Jones, *The Trade in Lunacy*, 116 f.; *Report from the Committee
      on Madhouses in England* (1815), 314-20. Edward Wakefield told the
      Committee, 279: 'The 25th September I called upon Mr Finch,
      Surgeon, at Laverstock near Salisbury. This gentleman appears to me
      to be a humane man; a man of sense, and conducts his house in an
      admirable manner. He has 120 patients... He had not a single patient
      in a strait-waistcoat or in chains; and states that the proportion of
      dirty patients, through attention, is very small... Every possible kind
      of amusement was provided for them; billiards, backgammon, cards,
      books, &c. &c. in doors; a chapel on a Sunday; two distinct and
      separate houses within 500 yards for those patients whose friends are
      fearful of their being placed in a large establishment.'
32   Faulkner, *Observations on… Insanity*, 8-9.
33   Ibid., 18. Medically qualified madhouse-keepers felt entitled to refuse
      access to other physicians. This led, for example, to a bitter contro-
      versy at Dr Hall's Newcastle Asylum. Horsley, *Eighteenth Century
      Newcastle*, 126. See the discussion in Macalpine and Hunter, *George III
      and the Mad Business*, 328 f.
34   Hunter and Macalpine, *Three Hundred Years*, 200.
35   Irish, *Levamen Infirmi*, 53.
36   Faulkner, *Observations on… Insanity*, 24. Occasionally other amenities

were trumpeted. Thus an advertisement of 1797 for Middlesex House noted its shower bath.

37   Cowper's account is quoted in Ober, 'Madness and Poetry', 163. The comment on Smart is from Sherbo, quoted in Ober, ibid., 182.

38   Simond, *An American in Regency England*, 109.

39   Hunter and Macalpine, *Three Hundred Years*, 265.

40   Quoted in Hunter and Macalpine, *Three Hundred Years*, 366.

41   Ibid., 366.

42   Parry-Jones, *The Trade in Lunacy*, 225.

43   [Anon.] 'A Case Humbly Offered', 25.

44   Ibid.

45   Ibid.

46   Quoted in Byrd, *Visits to Bedlam*, 47.

47   Pargeter, *Observations on Maniacal Disorders*, 126.

48   Harper, *A Treatise on the Real Cause and Cure of Insanity*, 60.

49   Darwin, *Zoonomia*, ii, 352–53.

50   Burrows, *Commentaries on Insanity*, 696.

51   Ibid.

52   Browne, *What Asylums Were, Are and Ought to Be*, 229.

53   Craig, *The Legacy of Swift*, 20.

54   Smollett, *Sir Launcelot Greaves*, 190.

55   Faulkner, *Observations on… Insanity*; cf. Sekora, *Luxury*. Beddoes wrote of nations 'civilised enough to be capable of insanity': *Hygeia*, ii, 40.

56   Rowley, *A Treatise of Female Nervous, Hysterical, Hypochondriacal, Bilious, Convulsive Diseases*, 253–54.

57   Morison, *Outlines of Mental Diseases*, 73.

58   For social demonologies see Cohn, *The Pursuit of the Millennium*; idem, *Europe's Inner Demons*; Comfort, *The Anxiety Makers*; Delunieau, *Peur*.

59   Von Archenholz, *Picture*, ii, 156.

60   Faulkner, *Observations on…Insanity*, 8.

61   Latimer, *The Annals of Bristol in the Eighteenth Century*, 425. Cf. Malson, *Wolf Children*.

62   Latimer, *The Annals of Bristol in the Eighteenth Century*, ibid.

CHAPTER FOUR: THE MAKING OF PSYCHIATRY

1   Burton, *Anatomy of Melancholy*, 595. Burton comments, 'he that list may try it'.

2   Cobbett, *Advice to Young Men*, 253.

3   Wesley, *Primitive Physick*, 79–81.

4   Rogers, *A Discourse Concerning Trouble of the Mind and the Disease of Melancholy*, v.

5   Ibid.

6   Ibid., see also above, ch.2.

7   Rogers, *A Discourse of… Melancholy*, xi.

8   Boswell, *Life of Johnson*, ii, 440.

9   Ibid.

10   Matthews (ed.), *The Diary of Dudley Ryder*, 200 (20 March 1716).

11   Quoted in Ingram, *Boswell's Creative Gloom*, 104–05. Boswell wrote, 'I

have a kind of strange feeling as if wished nothing to be secret that concerns myself.' Quoted in ibid. Robert James noted pertinently in his *Medicinal Dictionary*: 'No disease is more troublesome, either to the Patient or Physician, than hypochondriac Disorders; and it often happens, that, thro' the Fault of both, the Cure is either unnecessarily protracted, or totally frustrated; for the Patients are so delighted, not only with a Variety of Medicines, but also of Physicians.' (Quoted in Ingram, ibid., 104)

12   Blackmore, *A Treatise of the Spleen and Vapours*, 92–93.

13   Ibid., 91.

14   Heberden, *Medical Commentaries*, 233. See also W. Smith, *A Sure Guide*, whose section on nervous complaints attributed them to fermentations in the stomach: Carlson and Simpson, 'Madness of the Nervous System'.

15   Cullen, *First Lines of the Practice of Physic*, ii, 121–22; Carlson and McFadden, 'Dr William Cullen on Mania'; Piñero, *Historical Origins of the Concept of Neurosis*, 11 f.

16   Cullen, *First Lines of the Practice of Physic*, iv, 126.

17   Trotter, *A View of the Nervous Temperament*, 1. Cf. Thomas Carlyle on the humbug of nervous complaints: 'Witchcraft, and all manner of Spectrework, and Demonology, we have now named Madness, and Diseases of the Nerves. Seldom reflecting that still the new question comes upon us: What is Madness, what are Nerves?' (Quoted in Harrison, *The Second Coming*, 217).

18   Adair, *Medical Cautions*, 13–14.

19   Smollett, *Sir Launcelot Greaves*, 187.

20   Beddoes, *Hygeia*, iii, Essay X, 27. Though favourable to nosology himself, Cullen was sceptical about such elaborate nosologies of madness as that advanced by Dr Thomas Arnold: 'The ingenious Dr Arnold has been commendably employed in distinguishing the different species of insanity as they appear with respect to the mind; and his labours may hereafter prove useful, when we shall come to know something more of the different states of the brain corresponding to these different states of the mind; but at present I can make little application of his numerous distinctions.' (*First Lines of the Practice of Physic*, quoted in Hunter and Macalpine, *Three Hundred Years*, 477).

21   Mortimer, *An Address to the Publick*, 28. Another respectable nostrum-monger was Dr Alexander Hunter, physician to the York Asylum, who sold 'green' and 'grey' powders as a 'sovereign remedy to cure the distempered brain'.

22   Ibid.

23   Young, *A Treatise on Opium*, 112–13; 114.

24   Ibid.

25   Ibid.

26   Locke, *Essay Concerning Human Understanding*, Bk II, xxxiii, 1.

27   Locke, *An Essay Concerning Human Understanding*, Bk II, ch. xxxiii, S.

28   Locke, quoted in Byrd, *Visits to Bedlam*, 51.

29   Harper, *A Treatise on the Real Cause and Cure of Insanity*, 27–28.

30   Hallaran, *An Enquiry Into the Causes Producing the Extraordinary Addition to the Number of Insane*, 2. Hallaran argued: 'I am aware of

exposing myself to animadversion, by seeming to admit the existence of insanity, independently of that intimate connexion which has been so generally supposed to prevail between it and the brain.'

31 Ibid, 2–3.

32 Sir George Baker, *De Aflectibus Animi et Morbis Inde Oriundis*, quoted in translation in Hunter and Macalpine, *Three Hundred Years*, 400.

33 Ibid.

34 Walker, *A Treatise on Nervous Diseases*, i, 212–13.

35 Ibid.

36 See Hartley's general view: *Observations on Man*, vol. i, 6: 'The Doctrine of Vibrations may appear at first Sight to have no Connexion with that of Association; however, if these Doctrines be found in fact to contain the Laws of the Bodily and Mental Powers respectively, they must be related to each other, since the Body and Mind are... I will endeavour... to trace out this mutual Relation.'

37 Bree, *A Practical Inquiry on Disordered Respiration*, quoted in Hunter and Macalpine, *Three Hundred Years*, 554–55. Bree explored asthma in the same light.

38 Bree, ibid.

39 Darwin, *Zoonomia*, i, 250–51.

40 Ferriar, *Medical Histories and Reflections*, ii, 119.

41 Arnold, *Observations on... Insanity*, ii, 126, ii, 129. Cf. Perfect, *Select Cases*, 293 ff.

42 Hill, *An Essay on the Prevention and Cure of Insanity*, 404.

43 Lettsom, 'Some Remarks on the Effects of *Lignum Quassiae Amarae*', 157; see also Rix, 'John Coakley Lettsom and Some of the Effects of Hard Drinking'. Cf. also Fothergill, *An Essay on the Abuse of Spiritous Liquors*, 19, 'The All-Conquering Power of Habit'.

44 Cheyne, *An Essay of Health and Long Life*, 49.

45 Mandeville, *Treatise on the Hypochondriack and Hysterick Passions*, 373–74.

46 Quoted in Wain, *Samuel Johnson*, 240.

47 Sibly, *Medical Mirror*, 80.

48 Foucault, *History of Sexuality*, 40.

49 Tissot, *Onanism*, 62.

50 Ibid., 40.

51 Ibid., 30–31.

52 Sibly, *Medical Mirror*, 144–45. The link between imagination and self-abuse was most explicitly made in Byron's mot about Keats frigging his imagination.

53 Buchan, *Domestic Medicine*, 112.

54 Pargeter, *Observations on Maniacal Disorders*, 129–30.

55 Gregory, *A Comparative View*, 22–23.

56 Battie, *A Treatise on Madness*, 68.

57 Battie, *A Treatise on Madness*, 93–94.

58 Robinson, *A New System of the Spleen*, 191.

59 Macalpine and Hunter, *George III and the Mad Business*, 282.

60 Quoted in Macalpine and Hunter, *George III and the Mad Business*, 271–72.

61 Pargeter, *Observations on Maniacal Disorders*, 50–51.

62   Ibid., 51-52.

63   Percival, *Medical Ethics*, quoted in Hunter and Macalpine, *Three Hundred Years*, 585.

64   Ibid.

65   Ferriar, *Medical Histories and Reflections*, ii, 136-37.

66   Ibid.

67   Pargeter, *Observations on Maniacal Disorders*, 52.

68   Ibid.

69   Ibid.

70   Faulkner, *Observations on... Insanity*, 15.

71   Cox, *Practical Observations on Insanity*, 42- 43.

72   Pargeter, *Observations on Maniacal Disorders*, 129-30.

73   Perfect, *Select Cases*, 131.

74   Ibid.

75   Darwin, *Zoonomia*, i, 352. For strait-waistcoats, see D. MacBride, *A Methodical Introduction to the Theory and Practice of Physick*, 591-92.

76   Darwin, *Zoonomia*, ibid.

77   Quoted in Macalpine and Hunter, *George III and the Mad Business*, 275.

78   Ibid.

79   Cox, *Practical Observations on Insanity*, 42-43.

80   Ibid., 43.

81   Ibid., 88.

82   Hallaran, *An Enquiry...*, 44-5. Compare T. Withers, *Observations on Chronic Weakness*, quoted in Hunter and Macalpine, *Three Hundred Years*, 464: 'The physician, therefore, should be a man of the world. He should be able to read internal characters from external signs... He should endeavour to penetrate at once into the mind, and to ascertain with a cautious exactness the ruling passion. He should observe countenances, gestures, words, and actions, and yet seem as perfectly regardless of these things as if he made no observations upon them.'

83   Hallaran, *An Enquiry...*, 45.

84   Ibid., 46.

85   Bakewell was a follower of Locke. See Bakewell, *A Letter Addressed*, quoted in Hunter and Macalpine, *Three Hundred Years*, 708: 'It must be admitted, that in those confirmed cases, where the suggestions of erroneous or visionary thoughts, are insisted upon as realities and rational facts, that the power or faculty of the mind, by which we are enabled to judge of the correctness of our own thoughts, is suspended; but the most common symptom is the excess of action in the thinking principle; the Patient being, at times, conscious of this excess.'

86   Ibid., 709.

87   Ibid.

88   Perfect, *Select Cases*, 1-2, 3-4, 6.

89   Ibid.

90   Ibid.

91   Ibid.

92   Ibid.

93 Battie, *Treatise on Madness*, 68-9.
94 Cox, *Practical Observations on Insanity*, 140-1.
95 Ibid.
96 Tuke, *A Description of the York Retreat*, 141-42.
97 Hibbert (ed.), *An American in Regency England*, 109-10.
98 Quoted in Walk, 'Some Aspects of the "Moral Treatment" of the Insane up to 1845', 817.
99 Baglivi, *The Practice of Physick*, 189.
100 Tuke, *A Description of the Retreat*, 151-2.
101 Hallaran, *An Enquiry*, 48.
102 Perceval, *A Narrative of the Treatment*, 174.

CHAPTER FIVE: THE VOICE OF THE MAD

1 Turner, *A Compleat History of the Most Remarkable Providences*, 110, quoted in Hunter and Macalpine, *Three Hundred Years*, 271-72.
2 Ibid.
3 Tuke, *Description of the Retreat*, 146-47. Nevertheless, case-notes form an invaluable source of information – as Thomas Percival argued at the beginning of the nineteenth century: 'The synthetic plan should be adopted; and a regular journal should be kept of every species of the malady which occurs, arranged under proper heads, with a full detail of its rise, progress, and termination; of the remedies administered, and of their effects in its several stages. The age, sex, occupation, mode of life, and if possible hereditary constitution of each patient should be noted: And, when the even proves fatal, the brain, and other organs affected should be carefully examined and the appearances on dissection minutely inserted in the journal. A register like this, in the course of a few years, would afford the most interesting and authentic documents, the want of which, on a late melancholy occasion, was felt and regretted by the whole kingdom.' (Quoted from Percival, *Medical Ethics*, in Hunter and Macalpine, *Three Hundred Years*, 586).
4 Tuke, *Description of the Retreat*, 146.
5 Matthews (ed.), *The Diary of Dudley Ryder*, 294.
6 Ibid, 363.
7 For Chatham, see Hack Tuke, *Chapters in the History of the Insane*, 105-07. Chatham was treated by the former madhouse-keeper, Anthony Addington.
8 Kramnick, *The Rage of Edmund Burke*,181
9 Darwin, quoted in Hunter and Macalpine, *Three Hundred Years*, 550.
10 Haslam, *Illustrations of Madness*, 61.
11 Ibid.,54-5.
12 Ibid., 68.
13 Ibid., BL Add. MSS 38231.
14 Climenson, *Elizabeth Montagu*, 1, 67.
15 Bettany (ed.), *Diaries of William Johnston Temple*, 46.
16 Ibid., 23.
17 Ibid., 24.
18 Ibid., 10.

19   Ibid., lxxix. For interpretations of dreams see Powell, Fuseli's 'The
        Nightmare'.

20   Millard (ed.), *Roger North*. 139

21   Neville, 156.

22   Ibid., 146.

23   Griggs (ed.), *Collected Letters of Samuel Taylor Coleridge*, i, 123 (letter 68).

24   Griggs, *Collected Letters*, i, 188 (letter 108).

25   Ibid., i, 128 (letter 68).

26   Wharton, 'Autobiography', i, 205.

27   Ibid., i, 214.

28   Ibid., i, 292.

29   Carkesse, *Lucida Intervalla*; Cunningham, 'Bedlam and Parnassus'; Porter,
        'Bedlam and Parnassus'.

30   Cowper, *Memoir*, 56, 57.

31   Cowper, *Memoir*, 44.

32   Illuminatingly discussed in Byrd, *Visits to Bedlam*, 151.

33   Oliver, *The Eccentric Life*. Similar protests of outrage at being held
        'prisoner' in Bethlem were made by Richard Stafford (1663-1703), a
        Jacobite pamphleteer. Stafford seems to have been able to publish
        Jacobite writings during his confinement at Bethlem, despite a
        request from the Speaker of the House of Commons to the gov-
        ernors of Bethlem to deprive him of access to pen and paper. See
        his *The Printed Sayings of Richard Stafford a Prisoner in Bethlem* (1692).
        For later protests against a wrongful confinement see McCandless,
        'Liberty and Lunacy'.

34   Peterson, *A Mad People's History*, 91; compare Mitford, *A Description of
        the Crimes and Horrors*; idem, *Part the Second of the Crimes and Horrors*;
        Porter, 'The History of Institutional Psychiatry in Europe'.

35   Perceval, *A Narrative of the Treatment*, 175-76, 179.

36   Ibid., 52, 208.

Illustrations

All illustrations courtesy of the Wellcome Library, London.

Acknowledgements

So many and so great are the debts which I have incurred while writing
this book that I feel doomed to be the ultimate undischarged academic
bankrupt. It would be quite impossible to thank here, individually, all the
scholars who by their conversations, criticisms and suggestions have helped
this book to come together, as also the hundreds of students who have been
on the receiving end of the lecture course from which it has emerged. My
thanks, collectively, to all. Some particular thanks, however, must be made.
First to everyone connected with the Wellcome Institute for the History of
Medicine for their unfailing kindness, immense expertise and services, and for
generally making it the most perfect of environments in which to work. Ben
Barkow has laboured like a Trojan as research assistant, and Betty Kingston
and Verna Cole have typed large sections of this book with unfailing accuracy
and patience. Many people have been exceptionally generous of their time in
reading and commenting upon earlier drafts of this book; I am in particular
indebted to William E. Bynum, Michael Dols, David Harley, Margaret Kinnell,
Christopher Lawrence, Sue Limb, Michael Neve, Sylvana Tomaselli, Jane Walsh
and Andrew Wear, and two anonymous publisher's referees, though errors of
fact and judgement which still remain after their stimulating suggestions are,
of course, my own. Lastly, and most vastly, thanks to Dorothy Watkins, who
has worked like crazy in helping during the last months to turn a mess of a
manuscript into a finished book. Only she knows how much is due to her.

Wellcome Institute for the History of Medicine, London, 1987

Bibliography

M.H. Abrams, *The Mirror and the Lamp* (New York, Oxford University Press, 1953)
— *Natural Supernaturalism* (London, Oxford University Press, 1971)
E.H. Ackerknecht, 'History of Legal Medicine', *Ciba Symposia* 11 (1950), 1286–304
— *A Short History of Psychiatry*, 2nd edn, trans. Sula Wolff (New York, Hafner, 1968)
J.M. Adair, *Medical Cautions, for the Consideration of Invalids* (Bath, Dodsley & Dilly, 1786)
— *A Philosophical and Medical Sketch of the Natural History of the Human Body and Mind* (Bath, Crutwell, 1787)
T.W. Adorno and M. Horkheimer, *The Dialectics of Enlightenment*, trans. J. Cummings (London, Verso Editions, 1979)
John Aikin, *Thoughts on Hospitals* (London, Johnson, 1771)
Mark Akenside, *The Pleasures of Imagination. A Poem in Three Books* (London, R. Dodsley, 1744)
Franz G. Alexander and Sheldon T. Selesnick, *The History of Psychiatry: an Evaluation of Psychiatric Thought and Practice from Prehistoric Times to the Present* (London, George Allen & Unwin, 1967)
P.K. Alkon, *Samuel Johnson and Moral Discipline* (Northwestern University Press, Evanston, Ill., 1967)
Patricia H. Allderidge, 'Criminal Insanity: Bethlem to Broadmoor', *Proceedings of the Royal Society of Medicine* 67 (1974), 897–904
— 'Management and Mismanagement at Bedlam, 1547–1633', in Charles Webster (ed.), *Health, Medicine and Mortality in the Sixteenth Century* (Cambridge, Cambridge University Press, 1979), 141–64
'Bedlam: Fact or Fantasy?', in W. F. Bynum, Roy Porter and Michael Shepherd (eds), *The Anatomy of Madness*, 2 vols (London, Tavistock, 1985), ii, 17–33
Don Cameron Allen, 'The Degeneration of Man and Renaissance Pessimism', *Studies in Philology* 35 (1938), 202–27

H.E. Allison, 'Locke's Theory of Personal Identity: a Re-Examination', in I. C. Tifton (ed.), *Locke on Human Understanding: Selected Essays* (Oxford, Clarendon Press, 1977)

M.D. Altschule, *Origin of Concepts in Human Behaviour: Social and Cultural Factors* (New York, Haistead Press, 1977)

A. Alvarez, *The Savage God* (London, Weidenfeld & Nicolson, 1972)

M. Anderson, *Family Structure in Nineteenth Century Lancashire* (London, Cambridge University Press, 1971)

J. Andrews, 'A History of Bethlem Hospital *c.*1600–*c.*1750' (London University PhD thesis, forthcoming)

S. Anglo, 'Reginald Scot's Discoverie of Witchcraft: Scepticism and Sadducceeism', in S. Anglo (ed.) ,*The Damned Art. Essays in the Literature of Witchcraft* (London, Routledge & Kegan Paul, 1977), 106–39

Anon., *Mrs Clark's Case* (London, Roberts, 1718)

— *The Ladies Dispensatory* (London, J. Hodges & J. James, 1740)

— *The Case of Henry Roberts, Esq; a Gentleman, who, by Unparalleled Cruelty was Deprived of his Estate under Pretence of Idiocy* (London, no publisher, 1747)

— 'A Case Humbly Offered to the Consideration of Parliament', *Gentleman's Magazine* 33 (1763), 25–26

— *Sketches in Bedlam* (London, Sherwood, Jones and Co., 1823)

— 'Richard Henderson and his Private Asylum at Hanham', Proceedings of *the Wesley Historical Society 3* (1902), 367–8

John Arbuthnot, *An Essay Concerning the Nature of Aliments and the Choice of Them According to the Different Constitutions of the Human Bodies* (London, J. Tonson, 1731)

J.W. von Archenholz, *A Picture of England: Containing a Description of the Laws, Customs and Manners of England* (trans., London, for the booksellers, 1797)

J. Archer, *Every Man his own Doctor...the Second Edition with Additions* (1st ed., London, Peter Lillicrap, 1671; 2nd ed., London, for the author, 1673)

Aristotle (pseud.), *Aristotle's Master-Piece: or the Secrets of Generation Displayed in all the Parts Thereof etc.* (London, W.B., 1694)

T. Arnold, *Observations on the Nature, Kinds, Causes and Prevention of Insanity*, 2 vols (1st edn, Leicester, Robinson and Cadell, 1782–86; 2nd edn used, London, Phillips, 1806)

M.P. Ashley, *John Wildman. Plotter and Postmaster* (London, Jonathan Cape, 1947)

J. Axtell (ed.), *The Educational Writings of John Locke* (Cambridge, Cambridge University Press, 1968)

L. Babb, *The Elizabethan Malady: A Study of Melancholia in English Literature from 1580 to 1640* (East Lansing, Michigan State University Press, 1951)

— *Sanity in Bedlam: A Study of Robert Burton's Anatomy of Melancholy* (East Lansing, Michigan State University Press, 1959)

G. Baglivi, *The Practice of Physick* (London, Midwinter, 1723)

M. Bailey (ed.), *Boswell's Column* (London, William Kimber, 1951)

F. Baker, '"Mad Grimshaw" and his Convenants with God: a Study in Eighteenth Century Psychology', *London Quarterly and Holborn Review* 182 (1952), 202–15, 270–9

Sir George Baker, *De Aflectibus Animi et Morbis Inde Oriundis* (Cambridge, Thurlbourn et al., 1755)

H.C. Baker, *The Wars of Truth* (Gloucester, Mass., P. Smith, 1969)

Thomas Bakewell, *The Domestic Guide in Cases of Insanity. Pointing out the Causes, Means of Preventing, and Proper Treatment, of that Disorder* (London, for the author, 1809)

— *Letters Addressed to the Chairman of the Select Committee of the House of Commons, Appointed to Enquire into the State of Madhouses* (Stafford, for the author, 1815)

K. Balderston (ed.), *Thraleana*, 2 vols (Oxford, Oxford University Press, 1941)

— 'Doctor Johnson and William Law', *Proceedings of the Modern Language Association* (1960), 382–94

— 'Johnson's Vile Melancholy', in F.B. Hilles and W.S. Lewis (eds), *The Age of Johnson* (New Haven, Yale University Press 1964), 3-14

J.B. Bamborough, *The Little World of Man* (London, Longman, Green & Co., 1952)

J. Barry, 'Cultural Habits of Illness: Medicine and Religion in Eighteenth Century Bristol', in Roy Porter (ed.), *Patients and Practitioners: Lay Perceptions of Medicine in Pre-Industrial Society* (Cambridge, Cambridge University Press, 1985), 177-204

R. Bartel, 'Suicide in Eighteenth Century England: the Myth of a Reputation', *Huntingdon Library Quarterly* 23 (1959), 145-55

W.J. Bate, 'The Sympathetic Imagination in Eighteenth Century English Criticism', *English Literary History* 12 (1945), 144-66

— *Samuel Johnson* (New York, Harcourt Brace Jovanovich, 1977)

— and A.B. Straus, *Samuel Johnson: The Rambler*, 3 vols (New Haven, Conn., The Yale Edition of the Works of Samuel Johnson, Yale University Press, 1969)

W.J. Bate, J.M. Bullit, and L.F. Powell (eds), *Samuel Johnson: The Idler and Adventurer* (New Haven, Conn., The Yale Edition of the Works of Samuel Johnson, Yale University Press, 1963)

Sir Frederic Bateman and W. Rye, *The History of Bethel Hospital at Norwich* (Norwich, Gibbs and Waller, 1906)

G. Bateson (ed.), *Perceval's Narrative: a Patient's Account of his Psychosis* (New York, Morrow Paperback Editions, 1974)

William Battie, *A Treatise on Madness, and John Monro, Remarks on Dr Battie's Treatise on Madness*, Introduction by R. Hunter and I. Macalpine (London, Dawsons, 1962, reprint of 1758 edn)

G. Battiscombe, *The Spencers of Althorp* (London, Constable, 1984)

C. Baxter, 'Johan Weyer's De Praestigiis Daemonium: Unsystematic Psychopathology', in S. Anglo (ed.), *The Damned Art* (London, Routledge & Kegan Paul, 1977) 53-75

Richard Baxter, *Reliquiae Baxterianae* (London, Parkhurst, Robinson, Laurence & Dunston, 1696)

— *The Signs and Causes of Melancholy* (London, Crutlenden & Cox, 1716)

G. Becker, *The Mad Genius Controversy* (Beverly Hills, Sage, 1978)

T. Beddoes, *Hygeia*, 3 vols (Bristol, J. Mills, 1802-03)

D.P. Behan, 'Locke on Persons and Personal Identity', *Canadian Journal of Philosophy* 9 (1979), 53-75

A.L. Beier, *Masterless Men: The Vagrancy Problem in England 1560-1640* (London, Methuen, 1985)

William Belcher, *Address to Humanity, Containing a Letter to Dr. Munro, a Receipt to Make a Lunatic, and Seize his Estates and a Sketch of a True Smiling Hyena*

(London, for the Author, 1796)

— *Intellectual Electricity* (London, Lee & Hurst (etc.), 1798)

C. Bell, *The Anatomy of Expression* (London, John Murray, 3rd edn, 1806)

J. Beresford (ed.), *The Diary of a Country Parson*, 5 vols (Oxford, Clarendon Press, 1981)

M. Berman, *The Re-enchantment of the World* (Ithaca, Cornell University Press, 1981)

L. Bettany (ed.), *The Diaries of William Johnston Temple, 1780-1796* (Oxford, Clarendon Press, 1929)

S. Billington, *The Social History of the Fool* (Brighton, Harvester Press, 1984)

John Birch, *A Letter to Mr George Adams, on the Subject of Medical Electricity* (London, for the author, 1792)

William Black, *Dissertation on Insanity* (London, Ridgway, 1810)

William George Black, *Folk Medicine: A Chapter in the History of Culture* (London, The Folk Lore Society, 1883)

Sir Richard Blackmore, *A Treatise of the Spleen and Vapours: or, Hypochondriacal and Hysterical Affections* (London, Pemberton, 1725)

E. Bladon (ed.), *The Hon. Robert Fulke Greville: Diaries* (London, John Lane, 1930)

Patrick Blair, 'Some Observations on the Cure of Mad Persons by the Fall of Water', Ms quoted in R. Hunter and I. Macalpine, *Three Hundred Years of Psychiatry 1535-1860* (London, Oxford University Press, 1963), 325-29

M.W. Bloomfield, *The Seven Deadly Sins* (Michigan, State University Press, 1967)

N. Blundell, *The Great Diurnal of Nicholas Blundell*, 3 vols, transcribed by Frank Tyrer, edited for the Record Society by J.J. Bagley (Chester, the Record Society of Lancashire and Cheshire, 1968-72)

M.P. Boddy, 'Burton in the Eighteenth Century', *Notes and Queries* 167 (1934), 206-08

H. Boerhaave, *Academical Lectures on the Theory of Physic*, 2nd edn (London, Innes, 1751)

J.S. Bolton, 'The Evolution of a Mental Hospital, Wakefield, 1818-1928', *Journal of Mental Science* 74 (1928), 587-633

D.F. Bond, '"Distrust" of Imagination in English Neoclassicism', *Philological Quarterly* 14 (1937), 54-69

— 'The Neoclassical Psychology of the Imagination', *English Literature and History* 4 (1937), 245-64

John Bond, *An Essay on the Incubus, or Night-Mare* (London, Wilson & Durham, 1753)

Jeffrey M.N. Boss, 'The Seventeenth Century Transformation of the Hysteric Affection', *Psychological Medicine* 9 (1979), 221-34

James Boswell, *Life of Johnson*, ed. G.B. Hill, 6 vols (Oxford, Clarendon, 1934)

— *The London Journal*, edited by F.A. Pottle (London, Heinemann, 1950)

— *Boswell's Column*, intro. and notes by Margery Bailey (London, Kimber, 1951)

P.G. Boucé (ed.), *Sexuality in Eighteenth Century Britain* (Manchester, Manchester University Press, 1982)

— 'Some Sexual Beliefs and Myths in Eighteenth Century England', in Boucé, ibid., 28-46

T. Bowen, *An Historical Account of the Origin, Progress and Present State of*

Bethlem Hospital (London, no publisher, 1784)

G. Bowles, 'Physical, Human and Divine Attraction in the Life and Thought of George Cheyne', *Annals of Science* 31(1974), 473-88

O.M. Brack Jr, *Journal Narrative Relative to Doctor Johnson's Last Illness* (Iowa City, Windhover Press, 1972)

W.R. Brain, 'The Great Convulsionary', and 'A Post-Mortem on Dr. Johnson', in *Some Reflections on Genius and Other Essays* (London, Pitman Medical Publishing, 1960), 69-71; 92-100

L. Bredvold, *The Natural History of Sensibility* (Detroit, Wayne State University Press, 1962)

Robert Bree, *A Practical Inquiry on Disordered Respiration* (London, R. Philips, 1807)

Timothy Bright, *A Treatise of Melancholie* (London, Thomas Vautrolier, 1586)

William Brockbank, *Portrait of a Hospital, 1752-1948* (London, Heinemann Medical Books, 1952)

Richard Brocklesby, *Reflections on Ancient and Modern Musick, with the Application to the Cure of Diseases* (London, Cooper, 1749)

W. Bromberg, *Man Above Humanity. A History of Psychotherapy* (Philadelphia, Lippincott, 1954)

J. Bronowski, *William Blake and the Age of Revolution* (London, Routledge & Kegan Paul, 1971)

B. Bronson (ed.), *Samuel Johnson, Rasselas, Poems and Selected Prose* (San Francisco, Ca., Rinehart Press, 1971)

John Brown, *Estimate of the Manners and Principles of the Times*, 2nd edn (London, L. Davis & C. Reymers, 1757)

T. Brown, 'Descartes, Dualism and Psychosomatic Medicine', in W.F. Bynum, Roy Porter and M. Shepherd (eds), *The Anatomy of Madness*, 2 vols (London, Tavistock, 1985), i, 151-65

Janet Browne, 'Darwin and the Face of Madness', in W.F. Bynum, Roy Porter and Michael Shepherd (eds), *The Anatomy of Madness*, 2 vols (London, Tavistock, 1985), i, 151-65

W.A.F. Browne, *What Asylums Were, Are and Ought to Be: Being the Substance of Five Lectures Delivered Before the Managers of the Montrose Royal Lunatic Asylum* (Edinburgh, Black, 1837)

Samuel Bruckshaw, *One More Proof of the Iniquitous Abuse of Private Madhouses* (London, the author, 1774)

— *The Case, Petition and Address of Samuel Bruckshaw, who Suffered a Most Severe Imprisonment for Very Near the Whole Year...* (London, the Author, 1774)

John Brydall, *Non Compos Mentis: or the Law Relating to Natural Fools, Mad-Folks and Lunatick Persons* (London, I. Cleave, 1700)

William Buchan, *Domestic Medicine* (Edinburgh, Balfour, Auld & Smellie, 1769)

Thomas Burgess, *The Physiology or Mechanism of Blushing* (London, John Churchill, 1828)

P. Burke, *Popular Culture in Early Modern Europe* (London, Maurice Temple Smith, 1978)

G.M. Burrows, *An Inquiry into Certain Errors Relative to Insanity; and their Consequences; Physical, Moral and Civil* (London, Underwood, 1820)

— *Commentaries on the Causes, Forms, Symptoms and Treatment, Moral and Medical, of Insanity* (London, Underwood, 1828)

Robert Burton, *The Anatomy of Melancholy*, edited by Floyd Dell and Paul

Jordan-Smith (New York, Tudor Publishing Company, 1927)

Joan Busfield, *Managing Madness. Changing Ideas and Practice* (London, Hutchinson, 1986)

M. Butler, *Romantics, Rebels and Reactionaries* (Oxford, Oxford University Press, 1981)

— 'English Romanticism', in Roy Porter and M. Teich (eds), *Romanticism in National Context* (Cambridge, Cambridge University Press, 1988)

T. Butler, *Mental Health, Social Policy and the Law* (London, Macmillan, 1985)

J. Butt, *The Poems of Alexander Pope* (London, Methuen, 1963)

John Byng, *The Torrington Diaries*, 4 vols, edited by C.B. Andrews (New York, Barnes & Noble, 1970)

William F. Bynum, 'Chronic Alcoholism in the First Half of the Nineteenth Century', *Bulletin of the History of Medicine*, 42 (1968), 160-85

— 'Time's Noblest Offspring: The Problem of Man in the British Natural Historical Sciences' (PhD Dissertation, University of Cambridge, 1974)

— 'Rationales for Therapy in British Psychiatry: 1780-1835', *Medical History* 18 (1974), 317-34

— 'Health, Disease and Medical Care', in G.S. Rousseau and Roy Porter (eds), *The Ferment of Knowledge* (Cambridge University Press, 1980), 211-54

— 'Theory and Practice in British Psychiatry from J.C. Prichard (1786-1848) to Henry Maudsley (1835-1918)', in T. Ogawa (ed.), *History of Psychiatry* (Osaka, Taniguchi Foundation, 1982), 196-216

— 'The Nervous Patient in Eighteenth and Nineteenth Century England: The Psychiatric Origins of British Neurology', in W.F. Bynum, Roy Porter and Michael Shepherd (eds), *The Anatomy of Madness*, 2 vols (London, Tavistock, 1985), i, 89-102

— and M.R. Neve, 'Hamlet on the Couch', in W.F. Bynum, Roy Porter, and Michael Shepherd (eds), *The Anatomy of Madness*, 2 vols (London, Tavistock, 1985), i, 289-304

— and Roy Porter (eds), *Medical Fringe and Medical Orthodoxy* (London, Croom Helm, 1986)

M. Byrd, *Visits to Bedlam* (Columbia, University of South Carolina Press, 1974)

H.C. Cameron, *Sir Joseph Banks; the Autocrat of the Philosophers* (London, Batchworth, 1956)

F. Capra, *The Turning Point: Science, Society and the Rising Culture* (New York, Simon & Shuster, 1982)

James Carkesse, *Lucida Intervalla: Containing Divers Miscellaneous Poems*, edited M.V. DePorte (Los Angeles, University of California Press, 1979, 1st edn, London, 1679)

Eric T. Carlson and Norman Dam, 'The Psychotherapy which was Moral Treatment', *American Journal of Psychiatry* 117 (1960), 519-24

— 'The Meaning of Moral Insanity', *Bulletin of the History of Medicine* 36 (1962), 130-40

Eric T. Carlson and B. McFadden, 'Dr William Cullen on Mania', *American Journal of Psychiatry* 117 (1960), 463-65

Eric T. Carlson and Meredith Simpson, 'Madness of the Nervous System in Eighteenth Century Psychiatry', *Bulletin of the History of Psychiatry* 43 (1969), 101-15

P.K. Carpenter, 'The Private Lunatic Asylums of Leicester' (forthcoming)

J. Carswell, *The South Sea Bubble* (London, Cresset Press, 1960)

P.L. Carver, *The Life of a Poet: a Biographical Sketch of William Collins* (London, Sidgwick & Jackson, 1967)

M. Casaubon, *A Treatise Concerning Enthusiasme as an Effect of Nature* (London, Roger Daniel, 1655)

E. and R. Castel and A. Lovell, *The Psychiatric Society* (Columbia, University Press, 1981)

Robert Castel, *Le Psychanalysme* (Paris, U.G.E. Collection, 1976)

J.E. Chamberlin and S.L. Gilman (eds), *Degeneration, The Dark Side of Progress* (New York, Columbia University Press, 1985)

E. Chambers, *Cyclopaedia*, 2 vols (London, Chambers, 1728)

C.F. Chapin, *The Religious Thought of Samuel Johnson* (Ann Arbor, Mich., University of Michigan Press, 1968)

P.P. Chase, 'The Ailments and Physicians of Dr. Johnson', *Yale Journal of Biology and Medicine* 23 (1951), 3 70-79

George Cheyne, *An Essay of Health and Long Life* (London, Strahan, 1724)

— *The English Malady: or, a Treatise of Nervous Diseases of All Kinds* (London, Strahan and Leake, 1733)

— *The Natural Method of Cureing the Diseases of the Body, and the Disorders of the Mind Depending on the Body* (London, Strahan & Knapton, 1742)

— *Dr. Cheyne's Own Account of Himself and his Writings* (London, J. Wilford, 1743).

Anthony Clare, *Psychiatry in Dissent. Controversial Issues in Thought and Practice* (London, Tavistock, 1976)

J.K. Clark, *Goodwin Wharton* (Oxford, Oxford University Press, 1984)

J.R. Clark, *Form and Frenzy in Swift's 'Tale of a Tub'* (Ithaca and London, Cornell University Press, 1970)

Michael J. Clark, 'The Rejection of Psychological Approaches to Mental Disorder in Late Nineteenth-Century British Psychiatry', in Andrew Scull (ed.), *Madhouses, Mad-Doctors, and Madmen* (London, Athlone Press, 1981), 271-312

Basil Clarke, *Mental Disorder in Earlier Britain* (Cardiff, University of Wales Press, 1975)

E.S. Clarke and Kenneth Dewhurst, *An Illustrated History of Brain Function* (Oxford, Sandford Publications, 1972)

E.S. Clarke and C.D. O'Malley, *The Human Brain and Spinal Cord* (Berkeley, University of California Press, 1968)

J.L. Clifford, *Dr Campbell's Diary* (Cambridge, Cambridge University Press, 1947)

— *Hester Lynch Piozzi — Mrs. Thrale*, 2nd edition (Oxford, Clarendon Press, 1952)

E.J. Climenson (ed.), *Elizabeth Montagu, the Queen of the Blue Stockings, Her Correspondence from 1720-1766*, 2 vols (London, John Murray, 1906)

J.J. Cobben, *Jan Wier, Devils, Witches and Magic*, trans. S.A. Prins (Philadelphia, Dorrance, 1976)

W. Cobbett, *Advice to Young Men*, ed. G. Spater (Oxford, Oxford University Press, 1980)

Stanley Cohen, *Folk Devils and Moral Panics* (London, MacGibbon and Kee, 1972)

Norman Cohn, *The Pursuit of the Millennium* (London, Paladin, 1970)

— *Europe's Inner Demons* (London, Paladin, 1976)

Rosalie Colie, *Paradoxia Epidemica* (Princeton, Princeton University Press, 1966)

R. Colp Jr, *To be an Invalid* (Chicago, University of Chicago Press, 1977)

Alex Comfort, *The Anxiety Makers* (London, Nelson, 1967)

John Conolly, *An Inquiry Concerning the Indications of Insanity* (London, Taylor, 1830)

— *The Construction and Government of Lunatic Asylums and Hospitals for the Insane* (London, Churchill, 1847)

— *The Treatment of the Insane Without Mechanical Restraint* (London, Smith and Elder, 1856)

M.D. Conway, *Demonology and Devil-Lore*, 2 vols (London, Chatto and Windus, 1879)

R.J. Cooter, 'Phrenology and British Alienists *circa* 1825–1845', *Medical History* 20 (1976), 135–51

I.P. Couliano, *Eros et Magie à la Renaissance* (Paris, Flammarion, 1984)

W.F. Courtney, *Young Charles Lamb, 1775–1802* (London, New York University Press, 1982)

W. Cowper, *Memoir of the Early Life of William Cowper, Esq.,* 2nd ed. (London, R. Edwards, 1816)

J.M. Cox, *Practical Observations on Insanity* (London, Baldwin and Murray, 1806)

S.D. Cox, *'The Stranger Within Thee': The Concept of the Self in Late Eighteenth Century Literature* (Pittsburgh, Pittsburgh University Press, 1980)

M. Craig, *The Legacy of Swift, A Bicentenary Record of St. Patrick's Hospital, Dublin* (Dublin, for the Governors, 1948)

R.S. Crane, 'Suggestions Towards the Genealogy of the Man of Feeling', in *The Idea of the Humanities and Other Essays* (Chicago, Chicago University Press, 1967), i, 188–213

P. Cranefield, 'A Seventeenth Century View of Mental Deficiency and Schizophrenia: Thomas Willis on "Stupidity and Foolishness"', *Bulletin of the History of Medicine* 35 (1961), 291–316

Sir Alexander Crichton, *An Inquiry into the Nature and Origin of Mental Derangement*, 2 vols (London, Cadell & Davis, 1798)

Nora Crook and Derek Guiton, *Shelley's Venomed Melody* (Cambridge, Cambridge University Press, 1986)

Bryan Crowther, *Practical Remarks on Insanity* (London, Thomas Underwood, 1811)

Alexander Cruden, *The London Citizen Exceedingly Injured* (London, for the author, 1739)

— *Mr Cruden Greatly Injured* (London, printed for A. Injured, 1739)

— *The Adventures of Alexander the Corrector* (London, for the author, 1754)

— 'Memoirs of Alexander Cruden', introducing *A Complete Concordance to the Holy Scriptures of the Old and New Testament; or, a Dictionary and Alphabetical Index to the Bible* (New York, Dodd, Mead, 1823)

W. Cullen, *First Lines of the Practice of Physic*, 4 vols (Edinburgh, William Creech, 1778–84)

— *Nosology: or, a Systematic Arrangement of Diseases* (Edinburgh, Creech, 1800)

S. Cunningham, 'Bedlam and Parnassus: Eighteenth Century Reflections', in B. Harris (ed.), *Eighteenth Century Studies*, 24 (1971), 35–55 James Currie, 'Two letters on the Establishment of a Lunatic Asylum at Liverpool', *The*

Liverpool Advertiser (29 August and 12 November, 1789)

— *Medical Reports on the Effect of Water, Cold and Warm, as A Remedy in Fever, and Febrile Diseases... With Observations on the Nature of Fever; and on the Effects of Opium, Alcohol, and Inanition* (London, Cadell and Davies, 1797)

C. Dainton, *The Story of England's Hospitals* (London, Museum Press, 1961)

B. Dale, *The Good Lord Wharton. His Family Life and Bible Charity,* new edition (London, Congregational Union of England and Wales, 1906)

Frances D'Arblay, *Diary and Letters,* ed. C.E Barrett, 7 vols (London, H. Colburn, 1842-46)

R. Darnton, *Mesmerism and the End of the Enlightenment in France* (Cambridge, Mass., Harvard University Press, 1968)

Erasmus Darwin, *Zoonomia,* 2 vols (London, Johnson, 1794 & 1796)

— *The Temple of Nature, or the Origin of Society – A Poem with Philosophical Notes* (London, J. Johnson, 1803)

A.G. Debus, *Man and Nature in the Renaissance* (Cambridge, Cambridge University Press, 1978)

D. Defoe, *An Essay Upon Projects* (London, Cockerill, 1697)

— *Augusta Triumphans: or, the Way to Make London the Most Flourishing City in the Universe* (London, Roberts, 1728)

— *A Tour Through the Whole Island of Great Britain,* ed. P. Rogers (Harmondsworth, Penguin, 1972)

M. DeLacy, *Prison Reform in Lancashire 1700-1850* (Manchester, Chetham Society, 1986)

P. Delany, *British Autobiography in the Seventeenth Century* (London, Routledge & Kegan Paul, 1969)

Michael V. DePorte, *Nightmares and Hobby Horses. Swift, Sterne and Augustan Ideas of Madness* (San Marino, California, Huntingdon Library, 1974)

— 'Digressions and Madness in "A Tale of Tub" and "Tristram Shandy"', *Huntingdon Library Quarterly* 34 (1970), 45-57

— (ed.), *James Carkesse: Lucida Intervalla* (Los Angeles, University of California Press, 1979)

R. Descartes, *Treatise on Man,* trans. and ed. T.S. Hall (Cambridge, Mass., Harvard University Press, 1974)

N. Dewey, 'Robert Burton and the Drama' (PhD thesis, Princeton University, 1969)

K. Dewhurst, *John Locke (1632-1704), Physician and Philosopher* (London, Wellcome Institute for the History of Medicine, 1963)

— *Dr Thomas Sydenham (1624-1689): His Life and Original Writings* (London, Wellcome Institute for the History of Medicine, 1966)

— (ed.), *Willis' Oxford Casebook (1650-52)* (Oxford, Sandford, 1981)

D. Diderot, *Rameau's Nephew; D'Alembert's Dream,* trans. L. W. Tancock (Harmondsworth, Penguin, 1966)

Georges Didi-Huberman, *Invention de l'Hysterie. Charcot et l'Iconon graphie de la Salpêtrière* (Paris, Editions Macula, 1982)

Oskar Dietheim, 'The Medical Teaching of Demonology in the Seventeenth and Eighteenth Centuries', *Journal of the History of the Behavioural Sciences* 6 (1970), 3-15

Anne Digby, 'Changes in the Asylum: The Case of York, 1777-1815', *Economic History Review,* second series 37 (1983), 218-39

— 'The Changing Profile of a Nineteenth-Century Asylum: the York

Retreat', *Psychological Medicine* 14 (1984), 739–48

— 'Moral Treatment at the York Retreat', in W.F. Bynum, Roy Porter and Michael Shepherd (eds), *The Anatomy of Madness*, 2 vols (London, Tavistock, 1985), ii, 52–72

— *Madness, Morality and Medicine* (Cambridge, Cambridge University Press, 1985)

— *From York Lunatic Asylum to Bootham Park Hospital* (York, Borthwick Papers, No.69, 1986)

— 'Quantitative and Qualitative Perspectives on the Asylum', in R. Porter and A. Wear (eds), *Problems and Methods in the History of Medicine* (London, Croom Helm, 1987), 153–74

K.S. Dix, 'Madness in Russia: 1775–1864, Official Attitudes and Institutions for the Insane' (University of California, Los Angeles, PhD, 1977)

E.R. Dodds, *The Greeks and the Irrational* (Berkeley and London, University of California Press, 1951)

K. Doerner, *Madmen and the Bourgeoisie*, trans. J. Neugroschel and J. Steinberg (Oxford, Basil Blackwell, 1981)

M. Dols, 'Insanity and its Treatment in Islamic Society', *Medical History* 31 (1987), 1–14

M. Donnelly, *Managing the Mind* (London, Tavistock, 1983)

Penelope E.R. Doob, *Nebuchadnezzar's Children. Conventions of Madness in Middle English Literature* (New Haven and London, Yale University Press, 1974)

O. Doughty, 'The English Malady of the Eighteenth Century', *The Review of English Studies* 2 (1926), 257–69

E. Dudley and M.E. Novak (eds), *The Wild Man Within* (Pittsburgh, University of Pittsburgh Press, 1972)

A. Duncan, Sen., *Observations on the Structure of Hospitals for the Treatment of Lunatics* (Edinburgh, Ballantyne, 1809)

J. Eigen, 'Intentionality and Insanity: What the Eighteenth Century Juror Heard', in W.F. Bynum, Roy Porter and Michael Shepherd (eds), *The Anatomy of Madness*, 2 vols (London, Tavistock, 1985), ii, 34–51

Henri F. Ellenberger, The *Discovery of the Unconscious: The History and Evolution of Dynamic Psychiatry* (New York, Basic Books, 1971)

J. Engell, *The Creative Imagination* (Cambridge Mass., Harvard University Press, 1981)

Pedro Lain Entralgo, *Mind and Body. Psychosomatic Pathology*, trans. A.M. Espinosa (London, Harvill, 1955)

— *The Therapy of the Word in Classical Antiquity*, L.J. Rather and John M. Sharp (trans. & eds) (New Haven, Yale University Press, 1970)

J.E.D. Esquirol, *Mental Maladies: A Treatise on Insanity*, Facsimile of English Edition, 1845, published by the Library of the New York Academy of Medicine (New York, Hafner Publishing Company, 1965)

Berger Evans, *The Psychiatry of Robert Burton* (New York, Octagon Books, 1972)

Robin Evans, *The Fabrication of Virtue. English Prison Architecture, 1750-1840* (Cambridge, Cambridge University Press, 1982)

S.B. Ewing, *Burtonian Melancholy in the Plays of John Ford* (New York, Octagon, 1969)

William Falconer, *A Dissertation on the Influence of the Passions upon Disorders of the Body* (London, C. Dilly, 1788)

T. Fallowes, *The Best Method for the Cure of Lunaticks* (London, for the author, 1705)

Hugh Farmer, *An Essay on the Demoniacs of the New Testament* (London, Robinson, 1775)

B. Faulkner, *Observations on the General and Improper Treatment of Insanity* (London, for the author, 1789)

M. Fears, 'Therapeutic Optimism and the Treatment of the Insane' in R. Dingwall (ed.), *Health Care and Health Knowledge* (London, Croom Helm, 1977), 66–81

— 'The "Moral Treatment" of Insanity: A Study in the Social Construction of Human Nature' (University of Edinburgh PhD Thesis, 1978)

L. Feder, *Madness in Literature* (Princeton, Princeton University Press, 1980)

H.M. Feinstein, 'The Prepared Heart; a Comparative Study of Puritan Theology and Psychoanalysis', *American Quarterly* 22 (1970), 166–76

K. Fenwick (ed.), *Ned Ward: The London Spy* (London, Folio Society, 1950)

John Ferriar, *Medical Histories and Reflections*, 3 vols (London, Cadell & Davies, 1795)

A. Fessler, 'The Management of Lunacy in Seventeenth Century England. An Investigation of Quarter Session Records', *Proceedings of the Royal Society of Medicine* 49 (1956), 901–07

Henry Fielding, *Amelia*, edited by M.C. Battestin (Oxford, Clarendon Press, 1983; 1st edn, London, 1752)

Mark Finnane, *Insanity and the Insane in Post-Famine Ireland* (London, Croom Helm, 1981)

E. Fischer-Hombergei, *Hypochrondie, Melancholia bis Neurose, Kran kenheit und Zustandsbilder* (Bern, Hans Huber, 1970)

— 'Hypochondriasis of the Eighteenth Century: Neurosis of the Present . Century', *Bulletin of the History of Medicine* 46 (1972), 391–401

— *Die Traumatische Neurose. Vom Somatischen zum Sozialen Leiden* (Bern, Hans Huber, 1975)

S. Fish, *Self-Consuming Artifacts* (Berkeley, University of California Press, 1972)

Thomas Fitzgerald, 'Bedlam', in *Poems on Several Occasions* (London, Watts, 1733)

H. Flasher, *Melancholie und Melancholiker in den Medisinischen Theorien der Antike* (Berlin, de Gruyter, 1966)

T.R. Forbes, *Surgeons at the Bailey. English Forensic Medicine to 1878* (London, Yale University Press, 1985)

A. Fothergill, *An Essay on the Abuse of Spiritous Liquors* (Bath, Crutwell, 1796)

Michael Foucault, *Folie et Déraison: Histoire de la Folie a l'Age Classique* (Paris, Librairie Plon, 1961); trans. and abridged as *Madness and Civilisation, A History of Insanity in the Age of Reason*, trans. Richard Howard (New York, Random House, 1965)

— *Discipline and Punish*, trans. A. Sheridan (London, Allen Lane, 1977)

— *The History of Sexuality*, vol. i (London, Allen Lane, 1979)

— and R. Sennett, 'Sexuality and Solitude', *London Review of Books* (21 May 1981), 3–5

Edward Long Fox, *Brislington House, an Asylum for Lunatics, Situated Near Bristol* (Bristol, for the author, 1806)

F.K. & C.J. Fox, 'History and Present State of Brislington House, near Bristol', reprinted in *Brislington House Quarterly News Centenary Number* (1906), 16–23

G. Fox, *Book of Miracles*, ed. M.J. Cadbury (Cambridge, Cambridge University Press, 1948)

C.N. French, *The Story of St. Luke's Hospital* (London, Heinemann Medical Books, 1951)

R. French, *Robert Whytt, the Soul and Medicine* (London, Wellcome Institute for the History of Medicine, 1969)

P. Frings, *A Treatise on Phrenzy* (London, Gardner, 1746)

N. Fruman, *Coleridge, The Damaged Archangel* (London, Allen & Unwin, 1971)

S.P. Fullinwider, 'Insanity and the Loss of Self: the Moral Insanity Controversy Revisited', *Bulletin of the History of Medicine* 49 (1975), 87–101

—— *Technicians of the Finite* (Westpoint, Conn., Greenwood Press, 1982)

P. Fussell, *The Rhetorical World of Augustan Humanism* (Oxford, Clarendon Press, 1965)

I. Galdston (ed.), *Historic Derivations of Modern Psychiatry* (New York, McGraw-Hill, 1967)

J.K. Gardiner, 'Elizabethan Psychology and Burton's Anatomy of Melancholy', *Journal of the History of Ideas* 38 (1977), 373–88

D. Garnett (ed.), *The Novels of Thomas Love Peacock* (London, Rupert Hart-Davis, 1948)

C. Garrett, *Respectable Folly: Millenarians and the French Revolution in France and England* (Baltimore, Johns Hopkins University Press, 1975)

M.D. George, *English Political Caricature to 1792* (Oxford, Clarendon Press, 1959)

—— *London Life in the Eighteenth Century* (Harmondsworth, Penguin, 1965)

Johanna Geyer-Kordesch, 'Cultural Habits of Illness: The Enlightened and the Pious in Eighteenth Century Germany', in Roy Porter (ed.), *Patients and Practitioners* (Cambridge, Cambridge University Press, 1985), 177–204

Arthur N. Gilbert, 'Doctor, Patient and Onanist Diseases in the Nineteenth Century', *Journal of the History of Medicine and Allied Sciences* 30 (1975), 217–34

S. Gilbert and S. Gubarr, *The Madwoman in the Attic: The Woman Writer and the Nineteenth-Century Imagination* (New Haven, Yale University Press, 1979)

Mrs Gilchrist, *Mary Lamb* (London, W. H. Allen, 1893)

Sander L. Gilman, *The Face of Madness: Hugh W. Diamond and the Origin of Psychiatric Photography* (New York, Brunner, Mazel, 1976)

—— *Seeing the Insane* (New York, Brunner, Mazel, 1982)

—— *Difference and Pathology* (Ithaca and London, Cornell University Press, 1985)

E. Godlee, 'The Retreat and Quakerism', in W.E. Bynum, Roy Porter and Michael Shepherd (eds), *The Anatomy of Madness*, 2 vols (London, Tavistock, 1985), ii, 73–85

E. Goffman, *Asylums* (New York, Anchor Books, 1961)

M. Golden, *In Search of Stability: the Poetry of William Cowper* (New Haven, Yale University Press, 1969)

—— *The Self Observed* (Baltimore, Johns Hopkins University Press, 1972)

J. Goldstein, '"Moral Contagion". A Professional Ideology of Medicine and Psychiatry in Eighteenth and Nineteenth Century France', in G. Geison (ed.), *Professions and the French State, 1700-1900* (Philadelphia, University of Pennsylvania Press, 1984), 180–222

Philip Goodwin, *The Mystery of Dreams, Historically Discoursed* (London, Tyton, 1658)

Kathleen Grange, 'Pinel and Eighteenth Century Psychiatry', *Bulletin of the History of Medicine* 35 (1961), 442–53

— 'Dr. Samuel Johnson's Account of a Schizophrenic Illness in Rasselas (1759)', *Medical History* 6 (1962), 162–68

— 'Pinel or Chiarugi?', *Medical History* 7 (1963), 371–80

Jonathan Gray, *The History of the York Lunatic Asylum* (York, 1815)

John Gregory, *A Comparative View of the State and Faculties of Man with those of the Animal World* (London, Dodsley, 1765)

J.Y.T. Greig (ed.), *The Letters of David Hume* (Oxford, Clarendon Press, 1932)

Nehemiah Grew, *Cosmologia Sacra* (London, Rogers et al., 1701)

E.L. Griggs (ed.), *Collected Letters of Samuel Taylor Coleridge* (Oxford, Clarendon Press, 1956)

H. Gruber, *Darwin on Man* (London, University of Chicago Press, 1974)

J. Hall, *A Narrative of the Proceedings Relative to the Establishment etc. of St Luke's House* (Newcastle-upon-Tyne, for the author, 1767)

W.S. Hallaran, *An Enquiry into the Causes Producing the Extraordinary Addition to the Number of Insane* (Cork, Edwards & Savage, 1810)

R.C. Ham, *Otway and Lee* (New Haven, Conn., Yale University Press, 1931)

F.J. Harding, 'Dr Nathaniel Cotton of St Albans, Poet and Physician', *Herts. Countryside* 23 (1969), 46–48

B. Cozens Hardy (ed.), *The Diary of Sylas Neville* (London, Oxford University Press, 1950)

E.H. Hare, 'Masturbatory Insanity: the History of an Idea', *Journal of Mental Science* 106 (1962), 1–25

— 'Was Insanity on the Increase?', *British Journal of Psychiatry* 142 (1983), 439–55

D. Harley, 'Mental Illness, Magical Medicine and the Devil in the North of England, 1650–1700' (unpublished paper, 1986)

Andrew Harper, *A Treatise on the Real Cause and Cure of Insanity* (London, Stalker & Waltes, 1789)

V.I. Harris, *All Coherence Gone* (London, Frank Cass & Co., 1966)

Brian Harrison, *Drink and the Victorians. The Temperance Question in England, 1815–1872* (London, Longman, 1971)

J.F.C. Harrison, *The Second Coming* (London, Fontana, 1979)

David Hartley, *Observations on Man, his Frame, his Duty, and his Expectations* (London, Leake & Frederick, 1749)

E.R. Harvey, *The Inward Wits: Psychological Theory in the Middle Ages and the Renaissance* (London, The Warburg Institute, 1975)

John Haslam, *Observations on Madness and Melancholy*, 2nd edn (London, John Callow, 1809)

— *Illustrations of Madness* (London, Rivingtons, 1810)

— *Medical Jurisprudence as it Relates to Insanity According to the Laws of England* (London, C. Hunter, 1817)

— *Considerations on the Moral Management of Insane People* (London, no publisher, 1817)

M.G. Hay, 'Understanding Madness: Some Approaches to Mental Illness' (University of York, PhD thesis, 1979)

John Haygarth, *Of the Imagination, as a Cause and as a Cure of Disorders of the*

Body (Bath, Cadell & Davies, 1800)

W. Hazlitt, *Table Talk* (London, Everyman edn, 1936)

William Heberden, *Medical Commentaries on the History and Cure of Diseases* (London, T. Payne, 1802)

N. Hervey, 'A Slavish Bowing Down', in W.F. Bynum, Roy Porter and Michael Shepherd (eds), *The Anatomy of Madness*, 2 vols (London, Tavistock, 1985), ii, 98-131

— 'Advocacy or Folly? The Alleged Lunatics' Friends Society, 1845-63', *Medical History* 30 (1986), 254-75

H.M. Herwig, *The Art of Curing Sympathetically, or Magnetically* (London, T. Newborough, 1700)

M. Heyd, 'The Reaction to Enthusiasm', *Journal of Modern History* 53 (1981), 258-80

C. Hibbert (ed.), *An American in Regency England* (London, History Book Club, 1968)

A.W. Hill, *John Wesley Among the Physicians* (London, Epworth Press, 1958)

B. Hill, '"My Little Physician at St. Albans". Nathaniel Cotton 1705–1788', *Practitioner* 199 (1967), 363-67

Christopher Hill, *Antichrist in Seventeenth Century England* (London, Oxford University Press, 1971)

— *The World Turned Upside Down: Radical Ideas During the English Revolution* (Harmondsworth, Penguin, 1978)

— *Intellectual Consequences of the English Revolution* (London, Weidenfeld & Nicolson, 1980)

— 'God and the English Revolution', *History Workshop* 17 (1984), 19-31

— and Michael Shepherd, 'The Case of Arise Evans: a Historico-psychiatric Study', *Psychological Medicine* 6 (1976), 351-58

Draper Hill, *Mr Gillray, the Caricaturist* (London, Phaidon Press, 1966) G.B. Hill (ed.), *Boswell's Life of Johnson*, 6 vols (Oxford, Clarendon Press, 1887)

— *Letters of Samuel Johnson*, 2 vols (Oxford, Clarendon Press, 1892)

George Nesse Hill, *An Essay on the Prevention and Cure of Insanity* (London, Longman, 1814)

Sir John Hill, *Hypochondriasis, A Practical Treatise on the Nature and Cure of That Disorder Commonly Called the Hyp or Hypo* (London, for the author, 1766)

Robert Gardiner Hill, *Total Abolition of Personal Restraint in the Insane* (London, Simpkin, Marshall, 1839)

— *A Concise History of the Entire Abolition of Mechanical Restraint in the Treatment of the Insane and of the Introduction, Success and Final Triumph of the Non-Restraint System. Together with a Reprint of a Lecture Delivered on the Subject in the Year 1838* (London, Longman, 1857)

G. Himmelfarb, *The Idea of Poverty in the Industrial Revolution* (New York, Random House, 1984)

J. Hirsh, 'Enlightened 18th Century Views of the Alcohol Problem', *Journal of the History of Medicine* 4 (1949), 230-36

P.Q. Hirst and P. Woolley, *Social Relations and Human Attributes* (London, Tavistock, 1982)

Thomas Hobbes, *Leviathan*, edited by A.D. Lindsay (New York, Everyman Library, 1953; 1st edn, London, Crooke, 1651)

R.G. Hodgkinson, 'Provision for Pauper Lunatics 1834-1871', *Medical History* 10 (1966), 138-54

R. Hoeldtke, 'The History of Associationism and British Medical Psychology', *Medical History* 11(1967), 46-65

G. Holmes, *Augustan England, Professions, State, and Society, 1680-1730* (London, Allen & Unwin, 1982)

R. Holmes, *Shelley. The Pursuit* (London, Weidenfeld & Nicolson, 1974)

P.M. Horsley, *Eighteenth Century Newcastle* (Newcastle, Oriel Press, 1971)

John Howard, *The State of the Prisons* (Warrington, Lancashire, for the author, 1777)

J.G. Howells (ed.), *World History of Psychiatry* (New York, Brunner/Mazel, 1968)

Michael Hunter, *Science and Society in Restoration England* (Cambridge, Cambridge University Press, 1981)

Richard Hunter, 'A Brief Review of the Use of Electricity in Psychiatry', *British Journal of Physical Medicine* n.s. 20 (1957), 99

— 'Some Notes on the Importance of Manuscript Records for Psychiatric history', Archives 4 (1959), 9-11

— and Ida Macalpine, 'The Reverend William Pargeter, M.A., M.D. (1760-1810), Psychiatrist', *St Bart's Hospital Journal* 60 (Feb. 1956), 52-60

— *Schizophrenia 1677. A Psychiatric Study of An Illustrated Autobiographical Record of Demonical Possession* (London, Dawsons, 1956)

— 'John Thomas Perceval (1803-1876), Patient and Reformer', *Medical History* 6 (1961), 391-95

— *Three Hundred Years of Psychiatry, 1535-1860* (London, Oxford University Press, 1963)

— 'Samuel Tuke's First Publication on the Treatment of Patients at the Retreat, 1811', *British Journal of Psychiatry* 111 (1965), 771

— *Psychiatry for the Poor. 1851 Colney Hatch Asylum. Friern Hospital 1973: A Medical and Social History* (London, Dawsons, 1974)

Richard Hunter and L.M. Payne, 'The County Register of Houses for the Reception of "Lunatics", 1798-1812', *Journal of Mental Science* 102 (1956), 856-63

Richard Hunter and J.B. Wood, 'Nathaniel Cotton, M.D., Poet and Physician', *King's College Hospital Gazette* 36 (1957), 120

Michael Ignatieff, *A Just Measure of Pain: The Penitentiary in the Industrial Revolution, 1750-1850* (New York, Pantheon, 1978)

— 'Total Institutions and Working Classes: a Review Essay', *History Workshop Journal* 15 (1983), 169-72

David Ingleby (ed.), *Critical Psychiatry. The Politics of Mental Health* (Harmondsworth, Penguin, 1981)

— 'The Social Construction of Mental Illness', in P. Wright and A. Treacher (eds), *The Problem of Medical Knowledge* (Edinburgh, Edinburgh University Press, 1982), 123-43

A.M. Ingram, *Boswell's Creative Gloom* (London, Macmillan, 1982)

D. Irish, *Levamen Infirmi: or, Cordial Counsel to the Sick and Diseased* (London, for the author, 1700)

G. Irwin, *Samuel Johnson. A Personality in Conflict* (Auckland, Auckland University Press, 1971)

Hansruedi Isler, *Thomas Willis, 1621-1675, Doctor and Scientist* (New York, Hafner, 1968)

Stanley W. Jackson, 'Galen: On Mental Disorder', *Journal of the History of the*

Behavioural Sciences 5 (1969), 365-84

— 'Melancholia and the Waning of the Humoral Theory', *Journal of the History of Medicine and Allied Sciences*, 33 (1978), 367-76

— *Melancholia and Depression From Hippocratic Times to Modern Times* (New Haven, Yale University Press, 1986)

Robert James, *Medicinal Dictionary*, 3 vols (London, T. Osborne, 1743)

Nicholas Jewson, 'The Disappearance of the Sick Man from Medical Cosmology 1770-1870', *Sociology* 10 (1976), 225-44

M.A. Jimenez, 'Madness in Early American History: Insanity in Massachusetts from 1700 to 1830', *Journal of Social History* 20 (1986), 25-44

T.H. Jobe, 'Medical Theories of Melancholia in the Seventeenth and Early Eighteenth Centuries', *Clio Medica* 19 (1976), 217-31

R. Brimley Johnson (ed.), *Letters from Lady Mary Wortley Montagu* (London, Everyman edition, 1925)

Samuel Johnson, *Diaries, Prayers and Annals*, edited by E.L. McAdam Jr and D. and M. Hyde (New Haven, Yale University Press, 1958)

— *The Idler and Adventurer*, edited by W.J. Bate, J.M. Bullitt and L.F. Powell (New Haven, Conn., Yale University Press, 1963)

— 'A Review of Soame Jenyns' *A Free Enquiry into the Nature and Origin of Evil*', in B. Bronson (ed.), *Samuel Johnson, Rasselas, Poems and Selected Prose* (San Francisco, Calif., Rinehart Press, 1971)

— *Rasselas*, in B. H. Bronson (ed.), *Samuel Johnson, Rasselas, Poems and Selected Prose* (San Francisco, Rinehart Press, 1971)

John Johnston, *Medical Jurisprudence on Madness* (Birmingham, J. Beicher, 1800)

C. Jones, 'The Treatment of the Insane in Eighteenth and Early Nineteenth-Century Montpellier', *Medical History* 24 (1980), 371-90

G.F.T. Jones, *Sawpit Wharton. The Political Career from 1640-1691 of Philip, Fourth Lord Wharton* (Sydney, Sydney University Press, 1967)

John Jones, *The Mysteries of Opium Reveal'd* (London, R. Smith, 1700)

Kathleen Jones, *Lunacy, Law and Conscience, 1744-1845* (London, Routledge & Kegan Paul, 1955)

— *Mental Health and Social Policy, 1845-1959* (London, Routledge & Kegan Paul, 1960)

— *A History of the Mental Health Services* (London, Routledge & Kegan Paul, 1972)

— 'Scull's Dilemma', *British Journal of Psychiatry* 141 (1982), 221–6

W.L. Jones, *Ministering to Minds Diseased. A History of Psychiatric Treatment* (London, Heinemann, 1983)

Edward Jorden, *A Brief Discourse of a Disease called the Suffocation of the Mother* (London, Windet, 1603)

W. Kaiser, *Praisers of Folly* (London, Victor Gollancz, 1964)

M. Kallich, *The Association of Ideas and Critical Theory in Eighteenth Century England* (The Hague, Mouton, 1970)

G. Kelly, *The English Jacobin Novel, 1780-1805* (Oxford, Clarendon Press, 1976)

D. Kevies, *In the Name of Eugenics* (Harmondsworth, Pelican, 1986)

G. Keynes (ed.), *The Complete Writings of William Blake* (London, Oxford University Press, 1966)

A.D. King (ed.), *Buildings and Society* (London, Routledge & Kegan Paul, 1980)

J. King and C. Ryskamp (eds), *The Letters and Prose Writings of William Cowper*

(Oxford, Clarendon Press, 1979)

Lester S. King, *The Medical World of the Eighteenth Century* (Chicago, University of Chicago Press, 1958)

— *The Philosophy of Medicine. The Early Eighteenth Century* (Cambridge, Mass., Harvard University Press, 1978)

D. King-Hele (ed.), *The Essential Writings of Erasmus Darwin* (London, McGibbon and Kee, 1968)

— *Doctor of Revolution: The Life and Genius of Erasmus Darwin* (London, Faber, 1977)

— (ed.), *The Letters of Erasmus Darwin* (Cambridge, Cambridge University Press, 1981)

D. Bayne Kinneir, 'A Copy of a Letter from Dr. David Kinneir...to Dr Campbell...Touching the Efficacy of Camphire in Maniacal Disorders', *Philosophical Transactions* 35 (1717), 347–51

R.S. Kinsman, 'Folly, Melancholy and Madness: A Study in Shifting Styles of Medical Analysis and Treatment, 1450-1675', in R.S. Kinsman (ed.), *The Darker Vision of the Renaissance* (Berkeley, University of California Press, 1974)

A. Kleinman, *Social Origins of Distress and Disease: Depression, Neurasthenia, and Pain in Modern China* (New Haven, Yale University Press, 1986)

R. Klibansky, E. Panofsky and F. Saxl, *Saturn and Melancholy* (London, Nelson, 1964)

Paul Slade Knight, *Observations on the Causes, Symptoms and Treatment of Derangement* (London, Longman, 1827)

R.A. Knox, *Enthusiasm* (London, Oxford University Press, 1950)

P.H. Kocher, *Science and Religion in Elizabethan England* (San Marino, California, Huntingdon Library, 1953)

E. Kraepelin, *One Hundred Years of Psychiatry* (London, Peter Owen, 1962)

I. Kramnick, *The Rage of Edmund Burke* (New York, Basic Books, 1977)

J. Kromm, 'Studies in the Iconography of Madness, 1600-1900' (PhD thesis, Emory University, 1984)

R.G. Macdonald Ladell, 'The Neurosis of Dr. Samuel Johnson', *The British Journal of Medical Psychology* 9 (1929), 314–25

C. Lamb, 'The Sanity of True Genius', in G.E. Hollingsworth (ed.), *Lamb: The Last Essays of Elia* (London, n.d.)

Joan Lane, '"The Doctor Scolds Me". The Diaries and Correspondence of Patients in Eighteenth Century England', in Roy Porter (ed.), *Patients and Practitioners. Lay Perceptions of Medicine in Pre-Industrial Society* (Cambridge, Cambridge University Press, 1985), 204–48

Thomas Laqueur, 'Orgasm, Generation and the Politics of Reproductive Biology', *Representations* 14 (1986), 1–42

M.W. Latham, *The Elizabethan Fairies* (New York, Columbia University Studies in English and Comparative Literature, 1930)

R. Latham and W. Matthews (eds), *The Diary of Samuel Pepys*, 2 vols (London, Bell and Hyman, 1970-83)

J. Latimer, *The Annals of Bristol in the Eighteenth Century* (London, Butler and Tanner, 1893)

Andreas Laurentius, *A Discourse of the Preservation of Sight: of Melancholike Disease: and of Old Age*, trans. Richard Surphlet, 1599, reprinted with introduction by S.V. Larkey (Oxford, The Shakespeare Association Facsimiles,

1938; 1st edn, 1599)

C.J. Lawrence, 'The Nervous System and Society in the Scottish Enlightenment', in B. Barnes and S. Shapin (eds), *Natural Order: Historical Studies of Scientific Culture* (London, Sage Publications, 1979), 19-40

— 'Medicine as Culture: Edinburgh and the Scottish Enlightenment' (University of London, PhD thesis, 1984)

W. LeFanu (ed.), *Betsy Sheridan's Journal. Letters from Sheridan's Sister, 1784-1786 and 1788-1790* (London, Eyre and Spottiswoode, 1960)

M. Lefebure, *Samuel Taylor Coleridge: A Bondage of Opium* (London, Gollancz, 1974)

Denis Leigh, *The Historical Development of British Psychiatry*, vol. 1 (Oxford, Pergamon, 1961)

J.C. Lettsom, 'Some Remarks on the Effects of *Lignum Quassiae Amarae*', *Memoirs of the Medical Society of London* 1 (1787), 128-65

Sir Aubrey Lewis, 'British Psychiatry in the First Half of the Nineteenth Century: Philippe Pinel and the English', *Proceedings of the Royal Society of Medicine* 48 (1955), 581-86

— *The State of Psychiatry* (London, Routledge & Kegan Paul, 1967)

— *The Later Papers of Sir Aubrey Lewis* (Oxford University Press, 1979)

Jack Lindsay (ed.), *Loving Mad Tom. Bedlamite Verses of the Seventeenth and Eighteenth Centuries* (Welwyn Garden City, Seven Dials Press, 1969)

— *William Blake* (London, Canfrolico Press, 1978)

J. Locke, *An Essay Concerning Human Understanding* (1690), ed. by John Yolton (London, Everyman, 1961)

Louisa Lowe, *The Bastilles of England; or The Lunacy Laws at Work* (London, Crookenden, 1883)

E.V. Lucas (ed.), *The Works of Charles and Mary Lamb*, 7 vols (London, Methuen, 1903–05)

Bridget Gellert Lyons, *Voices of Melancholy. Studies in Literary Treatment of Melancholy in Renaissance England* (London, Routledge and Kegan Paul, 1971)

J.O. Lyons, *The Invention of the Self* (Carbondale, Southern Illinois University Press, 1978)

A. Lytes, *Methodism Mocked* (London, Epworth Press, 1960)

Richard Mabey, *Gilbert White* (London, Century, 1986)

E.L. McAdam Jr and D. and M. Hyde (eds), *Samuel Johnson, Diaries, Prayers and Annals* (New Haven, Yale University Press, 1958)

Ida Macalpine and Richard Hunter, 'The Schreber Case: A Contribution to Schizophrenia, Hypochondria and Psychosomatic Symptom Formation', *The Psychoanalytic Quarterly* 22 (1953), 328-71

— (eds), *Memoirs of My Nervous Illness*, by Daniel Paul Schreber (London, William Dawson & Sons, 1955)

— *A Psychiatric Study of an Illustrated Autobiographical Record of Demoniacal Possession* (London, Dawson and Sons, 1956)

— *George III and the Mad Business* (London, Allen Lane, 1969)

D. MacBride, *A Methodical Introduction on the Theory and Practice of Physick* (London, Strahan, 1772)

Peter McCandless, 'Build! Build! The Controversy over the Care of the Chronically Insane in England, 1855-1870', *Bulletin of the History of Medicine* 53 (1979), 553-74

— 'Liberty and Lunacy: The Victorians and Wrongful Confinement', in
   Andrew Scull (ed.), *Madhouses, Mad-Doctors and Madmen* (London, Athlone
   Press, 1981), 339-62
— 'Curses of Civilisation; Insanity and Drunkenness in Victorian Britain',
   British Journal of Addiction 79 (1984), 49-58
Michael MacDonald, 'The Inner Side of Wisdom: Suicide in Early Modern
   England', *Psychological Medicine* 7 (1977), 565-83
— *Mystical Bedlam: Madness, Anxiety and Healing in Seventeenth Century England*
   (Cambridge, Cambridge University Press, 1981)
— 'Insanity and the Realities of History in Early Modern England',
   Psychological Medicine 11 (1981), 11-25
— 'Religion, Social Change and Psychological Healing in England 1600-
   1800', in W. Sheils (ed.), *The Church and Healing* (Oxford, Basil Blackwell,
   1982), 101-26
— 'Popular Beliefs about Mental Disorder in Early Modern England', in
   W. Eckart and J. Geyer-Kordesch (eds), *Heilberufe und Kranke in 17 and 18
   Jahrhundert* (Munster, Burgverlag, 1982), 148-73
— 'The Secularisation of Suicide in England 1600-1800', *Past and Present* 111
   (1986), 50-100
— 'Madness, Suicide, and the Computer', in Roy Porter and Andrew Wear
   (eds), *Problems and Methods in the History of Medicine* (London, Croom
   Helm, 1987), 207-29
A.D.J. Macfarlane, *Witchcraft in Tudor and Stuart England* (London, Routledge
   & Kegan Paul, 1970)
N. McKendrick, John Brewer and J.H. Plumb, *The Birth of a Consumer Society*
   (London, Europa, 1982)
C. Mackenzie, 'Women and Psychiatric Professionalization 1780-1914', in
   London Feminist History Collective (eds), *The Sexual Dynamics of History*
   (London, Pluto Press, 1983), 107-19
— 'A Family Asylum: a History of the Private Madhouse at Ticehurst in
   Sussex, 1792–1917' (University of London, PhD thesis, 1987)
H. Mackenzie, *The Man of Feeling* (Oxford, Oxford University Press, 1970)
A. Maclaren, *Reproductive Rituals* (London, Methuen, 1984)
C.E. McMahon, 'The Role of Imagination in the Disease Process: Pre-
   Cartesian History', *Psychological Medicine* 6 (1976), 179-184
W.H. McMenemey, 'A Note on James Parkinson as a Reformer of the Lunacy
   Acts', *Proceedings of the Royal Society of Medicine* 48 (1955), 593-94
Lucien Malson, *Wolf Children* (London, New Left Books, 1972)
B. Mandeville, *A Treatise of Hypochondriack and Hysterick Passions* (London,
   Dryden Leech, W. Taylor, 1711, edn quoted, 1730)
T.A. Markus (ed.), *Order in Space and Society* (Edinburgh, Mainstream
   Publishing Co., 1982)
Otto M. Marx, 'Descriptions of Psychiatric Care in Some Hospitals During
   the First Half of the 19th-Century', *Bulletin of the History of Medicine* 41
   (1967), 208-14
A. Masters, *Bedlam* (London, Michael Joseph, 1972)
W. Matthews (ed.), *The Diary of Dudley Ryder (1715-1716)* (London, Methuen,
   1939)
H. Maudsley, *Body and Mind: An Inquiry into their Connection and Mutual
   Influence, Specially in Reference to Mental Disorders* (London, Guistonian

Lectures, 1870)

H. Mayer, *Outsiders. A Study in Life and Letters* (Cambridge, Mass., MIT Press, 1984)

Everard Maynwaring, *Tutela Sanitatis* (London, Thompson & Basset, 1664)

T. Mayo, *Remarks on Insanity* (London, Underwood, 1817)

Otto Mayr, *Authority, Liberty and Automatic Machines in Early Modern Europe* (Baltimore and London, The Johns Hopkins University Press, 1986)

Richard Mead, *Medical Precepts and Cautions*, trans. Thomas Stack (London, Brindley, 1751)

D.J. Mellett, 'Bureaucracy and Mental Illness: the Commissioners in Lunacy 1845-90', *Medical History* 25 (1981), 221-250

— *The Prerogative of Asylumdom* (New York, Garland, 1982)

L. Melville, *Lady Suffolk and Her Circle* (London, Hutchinson, 1924)

Urbane Metcalf, *The Interior of Bethlehem Hospital* (London, The Author, 1818)

E.H.W. Meyerstein, *A Life of Thomas Chatterton* (London, Ingpen and Grant, 1930)

Erik Midelfort, 'Madness and Civilisation in Early Modern Europe', in B. Malament (ed.), *After the Reformation. Essays in Honor of J.H. Hexter* (Philadelphia, University of Pennsylvania Press, 1980), 247-65

J. Midriff, *Observations on the Spleen and Vapours, Containing Remarkable Cases of Person of Both Sexes and All Ranks from the Aspiring Directors to the Humble Bubbler who have been Miserably Afflicted with these Melancholy Disorders Since the Fall of the South Sea and Other Public Stocks* (London, no publisher, 1721)

P. Millard (ed.), *Roger North: General Preface and Life of Dr. John North* (Toronto, University of Toronto Press, 1984)

C. Kerby Miller, *The Memoirs of Martin Scriblerus* (New York, Russell and Russell, 1966)

P. Miller and Nikolas Rose (eds), *The Power of Psychiatry* (London, Polity Press, 1986)

John Mitford, *A Description of the Crimes and Horrors in the Interior of Warburton's Private Madhouse at Hoxton, Commonly Called Whitmore House* (London, Benbow, 1825)

— *Part Second of the Crimes and Horrors of the Interior of Warburton 's Private Madhouses at Hoxton and Bethnal Green and of These Establishments in General with Reasons for Their Total Abolition* (London, Benbow, 1825)

Esther Moir, 'Sir George Onesiphorus Paul', in H.P.R. Finberg (ed.), *Gloucestershire Studies* (Leicester, Leicester University Press, 1957), 195–224

J. Moncrief, *The Poor Man's Physician, or the Receipts of the Famous Moncrief* (Edinburgh, G. Stewart, 1716)

John Monro, *Remarks on Dr. Battie's Treatise on Madness, reprinted with an introduction by Richard Hunter and Ida Macalpine* (London, Dawsons, 1962; 1st edn London, Clarke, 1758)

C.A. Moore, 'The English Malady', in *Backgrounds of English Literature, 1700-1760* (Minneapolis, University of Minnesota Press, 1953)

John Moore, *Religious Melancholy* (London, no publisher, 1692)

E. William Monter, 'The Historiography of European Witchcraft: Progress and Prospects', *Journal of Interdisciplinary History* 2 (1972), 435-51

— *Ritual, Myth and Magic in Early Modern Europe* (Brighton, Harvester Press, 1983)

George Mora, 'The History of Psychiatry: A Cultural and Bibliographic Survey', *The Psychoanalytic Review* 52 (1966), 335-56

— 'The Psychiatrist's Approach to the History of Psychiatry', in George Mora and Jeanne L. Brand (eds), *Psychiatry and its History. Methodological Problems in Research* (Springfield, Charles C. Thomas, 1970)

— 'Historical and Theoretical Trends in Psychiatry', in H.I. Kaplan and B.J. Sadock (ed.), *Comprehensive Textbook of Psychiatry,* 2nd edn (Baltimore, Williams and Wilkins Company, 1978), 2034–54

Henry More, *Enthusiasmus Triumphatus, or, a Discourse of the Nature, Causes, Kinds, and Cure, of Enthusiasme; written by Philophilus Parresiastes* (London, Morden, 1656)

Sir Alexander Morison, *Outlines of Lectures on Mental Diseases* (Edinburgh, Lisars, 1825)

A.D. Morris, *The Hoxton Madhouses* (March, Cambridgeshire, for the Author, 1958)

D.B. Morris, 'The Kinship of Madness in Pope's "Dunciad"', *Philological Quarterly* 1 (1927), 813–31

J.N. Morris, *Versions of the Self* (New York, Basic Books, 1966)

Cromwell Mortimer, *An Address to the Publick, Containing Narratives of the Effects of Certain Chemical Remedies in most Diseases* (London, C. Davis, 1745)

E.C. Mossner, *The Life of David Hume* (London, Nelson, 1954)

H.B.M. Murphy, 'The Advent of Guilt Feelings as a Common Depressive Symptom: A Historical Comparison on Two Continents', *Psychiatry* 41 (1978), 229–42

T.J. Murray, 'Doctor Samuel Johnson's Abnormal Movements', in A.J. Friedhoff and T.N. Chase (eds), *Gilles de la Tourette Syndrome* (New York, Raven Press, 1982), 25-30

V. Grosvenor Myer 'Tristram and the Animal Spirits', in V. Grosvenor Myer (ed.), *Laurence Sterne: Riddles and Mysteries* (London, Vision, 1984), 99-114

Judith S. Neaman, *Suggestion of the Devil: the Origin of Madness* (New York, Anchor Books, 1975)

Jerome Neu, *Emotion, Thought and Therapy* (London, Routledge & Kegan Paul, 1977)

Max Neuberger, *The Doctrine of the Healing Power of Nature*, trans. L. J. Boyd (New York, 1943)

Richard Neugebauer, 'Mental Illness and Government Policy in Sixteenth and Seventeenth Century England' (New York, University of Columbia PhD, 1976)

— 'Treatment of the Mentally Ill in Medieval and Early Modern England', Journal of the History of the Behavioral Sciences 14 (1978), 158-69

— 'Medieval and Early Modern Theories of Mental Illness', *Archives of General Psychiatry* 36 (1979), 477–83

M.H. Nicolson, *A World in the Moon* (Northampton, Mass., Smith College, 1936)

— and G. S. Rousseau, *This Long Disease my Life. Alexander Pope and the Sciences* (Princeton, Princeton University Press, 1968)

D. Nokes, *Jonathan Swift, A Hypocrite Reversed: A Critical Biography* (Oxford, Oxford University Press, 1985)

C. Noon, 'On Suicide', *Journal of the History of Ideas* 39 (1978), 371-86

William B. Ober, 'Madness and Poetry: A Note on Collins, Cowper and
    Smart', in *Boswell's Clap and Other Essays* (Carbondale, Illinois, Southern
    Illinois University Press, 1979)

E.G. O'Donoghue, *The Story of Bethlem Hospital from its Foundation in 1247*
    (London, T. Fisher & Unwin, 1914)

— *Bridewell: Hospital, Palace, Prison Schools from the Earliest Times to the End of
    the Reign of Elizabeth* (London, Bodley Head, 1923)

E. Oliver, *The Eccentric Life of Alexander Cruden* (London, Faber, 1934)

W.H. Oliver, *Prophets and Millennialists* (Auckland, New Zealand, 1978)

A.P Oppé, *Alexander and John Robert Cozens* (London, Adam and Charles
    Black, 1952)

David Owen, *Philanthropy in England, 1660-1960* (Cambridge, Mass., Harvard
    University Press, 1965)

W. Pargeter, *Observations on Maniacal Disorders* (Reading, for the author, 1792)

J. Parkinson, *Madhouses. Observations on the Act for Regulation of Mad-Houses,
    and A Correction of the Statements of the Case of Benjamin Elliott, Convicted
    of Illegally Confining Mary Daintree: With Remarks Addressed to the Friends of
    Insane Persons* (London, Sherwood, Neeley and Jones, 1811)

Parliamentary Papers Reports, Report from the Committee Appointed to
    Enquire into the State of Private Madhouses, *House of Commons Journal* 29
    (1763), 486-89

— Reports (4) from the Committee on Madhouses in England, *House of
    Commons* (1815)

— Reports (3) from the Committee on Madhouses in England, *House of
    Commons* (1816)

Parliamentary Papers, Returns, A Return of the Number of Houses in
    Each County, or Division of the County, Licensed for the Reception of
    Lunatics, *House of Commons* (1819)

— A Return of the Number of Lunatics Confirmed in the Different Gaols,
    Hospitals and Lunatic Asylums, *House of Commons* (1819)

William Llewellyn Parry-Jones, *The Trade in Lunacy, A Study of Private
    Madhouses in England in the Eighteenth and Nineteenth Centuries* (London,
    Routledge & Kegan Paul, 1971)

— 'The Model of Geel Lunatic Colony and its Influence on the Nineteenth
    Century Asylum System in Britain', in Andrew Scull (ed.), *Madhouses,
    Mad-Doctors and Madmen* (London, Athlone Press, 1981), 201-17

J. Passmore, *The Perfectibility of Man* (London, Duckworth, 1970)

Richard Paternoster, *The Madhouse System* (1841)

G.O. Paul, *Observations on the Subject of Lunatic Asylums* (Gloucester, for the
    Author, 1812)

R. Paulson, *Theme and Structure in Swift's Tale of a Tub* (New Haven, Conn.,
    Yale University Press, 1960)

— *Representations of Revolution* (New Haven, Conn., Yale University Press,
    1983)

M. Pelling, 'Healing the Sick Poor: Social Policy and Disability in Norwich,
    1550-1640', *Medical History* 29 (1985), 115-37

S. Pepys, *The Diary of Samuel Pepys*, 11 vols, ed. by R. Latham and W.
    Matthews (London, Bell and Hyman, 1970-83)

J.T. Perceval, *A Narrative of the Treatment Received by a Gentleman, During a State
    of Mental Derangement* (London, Effingham Wilson, 1838)

— (ed.), *Poems by a Prisoner in Bethlehem* (London, Effingham and Wilson, 1851)

Thomas Percival, *Medical Ethics* (Manchester, Johnson & Bickerstaff, 1803)

T. Percy, *Reliques of Ancient English Poetry* (London, J. Dodsley, 1765)

Edgar Allison Peers, *Elizabethan Drama and its Mad Folk* (Cambridge, Heffer, 1914)

W. Perfect, *Select Cases in the Different Species of Insanity* (Rochestei Gillman, 1787)

— *A Remarkable Case of Madness, with the Diet and Medicine used in the Cure* (Rochester, for the Author, 1791)

D.A. Peterson, 'The Literature of Madness: Autobiographical Writings by Mad People and Mental Patients in England and America from 143 6– 1975' (Stanford University PhD, 1977)

— (ed.), *A Mad People's History of Madness* (Pittsburgh, University of Pittsburgh Press, 1982)

H. Petit (ed.), *The Correspondence of Edward Young, 1683–1795* (Oxford, Clarendon Press, 1971)

Charles Palmer Phillips, *The Law Concerning Lunatics, Idiots and Persons of Unsound Mind* (London, Butterworths, 1858)

H. Temple Phillips, 'The Old Private Lunatic Asylum at Fishponds', *Bristol Medico-Chirurgical Journal 85* (1970), 41-44

— 'The History of the Old Private Lunatic Asylum at Fishponds Bristol, 1740-1859' (Bristol, University of Bristol MSc. thesis, 1973)

J.V. Pickstone, *Medicine and Industrial Society: A History of Hospital Development in Manchester and its Region 1752-1946* (Manchester, Manchester University Press, 1985)

C. Pierce, *The Religious Life of Samuel Johnson* (London, Athlone, 1983)

S. Piggott, *William Stukeley* (Oxford, Clarendon Press, 1950)

P. Pinel, *A Treatise on Insanity*, ed. P.E Cranefield (New York, Hafner, 1962)

S. Pollard, *The Genesis of Modern Management* (London, Edward Arnold, 1965)

A. Ponsonby (ed.), *More English Diaries* (London, Methuen, 1927)

Roy Porter, 'Medicine and the Enlightenment in Eighteenth Century England', *Bulletin of the Society for the Social History of Medicine* 25 (1979), 27-41

— 'Being Mad in Eighteenth Century England', *History Today* (December, 1981), 42–8

— 'Was There a Moral Therapy in the Eighteenth Century?', *Lychnos* (1981-82), 12-26

— 'Sex and the Enlightenment in Britain', in P. Boucé (ed.), *Sexuality in Eighteenth Century Britain* (Manchester, Manchester University Press, 1982), 1-27

— *English Society in the Eighteenth Century* (Harmondsworth, Penguin, 1982)

— 'The Sexual Politics of James Graham', *British Journal for Eighteenth Century Studies*, 5 (1982), 201-6

— 'Shutting People Up', *Social Studies of Science* 12 (1982), 467-76

— 'The Rage of Party: A Glorious Revolution in English Psychiatry?', *Medical History* 29 (1983), 35-50

— 'The Doctor and the Word', *Medical Sociology News* 9 (1983), 21-8

— 'In the 18th Century Were Lunatic Asylums Total Institutions?', *Ego* 4 (1983), 12-34

— 'Against the Spleen', in Valerie Grosvenor Myer (ed.), *Laurence Sterne: Riddles and Mysteries* (London & New York, Vision Press, 1984), 84–99
— 'The Dark Side of Samuel Johnson', *History Today* (December, 1984), 43-46
— 'Sex and the Singular Man: the Seminal Ideas of James Graham', *Studies on Voltaire and the Eighteenth Century* 228 (1984), 1-24
— '"Under the Influence": Mesmerism in England', *History Today* (September, 1985), 22-9
— 'Making Faces: Physiognomy and Fashion in Eighteenth Century England', *Études Anglaises* 38 (1985), 385-96
— '"The Secrets of Generation Displayed"; Aristotle's Master-Piece in Eighteenth Century England', in R.P. Maccubbin (ed.), *Unauthorised Sexual Behaviour During the Enlightenment* (Eighteenth Century Life special issue, vol. ix, 1985), 1-21
— '"The Hunger of Imagination": Approaching Samuel Johnson's Melancholy', in W.F. Bynum, Roy Porter and Michael Shepherd (eds), *The Anatomy of Madness*, 2 vols (London, Tavistock, 1985) i, 63-88
— (ed.), *Patients and Practitioners. Lay Perceptions of Medicine in Pre Industrial Society* (Cambridge, Cambridge University Press, 1985)
— 'The Drinking Man's Disease: The Prehistory of Alcoholism in Georgian Britain', *British Journal of Addiction* 80 (1985), 385-96
— 'The Diary of a Madman, 17th Century Style: Goodwin Wharton, M.P. and Communer with the Fairy World', *Psychological Medicine* 16 (1986), 503-18
— 'Love, Sex, and Madness in Eighteenth Century England', *Social Research* 53 (1986), 211-42
— and A. Wear (eds), *Problems and Methods in the History of Medicine* (London, Croom Helm, 1987)
— *The Social History of Madness* (London, Weidenfeld & Nicolson, 1987)
— 'Cleaning up the Great Wen', in F. Bynum (ed.), *Living and Dying in London* (London, Croom Helm, forthcoming)
— 'Erasmus Darwin, Doctor of Evolution?' in J. Moore (ed.), *Festschrift for John Greene* (Cambridge University Press, forthcoming)
— 'The History of Institutional Psychiatry in Europe', in *The Yale Hand book of the History of Psychiatry* (forthcoming)
— 'Anglicanism and Psychiatry: The case of Robert Burton and Sir Thomas Browne', in *The History of Psychiatry and Psychoanalysis* (forthcoming).
— 'Bedlam and Parnassus: Mad People's Writing in Georgian England', in G. Levine (ed.), *One Culture* (Madison, University of Wisconsin Press, forthcoming)
E.A. Pottle (ed.), *Boswell's London Journal 1762-1763* (London, Heinemann, 1950)
— *James Boswell: The Earlier Years* (London, Heinemann, 1966)
N. Powell, *Fuseli's 'The Nightmare'* (London, Allen Lane, 1973)
R. Powell, 'Observations on the Comparative Prevalence of Insanity at Different Periods', *Medical Transactions* 4 (1813), 131-59
John Purcell, *A Treatise of Vapours, or Hysterick Fits* (London, E. Place, 1707)
M. Quinlan, 'Memoir of William Cowper: An Autobiography', *Proceedings of the American Philosophical Society* 97 (1953), 359-82
— *William Cowper* (Minneapolis, Minn., University of Minnesota Press, 1953)
— *Samuel Johnson, a Layman's Religion* (Madison, Wis., University of Wisconsin

Press, 1964)

Theodore K. Rabb, *The Struggle for Stability in Early Modern Europe* (New York, Oxford University Press, 1975)

H.D. Rack, 'Doctors, Demons and Early Methodist Healing', in W.J. Sheils (ed.), *The Church and Healing* (Oxford, Basil Blackwell, 1982), 137-52

L.J. Rather, 'Old and New Views of the Emotions and Bodily Changes', *Clio Medica* 1 (1965), 1-25

— *Mind and Body in Eighteenth Century Medicine* (Berkeley, University of California Press, 196S)

C. Reade, *Hard Cash. A Matter of Fact Romance*, 3 vols (London, Sampson Low et al., 1863)

Barry Reay, *The Quakers and the English Revolution* (London, Temple Smith, 1985)

A.L. Reed, *The Background of Gray's Elegy: A Study in the Taste for Melancholy Poetry*, 1700-51 (New York, Columbia University Press, 1924)

K.T. Reed, 'This Tasteless Tranquillity: A Freudian Note on Johnson's *Rasselas*', *Literature and Psychology* 19 (1969), 61-2

R.R. Reed, *Bedlam on the Jacobean Stage* (Cambridge, Mass., Harvard University Press, 1952)

M. Regan, *A Caring Society. A Study of Lunacy in Liverpool and South West Lancashire from 1650 to 1948* (Merseyside, St. Helens & Knowsley Health Authority, 1986)

J. Reid, 'Report of Diseases', *The Monthly Magazine* 25 (1808), 166-7, 374-5

— *Essays on Hypochondriacal and Other Nervous Affections* (London, Longman et al., 1816)

Frederick Reynolds, *The Life and Times of Frederick Reynolds by Himself* (London, H. Colburn, 1826)

Francis J. Rice, 'Madness and Industrial Society. A Study of the Origins and Early Growth of the Organisation of Insanity in Nineteenth Century Scotland c.1830-70' (University of Strathclyde PhD thesis, 2 vols, 1981)

C. Ricks (ed.), *Laurence Sterne: Tristram Shandy* (Harmondsworth, Penguin, 1967)

Walter Riese, 'Descartes as a Psychotherapist', *Medical History* 10 (1966), 237-44

B. Hill Rigney, *Madness and Sexual Politics in the Feminist Novel* (Madison, Wisc., University of Wisconsin Press, 1978)

G.B. Risse, 'The Brownian System of Medicine: its Theoretical and Practical Implications', *Clio Medica* 5 (1970), 45-51

— *Hospital Life in Enlightenment Scotland* (Cambridge, Cambridge University Press, 1985)

K.B. Rix, 'John Coakley Lettsom and Some of the Effects of Hard Drinking', *Journal of Alcoholism* 11(1976), 98-103

B. Robinson and C.R. Hudleston, 'Two Vanished Fishponds Houses', *Transactions of the Bristol and Gloucester Archaeological Society* 60 (1938), 238-59

E. Robinson (ed.), *John Clare's Autobiographical Writings* (Oxford, Oxford University Press, 1983)

H.W. Robinson and W. Adams (eds), *The Diary of Robert Hooke* (London, Taylor & Francis, 1935)

N. Robinson, *A New System of the Spleen* (London, A. Bettesworth, 1729)

J. Rodgers, 'Ideas of Life in Tristram Shandy' (PhD thesis, University of East
    Anglia, 1978)

T. Rogers, *A Discourse Concerning Trouble of Mind and the Disease of Melancholy*
    (London, Thomas Parkhurst and Thomas Cockerill, 1691)

J. Rollo, 'Two Instances of the Effects of Drinking Pure Spirits, in Repeated
    and Large Quantities. Communicated in a Letter to Dr Simons, F.R.S.',
    London Medical Journal 7 (1786), 33-54

M. Rose, *The English Poor Law 1780-1930* (Newton Abbot, David and Charles,
    1971)

George Rosen, 'Social Attitudes to Irrationality and Madness in Seventeenth
    and Eighteenth Century Europe', *Journal of the History of Medicine and
    Allied Sciences* 18 (1963), 220-40

— 'The Mentally Ill and the Community in Western and Central Europe
    During the Late Middle Ages and the Renaissance', *Journal of the History of
    Medicine* 19 (1964), 377-88

— 'Emotion and Sensibility in Ages of Anxiety: A Comparative Historical
    Review', *American Journal of Psychiatry* 124 (1967), 771-84

— *Madness in Society. Chapters in the Historical Sociology of Mental Illness*
    (London, Routledge & Kegan Paul, 1968)

— 'Enthusiasm', *Bulletin of the History of Medicine* 42 (1968), 393–421

— 'Forms of Irrationality in the Eighteenth Century', in H.E. Pagliaro (ed.),
    Studies in Eighteenth Century Culture (Cleveland, Ohio, Case Western
    Reserve University, 1972)

W. Rossky, 'Imagination in the English Renaissance: Psychology and Poetic',
    in *Studies in the Renaissance* 4, edited by M.A. Shaaber (New York,
    Renaissance Society of America, 1954)

Martin Roth and Jerome Kroll, *The Reality of Mental Illness* (Cambridge,
    Cambridge University Press, 1986)

David Rorhman, *The Discovery of the Asylum* (Boston, Little, Brown, 1971)

G.S. Rousseau, 'John Wesley's Primitive Physick (1747)', *Harvard Library
    Bulletin* 16 (1968), 242-56

— 'Science and the Discovery of the Imagination in Enlightenment England',
    Eighteenth Century Studies 3 (1969), 108-35

— 'Nerves, Spirits and Fibres: Towards Defining the Origins of Sensibility;
    with a Postscript', *The Blue Guitar* 2 (1976), 125-53

— 'Science', in P. Rogers (ed.), *The Context of English Literature: The Eighteenth
    Century* (London, Methuen, 1978), 153-207

'Psychology', in G.S. Rousseau and Roy Porter (eds), *The Ferment of
    Knowledge* (Cambridge, Cambridge University Press, 1980), 143-210

— 'Medicine and Millenarianism: Immortal Dr. Cheyne', in R. Popkin (ed.),
    Millenarianism and Messianism in the Enlightenment (Berkeley, University of
    California Press, 1987)

William Rowley, *A Treatise of Female Nervous, Hysterical, Hypochondriacal, Bilious,
    Convulsive Diseases* (London, C. Nourse & E. Newbery, 1788)

B. Rush, *An Inquiry into the Effects of Spiritous Liquors on the Human Body*
    (Edinburgh, no publisher, 1791)

P. Rushton, 'Lunatics and Ideots: Mental Disability the Community and the
    Poor Law in North-East England, 1600-1800', *Medical History* vol. 32,
    (forthcoming, 1988)

R. Russell, 'Mental Physicians and their Patients; Psychological Medicine in

the English Pauper Lunatic Asylums of the Later Ninetenth-Century'
(Sheffield University PhD, 1983)

C.A. Ryskamp, *William Cowper of the Inner Temple, Esq.* (Cambridge,
Cambridge University Press, 1959)

— *Johnson and Cowper* (London, 1965)

A. Sachs, *Passionate Intelligence* (Baltimore, Md, Johns Hopkins University Press,
1967)

W. Sandford, *A Few Practical Remarks on the Medicinal Effects of Wine and Spirits*
(Worcester, Tymbs, 1799)

C. de Saussure, *A Foreign View of England in the Reign of George I and George II,
trans. and ed. by Madame Van Muyden* (London, J. Murray, 1902)

Simon Schaffer, 'Herschel in Bedlam: Natural History and Stellar Astronomy',
British Journal for the History of Science 12(1980), 211-39

Hans-Jurgen Schings, *Melancholie und Aufklarung: Melancholiker und ihre Df
Kritiker in Erfahrungsseelenkunde und Literatur des 18. Jahrhunderts* (Stuttgart,
Metzer, 1977)

J.M. Schneck, 'Insanity and Criminality in Tobias Smollett's "Roderick
Random"', *New York State Journal of Medicine* 75 (1975), 926-8

T.J. Schoeneman, 'The Role of Mental Illness in the European Witch Hunts
of the Sixteenth and Seventeenth Centuries: An Assessment', *Journal of the
History of the Behavioral Sciences* 13 (1977), 337-51

Daniel Paul Schreber, *Memoirs of my Nervous Illness,* trans. and ed. by Ida
Macalpine and R. Hunter (London, William Dawson & Sons, 1955)

William Schupbach, 'John Monro, MD and Charles James Fox, an Etching by
Thomas Rowlandson', *Medical History* 27 (1983), 80-3

H. Schwartz, *Knaves, Fools, Madmen, and 'That Subtle Effluvium'. A Study of
the Opposition to the French Prophets in England, 1706-1710* (Gainesville, Fla,
University Presses of Florida, 1978)

Reginald Scot, *The Discoverie of Witchcraft* (London, Brome, 1584)

M. Screech, *Rabelais* (London, Duckworth, 1979)

— *Ecstasy and the Praise of Folly* (London, Duckworth, 1980)

— 'The Mad "Christ" of Erasmus and the Legal Duties of his Brethren', in
N.J. Lacy and J.C. Nash (eds), *Essays in Early French Literature Presented to
Barbara M. Craig* (York, South Carolina, French Literature Publications
Company, 1982), 119-27

— *Montaigne and Melancholy* (London, Duckworth, 1983)

— 'Good Madness in Christendom', in W.E. Bynum, Roy Porter and Michael
Shepherd (eds), *The Anatomy of Madness*, 2 vols (London, 1985), i, 25-39

Andrew Scull, 'From Madness to Mental Illness: Medical Men as Moral
Entrepreneurs', *European Journal of Sociology* 16 (1975), 219-61– 'Mad-
doctors and Magistrates: English Psychiatry's Struggle for Professional
Autonomy in the Nineteenth Century', *European Journal of Sociology* 17
(1976), 279-305

— 'Madness and Segregative Control: The Rise of the Insane Asylum', *Social
Problems* 24 (1977), 338-51

— *Museums of Madness* (London, Allen Lane, 1979)

— 'A Convenient Place to Get Rid of Inconvenient People: the Victorian
Lunatic Asylum', in A.D. King (ed.), *Buildings and Society* (London,
Routledge & Kegan Paul, 1980), 37-60

— (ed.), *Madhouses, Mad-doctors, and Madmen: the Social History of Psychiatry in the Victorian Era* (London, Athlone Press, 1981)

— 'The Discovery of the Asylum Revisited: Lunacy Reform in the New American Republic'; 'The Social History of Psychiatry in the Victorian Era'; and 'Moral Treatment Reconsidered: Some Sociological Comments on an Episode in the History of British Psychiatry', in Andrew Scull (ed.), *Madhouses, Mad-Doctors and Madmen* (London, Athlone Press, 1981), 144-65; 5-26; 105-18

— 'Humanitarianism or Control? Some Observations on the Historiography of Anglo-American Psychiatry', *Rice University Studies* 67 (1981), 35-37

— 'The Domestication of Madness', *Medical History* 27 (1983), 233-48

— *Decarceration* (Englewood Cliffs, Prentice Hall, 1977; revised edition, Oxford, Polity Press, 1984)

— 'Was Insanity Increasing? A Response to Edward Hare', *British Journal of Psychiatry* 144 (1984), 432-36

— 'John Conolly: a Victorian Psychiatric Career', in W.F. Bynum, Roy Porter and Michael Shepherd (eds), *The Anatomy of Madness*, 2 vols (London, 1985), i, 103-50

Paul S. Seaver, *Wallington's World. A Puritan Artisan in Seventeenth Century London* (London, Methuen, 1985)

Peter Sedgwick, *Psycho Politics* (London, Pluto Press, 1982)

J. Sekora, *Luxury* (Baltimore, Johns Hopkins University Press, 1977)

R.R. Sellman, 'Note: Madness in an 18th-Century Village', *Devon and Cornwall Notes and Queries* 32 (1971), 2

A.L. Lytton Sells, *Thomas Gray: His Life and Works* (London, George Allen and Unwin, 1980)

J.F. Sena, 'The English Malady: The Idea of Melancholy from 1700 to 1760' (Princeton University PhD thesis, 1967)

— 'Swift, the Yahoos and the English Malady', *Papers in Language and Literature* 7 (1971), 300-03

P. Sérieux and L. Libert, 'Le Régime des Aliénés en France au 18ème Siècle d'après des Documents Inédits', *Annales Medico-Psychologiques* 6 (loème série) (1914) 43-76, 196-219, 311-24, 470-97, 598-627

W.K. and E.M. Sessions, *The Tukes of York* (London, The Friends Home Service Committee, 1971)

L.W. Sharp (ed.), *The Early Letters of Robert Wodrow* (Edinburgh, Scottish History Society 1937)

P. Shaw, *The Juice of the Grape; or, Wine Preferable to Water. A Treatise Wherein Wine is Shewn to be a Grand Preserver of Health, with a Word of Advice to the Vintners...By a Fellow of the College* (London, W. Lewis, 1724)

W. Sheils (ed.), *The Church and Healing* (Oxford, Basil Blackwell, 1982)

A. Sherbo, *Christopher Smart* (East Lansing, Michigan State University Press, 1967)

M. Shortland, 'The Body in Question; Some Perceptions, Problems and Perspectives of the Body in Relation to Character *c.*1750-1850' (University of Leeds, PhD thesis, 1985)

Elaine Showalter, 'Victorian Women and Insanity', in Andrew Scull (ed.), *Madhouses, Mad-Doctors and Madmen* (London, Athlone Press, 1981), 313-38

— *The Female Malady* (New York, Pantheon, 1986)

E. Sibly, *The Medical Mirror; or a Treatise on the Impregnation of the Human Female* (London, for the author, 1794)

L. Simond, *An American in Regency England*, ed. by C. Hibbert (London, History Book Club, 1968)

E.M. Sickels, *The Gloomy Egoist* (New York, Octagon Books, 1969)

Herbert Silvette, 'On Insanity in Seventeenth-Century England', *Bulletin of the Institute of the History of Medicine* 6 (1938), 22–33

Bennett Simon, *Mind and Madness in Ancient Greece* (Ithaca, Cornell University Press, 1978)

Vieda Skultans, *Madness and Morals* (London, Routledge & Kegan Paul, 1975)

— *English Madness: Ideas on Insanity, 1580–1890* (London, Routledge & Kegan Paul, 1979)

P. Slack, *The Impact of Plague* (London, Routledge & Kegan Paul, 1985)

Roger Smith, *Trial by Medicine: Insanity and Responsibility in Victorian Trials* (Edinburgh, Edinburgh University Press, 1981)

— 'The Boundary Between Insanity and Criminal Responsibility in Nineteenth Century England', in Andrew Scull (ed.), *Madhouses, Mad-Doctors and Madmen* (London, Athlone Press, 1981), 363–84

Sydney Smith, 'An Account of the York Retreat', *Edinburgh Review* 23 (1814), 189–98

W. Smith, *A Sure Guide in Sickness and in Health* (London, Bew and Walter, 1776)

T. Smollett, *The Life and Adventures of Sir Launcelot Greaves*, ed. by David Evans (London, Oxford University Press, 1973)

S. Sontag, *Illness as Metaphor* (London, Allen Lane, 1979)

Lewis Southcomb, *Peace of Mind and Health of Body United* (London, Cooper, 1750)

Joanna Southcott, *The Strange Effects of Faith with Remarkable Prophecies* (Exeter, Brill, 1801)

— *The Second Book of Wonders* (London, Marchant and Galubin, 1813)

P.M. Spacks, *The Female Imagination* (London, Allen and Unwin, 1975)

— *Imagining a Self* (Cambridge, Mass., London, Harvard University Press, 1976)

W.A. Speck, *The Divided Society. Parties and Politics in England, 1694-1716* (London, Edward Arnold, 1967)

T. Spencer, *Shakespeare and the Nature of Man* (New York, Cambridge University Press, 1958)

J. Spillane, *The Doctrine of the Nerves* (London, Oxford University Press, 1981)

S.E. Sprott, *The English Debate on Suicide from Donne to Hume* (London, Open Court Publishing Co., 1961)

Richard Stafford, *Because That I Have Seemed to Falsify my Promis, which I Made upon My Being Discharged out of Bethlem Hospital* [*viz*. *His Petition to the Principal Secretary of State*]..., (London, no publisher, 1693)

D. Stansfield, *Thomas Beddoes* (Dordrecht, Holland, D. Reidel Publishing Company, 1984)

William Stark, *Remarks on the Construction of Public Hospitals* (Edinburgh, for the Committee, 1807)

Carol Zisowitz Stearns, 'A Second Opinion on MacDonald's Mystical Bedlam', *Journal of Social History* 16 (1983), 149–51

Richard Steele and Joseph Addison, *The Tatler* (London, 1709-11)

Laurence Sterne, *Tristram Shandy*, ed. C. Ricks (Harmondsworth, Penguin, 1970)

Lawrence Stone, *The Family, Sex and Marriage in England 1500-1800* (London, Weidenfeld and Nicolson, 1977)

John Strype, *A Survey of the Cities of London and Westminster... Written at First in the Year MDXCVIII. By John Stow... Corrected, Improved and Very Much Enlarged...to the Present Time* (London, A. Churchill, 1720)

R.D. Stock, *The Holy and the Daemonic from Sir Thomas Browne to William Blake* (Princeton, Princeton University Press, 1982)

M. Storey, *The Poetry of John Clare: a Critical Introduction* (London, Macmillan, 1974)

W. Stukeley, *Of the Spleen, its Description and History* (London, for the author, 1723)

E. Sunstein, *A Different Face: The Life of Mary Wollstonecraft* (Boston, Mass., Little, Brown, 1975)

J. Swift, *A Tale of a Tub and Other Satires*, ed. by K. Williams (London, Everyman, 1975)

Thomas Sydenham, *The Entire Works* (London, E. Cave, 1742)

Thomas S. Szasz, *Law, Liberty and Psychiatry* (New York, Macmillan, 1963)

— *The Manufacture of Madness* (London, Paladin, 1972)

— *The Myth of Mental Illness* (London, Granada, 1972)

— *The Age of Madness. The History of Involuntary Hospitalisation Presented in Selected Texts* (London, Routledge & Kegan Paul, 1975)

— *The Therapeutic State: Psychiatry in the Mirror of Current Events* (Buffalo, N.Y., Prometheus Books, 1984)

G. Taylor, *The Problem of Poverty, 1660-1834* (London, Longmans, 1969)

O. Temkin, *The Falling Sickness* (Baltimore, Johns Hopkins University Press, 1974)

J. Tempest, *Narrative of the Treatment Experienced by John Tempest, Esq., of Lincoln's Inn, Barrister of Law, During Fourteen Months Solitary Confinement under a False Imputation of Lunacy* (London, for the author, 1830)

R.C. Tennant, 'The Anglican Response to Locke's Theory of Personal Identity', *Journal of the History of Ideas* 43 (1982), 73-90

J. Texte, *Jean-Jacques Rousseau and the Cosmopolitan Spirit in Literature* (London, Duckworth, 1899)

Ernest Thomas, 'The Old Poor Law and Medicine', *Medical History* 24 (1980), 1-19

Keith Thomas, 'The Double Standard', *Journal of the History of Ideas* 20 (1959), 195-216

— *Religion and the Decline of Magic* (Harmondsworth, Penguin, 1973)

— *Man and the Natural World* (Harmondsworth, Penguin, 1983)

G.M. Thompson, *The First Churchill* (London, Secker & Warburg, 1979)

Hester Thrale (Piozzi), *Anecdotes of Samuel Johnson During the Last Years of His Life*, in G.B. Hill (ed.), *Johnsonian Miscellanies*, 2 vols (Oxford, Clarendon Press, 1887)

John Thurnam, *Observations and Essays on the Statistics of Insanity, Including an Inquiry into the Causes Influencing the Results of Treatment in Establishments for the Insane. To which are Added the Statistics of the Retreat, Near York* (London, Gilpin, 1845)

J.W. Tibble and A. Tibble, *John Clare: a Life* (London, Cobden Sanderson, 1972)

I.C. Tifton (ed.), *Locke on Human Understanding: Selected Essays* (London, Oxford University Press, 1977)

E. M. Tillyard, *The Elizabethan World Picture* (London, Chatto & Windus, 1934)

S. A. A. D. Tissot, *Onanism; or a Treatise upon the Disorders Produced by Masturbation; or the Dangerous Effects of Secret and Excessive Venery*, trans. A. Hume (London, for the translator, 1766)

Janet Todd, *Sensibility. An Introduction* (London, Methuen, 1986)

C. Tomalin, *The Life and Death of Mary Wollstonecraft* (Harmondsworth, Penguin, 1977)

S. Tomaselli, 'The Enlightenment Debate on Women', *History Workshop Journal* 20 (1985), 101-29

G. Tonelli, 'Genius: from the Renaissance to 1770', in *Dictionary of the History of Ideas*, (ed.) P. Weiner (New York, 1973), ii, 293-97

Mrs Paget Toynbee (ed.), *The Letters of Horace Walpole*, 16 vols (Oxford, Clarendon Press, 1903-25)

— and Leonard Whibley (eds), *Correspondence of Thomas Gray*, 3 vols (Oxford, Clarendon Press, 1935)

C. P. C. Chenevix Trench, *The Royal Malady* (London, Longman, 1964)

E. Trillat, *Histoire De L'Hystérie* (Paris, Seghers, 1986)

George Trosse, *The Life of the Reverend Mr. George Trosse, Late Minister of the Gospel in the City of Exon, Who Died January 11th, 1712-13. In the Eighty Second Year of His Age, Written by Himself and Publish'd According to His Order* (Exeter, Richard White, 1714)

Thomas Trotter, *An Essay, Medical, Philosophical, and Chemical, on Drunkenness, and its Effects on the Human Body* (London, Longman & Rees, 1804)

— *A View of the Nervous Temperament* (London, Longman, Hurst, Rees & Orme, 1807)

Thomas Tryon, *A Treatise of Dreams and Visions* (London, T. Sowle, 1700)

S. I. Tucker, *Enthusiasm: a Study in Semantic Change* (Cambridge, Cambridge University Press, 1972

D. H. Tuke, *Chapters in the History of the Insane in the British Isles* (London, Kegan Paul, Trench & Co., 1882)

Samuel Tuke, *Description of the Retreat, an Institution Near York*, reprint, edited by R. Hunter and I. Macalpine of the 1813 edition (London, Dawsons, 1964)

B. S. Turner, *The Body and Society* (Oxford, Basil Blackwell, 1984)

E. S. Turner, *Taking the Cure* (London, Michael Joseph, 1967)

William Turner, *A Compleat History of the Most Remarkable Providences, both of Judgement and of Mercy, which have Happened in this Present Age* (London, John Dunton, 1697)

Ernest Tuveson, *The Imagination as Means of Grace* (Los Angeles, University of California Press, 1960)

— 'Locke and Sterne', in J. A. Mazzeo (ed.), *Reason and the Imagination* (London, Routledge & Kegan Paul, 1962), 255-77

Ilza Veith, *Hysteria: the History of a Disease* (Chicago, University Press, 1945)

Henry R. Viets, 'George Cheyne 1673-1743', *Bulletin of the History of Medicine* 23 (1949), 435-52

M. Vogel and C. Rosenberg (eds), *The Therapeutic Revolution* (Philadelphia, University of Pennsylvania Press, 1979)

R. Voitle, *Samuel Johnson the Moralist* (Cambridge, Mass., Harvard University Press, 1961)

J. Wain, *Samuel Johnson* (London, Macmillan, 1980)

Alexander Walk, 'Some Aspects of the "Moral Treatment" of the Insane up to

1845', *Journal of Mental Science* 100 (1954), 807-37

D.P. Walkei, *Spiritual and Demonic Magic from Ficino to Campanella* (London, Warburg Institute, 1988)

— *The Decline of Hell* (London, Routledge & Kegan Paul, 1964)

— *Unclean spirits. Possession and Exorcism in France and England in the Late Sixteenth and Early Seventeenth Centuries* (London, Scolar Press, 1981)

Nigel Walker, *Crime and Insanity in England*, vol. 1, *The Historical Perspective* (Edinburgh, Edinburgh University Press, 1968)

Sayer Walker, *A Treatise on Nervous Diseases* (London, J. Philips, 1796)

H. Walpole, *Memoirs of the Reign of George II*, 3 vols (New Haven, Yale University Press, 1985)

John K. Walton, 'Lunacy in the Industrial Revolution: a Study of Asylum Admissions in Lancashire, 1848-50', *Journal of Social History* 13 (1979), 1-22

— 'The Treatment of Pauper Lunatics in Victorian England: The Case of Lancaster Asylum, 1816-70', in Andrew Scull (ed.), *Madhouses, Mad-Doctors and Madmen* (London, Athlone Press, 1981), 166-200

— 'Casting Out and Bringing Back in Victorian England', in W.F. Bynum, Roy Porter and Michael Shepherd (eds), *The Anatomy of Madness*, 2 vols (London, Tavistock, 1985), ii, 132-46

Ned Ward, *The London Spy*, ed. K. Fenwick (London, Folio Society, 1955)

R.M. Wardle (ed.), *Collected Letters of Mary Wolistonecraft* (Ithaca, Cornell University Press, 1979)

J. Wardroper, *Jest upon Jest* (London, Routledge & Kegan Paul, 1970)

Thomas Warton, *The Pleasures of Melancholy* (London, Dodsley, 1747)

W.B.C. Watkins, *Perilous Balance* (Princeton, N.J., Princeton University Press, 1939)

Andrew Wear, 'Puritan Perceptions of Illness in Seventeenth Century England', in Roy Porter (ed.), *Patients and Practitioners: Lay Perceptions of Medicine in Pre-Industrial Society* (Cambridge, Cambridge, 1985), 55-99

— 'Caring for the Sick Poor in St. Bartholomew Exchange: 1580-1676', in W.F Bynum (ed.), *Living and Dying in London* (London, Croom Helm, 1988)

M. Weidhorn, *Dreams in Seventeenth Century Literature* (The Hague, Mouton, 1970)

E. Welsford, *The Fool: his Social and Literary History* (London, Faber, 1935)

J. Wesley, *The Journal of John Wesley*, 4 vols, ed. by Ernest Rhys (London, Everyman, 1906)

J. Wesley, *Primitive Physick* (London, T. Trye, 1747)

R.S. Westfall, *Never at Rest. A Biography of Isaac Newton* (Cambridge, Cambridge University Press, 1980)

J. Weyer, *De Praestigiis Daemonium* (Basle, no publisher, 1568)

G. Wharton, 'The Autobiography of Goodwin Wharton', 2 vols, British Library Add. Mss., 20, 006-7

G. Whitefield, *George Whitefield's Journal* (Guildford, Banner of Truth, 1960)

Robert Whytt, *An Essay on the Vital and Other Involuntary Motions of Animals* (Edinburgh, Hamilton et al., 1751)

— *Observations on the Nature, Causes and Cure of those Disorders which have been called Nervous, Hypochondriac, or Hysteric* (Edinburgh, Becket & P. du Hondt, 1765)

N. Willard, *Le Genie et La Folie* (Paris, Presses Universitaires de France, 1963)

D. Williams, 'The Missions of David Williams and James Tilley Matthews to

England (1793)', *English Historical Review* 53 (1938), 651-68

K. Williams, *Jonathan Swift: A Tale of a Tub and Other Satires* (London, Everyman Edition, 1975)

G. Williamson, 'The Restoration Revolt Against Enthusiasm', *Studies in Philology* 30 (1933), 571-603

— 'Mutability, Decay and Seventeenth Century Melancholy', *Journal of English Literary History* 2 (1935), 121-50

K. Williamson, *The Poetic Works of Christopher Smart* (Oxford, Oxford University Press, 1980)

F. Willis, *A Treatise on Mental Derangement, Containing the Substance of the Gulstonian Lectures for May, 1822* (London, Longman et al., 1823)

T. Willis, *Two Discourses Concerning the Soul of Brutes*, trans. S. Pordage (London, Dring, 1683)

— *The Practice of Physick* (London, Dring, 1684)

T. Wilson, *Distilled Spiritous Liquors the Bane of the Nation* (London, J. Roberts 1736)

J.K. Wing, *Reasoning about Madness* (London, Oxford University Press, 1978)

William Withering, *An Account of the Foxglove, and Some of its Medical Uses* (Birmingham, Robinson, 1785)

T. Withers, *Observations on Chronic Weakness* (York, Ward, 1777)

R. and M. Wittkower, *Born under Saturn* (London, Weidenfeld & Nicolson, 1963)

E.A. Woods and E.T. Carlson, 'The Psychiatry of Philippe Pinel', *Bulletin of the History of Medicine* 35 (1961), 14-25

John Woodward, *Select Cases, and Consultations, in Physick* (London, Davis & Reymers, 1757)

John Woodward, *To Do the Sick No Harm: a Study of the British Voluntary Hospital System to 1875* (London, Routledge & Kegan Paul, 1974)

A. Wright, 'Medieval Attitudes Towards Mental Illness', *Bulletin of the History of Medicine* 7 (1939), 352-56

John P. Wright, 'Hysteria and Mechanical Man', *Journal of the History of Ideas* 41 (1980), 233-47

P. Wright and A. Treacher (eds), *The Problem of Medical Knowledge* (Edinburgh, Edinburgh University Press, 1982)

T. Wright, *The Passions of the Mind in General* (London, W. Burre, 1604)

E. Wylie, *Thomas Gray* (New York, Twayne, 1969)

J. Yokon, *John Locke and the Way of Ideas* (Oxford, Oxford University Press, 1956)

— *Perceptual Acquaintance* (Oxford, Blackwell, 1984)

— *Thinking Matter* (Minneapolis, Minneapolis University Press, 1984)

George Young, *A Treatise on Opium, Founded upon Practical Observation* (London, Millar, 1753)

Robert M. Young, *Mind, Brain and Adaptation in the Nineteenth Century* (Oxford, Clarendon Press, 1970)

— 'Association of Ideas', in P.P. Wiener (ed.), *Dictionary of the History of Ideas*, 4 vols (New York, Scribner's Sons, 1973) i, 111-17

Zainoldin and Peter L. Tyor, 'Asylum and Society: An Approach to Industrial Change', *Journal of Soical History* 73 (1979), 23-48

G. Zilboorg, *The Medical Man and the Witch in the Renaissance* (Baltimore, Johns Hopkins University Press, 1935)

— *A History of Medical Psychology* (New York, W.W. Norton, 1941)

Index

TEMPUS – REVEALING HISTORY

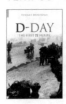

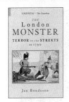

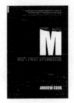

D-Day
The First 72 Hours
WILLIAM F. BUCKINGHAM
'A compelling narrative'
The Observer
£9.99
0 7524 2842 X

The London Monster
Terror on the Streets in 1790
JAN BONDESON
'Gripping'
The Guardian
£9.99
0 7524 3327 X

London
A Historical Companion
KENNETH PANTON
'A readable and reliable work of reference that deserves a place on every Londoner's bookshelf'
Stephen Inwood
£20
0 7524 3434 9

M: MI5's First Spymaster
ANDREW COOK
'Well-researched, penetrating and engagingly written'
Andrew Roberts
£20
0 7524 2896 9

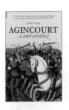

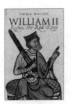

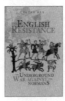

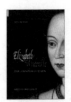

Agincourt: A New History
ANNE CURRY
'A highly distinguished and convincing account of one of the decisive battles of the Western world'
Christopher Hibbert
£25
0 7524 2828 4

William II
Rufus, the Red King
EMMA MASON
'A thoroughly new re-appraisal of a much maligned king. The dramatic story of his life is told with great pace and insight'
John Gillingham
£25
0 7524 3528 0

The English Resistance
The Underground War Against the Normans
PETER REX
'An invaluable rehabilitation of an ignored resistance movement'
The Sunday Times
£17.99
0 7524 2827 6

Elizabeth Wydeville
The Slandered Queen
ARLENE OKERLUND
'A penetrating, thorough and wholly convincing vindication of this unlucky queen'
Sarah Gristwood
£18.99
0 7524 3384 9

If you are interested in purchasing other books published by Tempus, or in case you have difficulty finding any Tempus books in your local bookshop, you can also place orders directly through our website

www.tempus-publishing.com

TEMPUS – REVEALING HISTORY

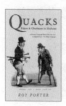 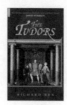

Quacks
Fakers and Charlatans in Medicine
ROY PORTER

'A delightful book'
The Daily Telegraph

£12.99

0 7524 2590 0

The Tudors
RICHARD REX

'Up-to-date, readable and reliable. The best introduction to England's most important dynasty'
David Starkey

£9.99

0 7524 3333 4

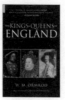 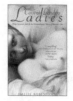

The Kings & Queens of England
MARK ORMROD

'Of the numerous books on the kings and queens of England, this is the best'
Alison Weir

£9.99

0 7524 2598 6

The Covent Garden Ladies
Pimp General Jack & the Extraordinary Story of Harris's List
HALLIE RUBENHOLD

'Has all the atmosphere and edge of a good novel… magnificent'
Frances Wilson

£9.99

0 7524 3739 9

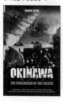 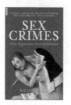

Okinawa 1945
GEORGE FEIFER

'A great book… Feifer's account of the three sides and their experiences far surpasses most books about war'
Stephen Ambrose

£17.99

0 7524 3324 5

Sex Crimes
From Renaissance to Enlightenment
W.M. NAPHY

'Wonderfully scandalous'
Diarmaid MacCulloch

£10.99

0 7524 2977 9

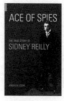 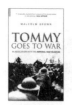

Ace of Spies The True Story of Sidney Reilly
ANDREW COOK

'The most definitive biography of the spying ace yet written… both a compelling narrative and a myth-shattering *tour de force*'
Simon Sebag Montefiore

£12.99

0 7524 2959 0

Tommy Goes To War
MALCOLM BROWN

'A remarkably vivid and frank account of the British soldier in the trenches'
Max Arthur

£12.99

0 7524 2980 4

If you are interested in purchasing other books published by Tempus, or in case you have difficulty finding any Tempus books in your local bookshop, you can also place orders directly through our website

www.tempus-publishing.com

ABOUT THE AUTHOR

Until his untimely death, Roy Porter was one of Britain's most revered social historians. His other books include *Enlightenment*, *London: A Social History*, *The Greatest Benefit to Mankind: A Medical History of Humanity*, *Blood and Guts: A Short History of Medicine*, *Flesh in the Age of Reason* and *Quacks: Fakers and Charlatans in Medicine*, also published by Tempus.

PRAISE FOR ROY PORTER

Quacks: Fakers & Charlatans in Medicine

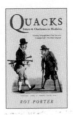

A *SUNDAY TELEGRAPH BOOK OF THE YEAR*

'A delightful book' *THE DAILY TELEGRAPH*

'Hugely entertaining' *BBC HISTORY MAGAZINE*

'The joy of this book lies in the colourful characters. My favourite is James Graham, a sex guru who guaranteed bliss and fertility in his patent 'Grand Celestial Bed' in return for what was then the vast sum of £50. He had no shortage of takers' *THE MAIL ON SUNDAY*

MADMEN